The Neurology of Autism

The Neurology of Autism

Edited by Mary Coleman

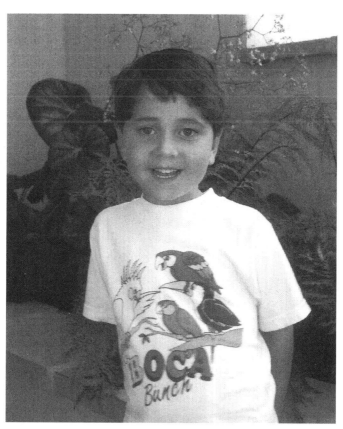

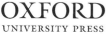
UNIVERSITY PRESS

OXFORD
UNIVERSITY PRESS

Oxford University Press, Inc., publishes works that further
Oxford University's objective of excellence
in research, scholarship, and education.

Oxford   New York
Auckland   Cape Town   Dar es Salaam   Hong Kong   Karachi
Kuala Lumpur   Madrid   Melbourne   Mexico City   Nairobi
New Delhi   Shanghai   Taipei   Toronto

With offices in
Argentina   Austria   Brazil   Chile   Czech Republic   France   Greece
Guatemala   Hungary   Italy   Japan   Poland   Portugal   Singapore
South Korea   Switzerland   Thailand   Turkey   Ukraine   Vietnam

Published by Oxford University Press, Inc.
198 Madison Avenue, New York, New York 10016
www.oup.com

First issued as an Oxford University Press paperback, 2009

Oxford is a registered trademark of Oxford University Press

Library of Congress Cataloging-in-Publication Data
The neurology of autism / edited by Mary Coleman.
p.   cm.
Includes bibliographical references and index.
ISBN 978-0-19-538776-6
1. Autism—Pathophysiology.   I. Coleman, Mary, 1928-
RC553.A88N53 2005
616.85'882—dc22   2004020708

9 8 7 6 5 4 3 2 1

Printed in the United States of America
on acid-free paper

This book is dedicated to Richmond S. Paine

Richmond S. Paine, M.D., was a giant of pediatric neurology. He formed a large department of pediatric neurology at the Children's Hospital of Washington, D.C., in the early 1960s. Before that, he had been in close touch with those in Europe—people like André Thomas, Albrecht Peiper, and Ronnie Mac Keith—who were contributing as pioneers to the field of child neurology. As a teacher, he was a splendid example of how a professional should be rich with curiosity yet rigorous about the scientific approach. To study with him was a constant intellectual adventure; he had the gifts of clarity and patience. To his patients, he brought the best in diagnosis and treatment. He was gentle with the children and much appreciated by their parents.

His distinguished teaching attracted students from around the world. Three of the authors of this book—Mary Coleman, Michele Zappella, and Yoshiko Nomura—benefited from his creative erudition.

In the case of Mary Coleman, the brilliant teaching of Richmond Paine changed her planned specialty from adult to pediatric neurology. He also handed her Bernard Rimland's book on autism with a recommendation to read it, sparking a lifelong interest in this subject.

Michele Zappella entered the department as a fellow in Neurology. He remembers how generous Paine was with him: for example, initially, until Zappella could find a place to live in town, Paine took him into his home for several days as if he were a son. Subsequently, Paine favored Zappella's research in all possible ways, allowing him to write various articles and a book on congenital encephalopathies, the first one written in Italian in which Richmond Paine wrote a good introduction. He also supported Zappella's initial interest in child psychiatry and allowed him to attend the corresponding department in the afternoons. In the following years, when Zappella began to deal with children with autism, Richmond's teaching was the basis upon which it was possible to imagine new sub-groups and syndromes.

Yoshiko Nomura came to Children's Hospital of Washington, D.C., with the dream of learning from Richmond Paine after having been fascinated by his original works. Although greatly disappointed that he was gone when she arrived, her learning from the team left behind by Richmond Paine determined her career.

Acknowledgments

The authors wish to thank the Morton B. and Blanche S. Prince Philanthropic Fund; Carol and Harvey Eisenberg; Tahma Metz, Executive Director of the Purine Research Society; Dr. Phillip L. Pearl; and Dr. Masaya Segawa, Director of the Segawa Neurological Clinic for Children. They also wish to thank Catharine Carlin and Jennifer Rappaport of Oxford University Press.

Preface

"Costumeless consciousness, that is he" said Emily Dickinson (Johnson 1963). Was she thinking of a child with autism or Asperger syndrome? These beautiful children may indeed reveal their feelings for all to see; they do share an incompetence for being deceitful. But in many other ways, they can be quite different. Some are gentle and passive while others can become angry or hyperactive; some are quite clumsy and while others are astonishingly graceful and balanced; some stun us with their brilliant savant skills even while otherwise functioning at much lower cognitive levels. Who are these enigmatic children?

To address this and other questions regarding the children who have been given the diagnosis of autism or Asperger syndrome, this book turns to neurological analysis. As discussed in chapter 1, autism and Asperger syndrome appear to be variations of the same neurodevelopmental syndrome, a vast syndrome with many different etiological factors. Whether all the cases labeled as PDD-NOS belong inside this huge syndrome, however, is far from clear. Chapter 2 takes a look at the components of the impaired neural networks that might underlie the presentation of autistic symptoms. Of particular interest is the dysfunction of the cerebellum and its circuits in so many of these children (chapter 3). The neurological signs and symptoms that can be found in children with autism/Asperger include abnormal cranial circumferences (chapter 4), epilepsy, changes of muscle tone, stereotypies, and mutism (chapter 5). The appendix contains a neurological examination form specifically designed for the examination of patients with autism/Asperger.

The field of autism today is focused on several problem areas. One is whether autism has been increasing in recent years. The reasons for this perception and a review of the historical prevalence rates in chapter 6 suggest that autism has never been a very rare disorder. Another topic of great interest is whether autism is reversible. Chapter 7 looks at the natural course of those diseases that have a transient autistic phase, using Rett syndrome as an example. Chapter 8 then reviews reports of reversible autistic behavior.

Finally, there is a review of therapies, alternative (chapter 9) and educational/medical (chapter 10). As discussed in these treatment chapters, many different therapies fill the landscape of helping the appropriately worried parents of these children. Parents often are overwhelmed by information. When you have many medical therapies, often contradictory, two possibilities exist. One is that the correct therapy for that disease has yet to be identified. The history of medicine is replete with incidents in which multiple, unsatisfactory therapies are offered until the single effective treatment for a single disease is discovered. The second possibility is that there is no such thing as one medical treatment because autism is not one disease after all but a syndrome, a final, common pathway of many, many different diseases, each of which may require its own medical therapy. In such cases, accurate diagnosis must precede therapy.

The authors of this book wish to recognize that the present level of knowledge about autism has been greatly aided by the heroic parents of children with autism, who have kept pushing the professionals to do better. What strength so many of these parents have! Among the parents of children with the autistic syndrome are the parent professionals, individuals with graduate training in many scientific fields. There are many such parents; they have organized schools and centers actively involved in supporting research, as well as seeking better diagnosis and treatment. When the medical history of autism is written, an unusual historical development will be noted: that several of the most important and seminal intellectual contributions in the field have been made by the parents of the patients themselves. One such example is Bernard Rimland, Ph.D., of the United States, who wrote the first comprehensive book challenging the psychoanalytic theory that autism was caused by poor mothering (Rimland 1964). He presented the case for a biological dysfunction of the brain and deduced that autism was a cognitive dysfunction. He studied the genetic basis of autism by comparing monozygotic and dizygotic twins. Another such parent professional is Lorna Wing, Ph.D., of England who made major clinical contributions to both autism (the triad of social impairment [Wing & Gould 1979], DISCO [Wing et al. 2002]) and Asperger syndrome by helping pull it from the dustbins of medical history (Wing 1981). She also has done groundbreaking work on catatonia in autism (Wing & Shah 2000).

The quantity and quality of research into autism has increased dramatically in the past few years, concomitant with the development of technical advances in imaging the brain and in molecular genetics; many of the questions posed in this volume may be better understood soon.

REFERENCES

Johnson TH (1963) *The poems of Emily Dickinson.* Cambridge, Mass.: Belknap Press. Poem 1454.

Rimland B (1964) *Infantile Autism; The syndrome and its implications for a neural theory of behavior.* Englewood Cliffs, N.J.: Prentice Hall.

Wing L (1981) Asperger syndrome: a clinical account. *Psychological Medicine* 11:115–129.

Wing L, Gould J (1979) Severe impairments of social interaction and associated abnormalities in children: epidemiology and classification. *Journal of Autism and Developmental Disorders* 9:11–29.

Wing L, Leekam SR, Libby SJ, Gould J, Larcombe M (2002) The Diagnostic Interview for Social and Communication Disorders: background, inter-rater reliability, and clinical use. *Journal of Child Psychology and Psychiatry* 43:307–325.

Wing L, Shah A (2000) Catatonia in autistic spectrum disorders. *British Journal of Psychiatry* 176:357–362.

Contents

Contributors

Catalina Betancur, MD, PhD
Faculté de Médecine
Université Paris XII
Paris, France

Mary Coleman, MD
Emeritus Clinical Professor of
    Pediatrics (Neurology)
Georgetown University School of
    Medicine
Washington, D.C., USA

G. Robert DeLong, MD
Professor of Pediatrics (Neurology)
Duke University Medical Center
Durham, North Carolina, USA

Christopher Gillberg, MD, PhD
Professor of Child and Adolescent
    Psychiatry
University of Göteborg, Sweden and
    University of London, UK

Yoshiko Nomura, MD
Segawa Neurological Clinic for
    Children
Chiyoda-ku, Toyko, Japan

Lorenzo Pavone, MD
Professor and Chairman of Pediatrics
Department of Pediatrics
University of Catania
Catania, Italy

Martino Ruggieri, MD, PhD
Senior Lecturer
Institute of Neurological Science
Italian National Research Council
Assistant Professor of Pediatrics
Department of Pediatrics
University of Catania
Catania, Italy

Michele Zappella, MD
Director of the Clinic of
    Neuropsychiatry
General Hospital di Siena
Siena, Italy

The Neurology of Autism

Chapter 1

Introduction

Mary Coleman and Catalina Betancur

It was 1866 in Londontown. The doctors, coming into their own beside the surgeons, had begun to classify diseases of the brain and help create the specialty of neurology. However, many children were hard to classify because they had something terribly wrong in brain function; they had great difficulty learning and were called idiots. Idiocy was an epithet, barely a disease entity, and a neglected one at that. But all that began to change when Dr. John Langdon Down (1866) published a paper pointing out that children who were classified as idiots and had enlarged tongues protruding from their mouths did not necessarily all have the same form of idiocy. They might have had the same major symptom (mental retardation), be the same age when it became obvious that something was wrong (usually after 18 months of age), and share a striking feature (the appearance of macroglossia), but he announced that they did not all have the same disease. Dr. Langdon Down wrote that one group had mongolism, a name he chose because of the appearance of the children's eyelids, and the other group had cretinism, a disease known today as infant hypothyroidism. This paper ushered in a new era of medical interest in these children, which also led to more humane care.

Almost a century and a half later, in the twenty-first century, over 2000 different disease entities have been described in which patients have mental retardation. Mental retardation is a series of neurodevelopmental syndromes due to chromosomal, genetic, infectious, endocrine, and toxic etiologies; in almost all cases, the disease process is underway prior to birth. Regarding genetic disease, when mutation of a single gene is both necessary and sufficient to cause disease, it is called a monogenetic trait; it is now known that over 200 of the mental retardation diseases are classified as monogenetic diseases (Zechner et al. 2001). The disease entities of the mental retardation syndromes have been generally grouped together into two major categories: syndromic and nonsyndromic mental retardation. These categories refer to syndromes in which there are multiple congenital anomalies and mental retardation (the MCA/MR syndromes) versus those syndromes without either major congenital anomalies or facial and other stigmata.

Does this story have any relevance to autism? The history of autism does not cover as many years. It was first identified by Leo Kanner in 1943 and thought to be a single psychiatric disease; he defined it as a behavioral disease entity beginning when children are very young. A recent study has suggested that autism may be already underway at the time of birth in almost all the children. In a study of archived neonatal blood, Nelson and colleagues (2001) found that the levels of certain neurotrophins and certain neuropeptides were higher in 99% of the children who were later diagnosed as autistic than they were in control children. These molecules were brain-derived neurotrophic factor (BDNF), neurotrophin 4/5 (NT4/5), vasoactive intestinal peptide (VIP), and calcitonin gene-related peptide (CGRP). The study by Nelson and colleagues also found similar elevations of the neurotrophins and neuropeptides in 97% of children who later were diagnosed with mental retardation, including those with Down syndrome. *It is of great interest that no measurement distinguished the children with autism from those with mental retardation, although these measurements did distinguish them from children who later were diagnosed with cerebral palsy and from normal controls.*

This study suggests that the autistic syndromes, like the mental retardation syndromes, begin prior to birth in the overwhelming number of cases. It adds one more piece of evidence that autism is a member of the family of neurodevelopmental syndromes with maturational disturbances and may be the behavioral stepsister of the mental retardation syndromes.

In fact, the autistic syndromes share many of the characteristics of the mental retardation syndromes. Both groups of syndromes begin to impair the brain in almost all cases during the gestational neurodevelopmental time frame; they are both present at birth but are not usually clinically apparent. They both have family histories with inheritance patterns that sweep across the landscape of genetics, from classical Mendelian to maternal inheritance patterns to trinucleotide repeat disorders to large numbers of sporadic cases. Twin, family, and linkage data and case histories reveal that the inheritance pattern in autism is very complex (for review, see Folstein & Rosen-Sheidley 2001). Although a percentage of children in both groups of syndromes develop epilepsy, the autistic syndromes actually include a higher prevalence of children with seizure disorders than do the population with severe mental retardation syndromes (Gillberg & Coleman 2000a). Children with autism do not have the same neuropsychological profile as youngsters classified as retarded; nevertheless, IQ is the single best predictor of outcome in both syndromes (Gillberg & Coleman 2000b). And, most important, the two syndromes overlap in the majority of children who are classified as autistic (Jacobson & Janicki 1983; Bryson et al. 1988); in most studies IQ is below 70 in 70% of individuals who are defined as having autism.

THE TIMING OF AUTISM

If autistic traits develop because of neurodevelopmental missteps, when during gestation does that occur? Neuroembryology is a very complex phenomenon although neurodevelopment of the brain seems to occur gradually and seamlessly. Rice and Barone (2000) and many others have noted evidence of critical periods of vulnerability in the developing nervous system (these periods are topics of important future research). In the case of autism, data obtained from several groups of children with autistic characteristics show evidence that the disease process can be initiated in all three trimesters (Rodier et al. 1996; Coleman 1994; Yamashita et al. 2003). (There is some postnatal evidence, too [Minshew 1996].) As evidence from these trimesters is reviewed, one useful way to look at this neurodevelopmental problem might be to classify the autistic syndromes with the same general terms that are used to classify mental retardation syndromes, that is, syndromic or nonsyndromic. However, in both mental retardation and autism, the concept of stigmatized versus nonstigmatized children is in reality a bit too stark. Certainly in autism a continuum from minor to major physical stigmata can be seen. In syndromes with large numbers of patients, it often is apparent that the variable degree of phenotypic manifestation between individuals could be represented as a continuum from the full disease to even minor or undetectable expression. The concept of syndromic autism versus nonsyndromic autism will be presented here as a structural framework in which to tentatively place the disease entities.

The first trimester, primarily a time when the body and face are formed, would be the time of syndromic autism, the period when MCA/MR syndromes are initiated. It has been demonstrated that some of the MCA/MR syndromes that include an autistic subgroup, such as the Möbius sequence, thalidomide embryopathy, or the CHARGE association (coloboma, heart defect, atresia of the choanae, retarded growth and mental development, genital anomalies, and ear malformations and hearing loss), may begin as early as 20 to 24 days postfertilization. In addition, in an autism autopsy case, Rodier et al. (1996) identified a shortening of the brain stem, a defect that could have occurred only during neural tube closure. In the development of the cerebral cortex, 6 to 8 weeks of gestational age are called the embryonic period. Children with autism and a grossly abnormal stigmata examination are 10 times more likely to be diagnosed with a known genetic syndrome and are twice as likely to have structural abnormalities in their brains than children with autism without gross stigmata (Miles & Hillman 2000).

A large number of MCA/MR syndromes include a subgroup of children with autism (table 1-1A). Estimates of the number of children with autism who have these syndromes vary widely from 7% to 37%, indicating either a different pop-

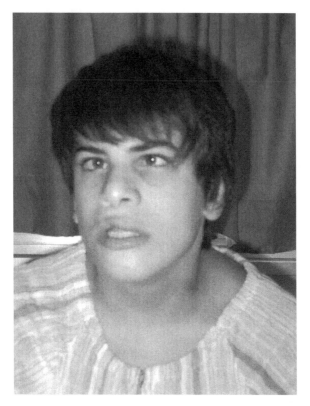

Figure 1.1   Fourteen-year-old girl with syndromic autism, ectodermal dysplasia, MR.

ulation mix, or a different method of selection by the investigators. Around 12% is a reasonable working estimate for population-based surveys (Kielinen et al. 2004). The relevant question in each MCA/MR syndrome is whether the syndrome is somehow related to autistic symptoms or whether the affected children have two completely separate syndromes, the MCA/MR syndrome and a second autistic syndrome. Each syndrome must be evaluated separately, because the majority of children in most of the MCA/MR syndromes in which autistic patients have been reported do *not* have autistic features.

In the MCA/MR syndromes that are very rare and include few cases of autism, a reasonable assumption could be that, in a coincidental double syndrome, an unlucky child described with autistic features perhaps did have the syndrome by chance. If the child also has established autism stigmata that differ from those of other children with the particular syndrome, this weighs in favor of coincidence instead of relevance; the unlucky patient likely has two separate disease entities.

Table 1-1   Some of the double syndromes in which a subgroup of patients meeting autistic criteria has been described

A. Multiple congenital anomalies/mental retardation (MCA/MR) syndromes

Angelman syndrome	Möbius sequence
CATCH 22	Neurofibromatosis 1
CHARGE association	Noonan syndrome
Cohen syndrome	Orstavik 1997 syndrome
Cole-Hughes macrocephaly syndrome	Rett syndrome
Cowden syndrome	Rubinstein-Taybi syndrome
15q11-q13 duplication syndrome	Smith-Lemli-Opitz syndrome
de Lange syndrome	Smith-Magenis syndrome
Down syndrome	Sotos syndrome
Ehlers-Danlos syndrome	Steinert's myotonic dystrophy
Fragile X syndrome	Timothy syndrome
Goldenhar syndrome	Tuberous sclerosis complex
Hypomelanosis of Ito	Turner syndrome
Lujan-Fryan syndrome	Williams syndrome

B. Neurological syndromes

Dysmaturational syndrome with familial complex tics
Joubert syndrome
Leber's congenital amaurosis
Mitochondrial syndromes, including the HEADD syndrome
Neuroaxonal dystrophy variant
Tourette syndrome/autism
X-linked creatine transporter defect

C. Psychiatric syndromes

Anorexia nervosa/autism
Infantile autistic bipolar subgroup

An example is the case of a boy with Myhre syndrome, who met the DMS-IV criteria of autism and exhibited several symptoms that are not usually found in the syndrome (Titomanlio et al. 2001). In addition to peculiar skin histology not typically described in Myhre syndrome, he also had hypertelorism and partial cutaneous syndactyly of the second and third toes. These are stigmata singled out in studies of minor physical anomalies in children with nonsyndromic autism. These facts weigh in favor of two separate disease entities in this boy.

However, other MCA/MR syndromes, such as the disease process of the tuberous sclerosis complex, may be more prone to creating autistic symptoms in their population. Epidemiological studies suggest that 43–86% of individuals with the tuberous sclerosis complex have a pervasive developmental disorder similar to autism (Harrison & Bolton 1997), and this disease alone may account for from 1% to 4% of children with autism in some series (Smalley 1998). It is possible

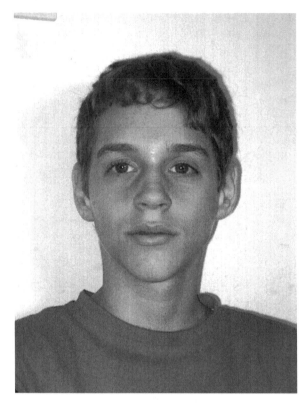

Figure 1.2   Fourteen-year-old boy with nonsyndromic, high-functioning autism.

that the autistic symptoms in some of these children may spring from the underlying disease process, such as the number, location, and size of the brain tubers of the tuberous sclerosis complex (Humphrey et al. 2004), which also can be a source of epileptic foci (Chugani et al 1998). Because they are much more thoroughly studied, the MCA/MR syndromes can be helpful in highlighting information that may underlie autistic symptoms. However, it must always be kept in mind that each of these syndromes has many other nonautistic symptoms, and it is only by putting together the information from many different disease entities that some form of standardized picture might come to light.

Several syndromes in which autistic features are part of the initial description of the syndrome have been reported. Examples are HEADD syndrome (hypotonia, epilepsy, autism, and developmental delay) and Orstvik 1997 syndrome (macrocephaly, epilepsy, autism, stigmata, and mental retardation) (Orstavik et al. 1997; Fillano et al. 2002; van Karnebeek et al. 2002). Evidence of mitochondrial dysfunction and mitochondrial DNA (mtDNA) deletions has been found in children with HEADD syndrome. It is too early to be sure, but apparently almost all patients diagnosed with these new syndromes would be considered autistic. Even so, each child with a double syndrome of both autism and any MCA/MR syndrome should be evaluated as an individual; this has both genetic counseling and treatment implications.

While on the topic of MCA/MR syndromes, it should be noted that a child with autism does not have to possess major anomalies or major stigmata to have a disease entity that began in the first trimester. Some minor stigmata can be traced to the first trimester (Rodier et al. 1997b). Sometimes the syndrome is missed because the stigmata and skin lesions that characterize the children's faces are not always apparent in infancy and early childhood. Examples of this delayed diagnostic phenomenon are reported in tuberous sclerosis, Cohen syndrome, and chromosome 22q11.2 deletion syndrome. Yet another possibility is the recent revelation that a child may be clinically classified as having nonsyndromic autism and also have a mutation on the same gene affected in a MCA/MR syndrome (Turner et al. 2002); this is the same phenomenon that is seen in syndromic and nonsyndromic forms of mental retardation (Nokelainen & Flint 2002).

The second trimester is believed to be a time when many of the neurodevelopmental errors that lead to nonsyndromic autism occur. The period from 8 to 20–24 weeks of gestational age including the end of the first as well as the second trimester is the fetal period of brain development. When autism was first being studied, it was noted how beautiful and unstigmatized many of these children were. This may even have been a factor in the initial blaming of the parents who were raising such normal-looking children. But as soon as any systematic research was conducted on this question, it became clear that children with autism who looked unstigmatized were more likely to have minor physical anomalies than control children matched for age, sex, and socioeconomic status (Steg & Rapoport 1975; Walker 1976; Campbell et al. 1978; Links et al. 1980; Rodier et al. 1997a). The timing of formation of these minor anomalies spans from the first trimester to the beginning of the second trimester. In these studies, the single most common minor anomaly in these studies found in autism was an ear anomaly characterized by particularly low seating and posterior rotation of the ears. This anomaly was even more common in children with autism than in children with mental retardation. Other minor anomalies found in children with autism by more than one of these studies were partial or full syndactyly of the second and third toes and a slight hypertelorism.

It is far from clear in which trimester to place the infantile forms of neurological (table 1-1B) and psychiatric disorders (table 1-1C) already defined in older populations. Because these beautiful children have so few stigmata, these categories temporarily go into the second trimester lists. The issue will become clearer disease by disease as the neuroanatomical and genetic basis of the primary disorders are better understood.

In a prospective study of prenatal factors comparing children who developed autism with normal and mentally retarded controls, statistically significant second-trimester bleeding was limited to the mothers of children with autism (Torrey et al. 1975). There are a few reported cases of accurately timed infections in mothers of children who later developed autism. In children with autism and congenital rubella (Chess 1977) or congenital cytomegalovirus (Ivarsson et al. 1990), the maternal infections occurred in the second trimester. Maternal auto-immune diseases in the second trimester also may increase risk (Croen et al. 2005).

Malformations of cortical development due to abnormal neuronal and glial proliferation are seen in neuroectodermal diseases, such as tuberous sclerosis. Evidence of neuronal migration aberrations is found in many MRIs of children with both autism and Asperger syndrome. (See chapter 2 for references.) Table 1-2 lists some of the diseases in which these neuroembryological errors are found. Both genetic and infectious etiologies can cause these aberrations. They are primarily second trimester phenomena.

Relatively few patients with autism are thought to have injuries to the central nervous system initiated during the third trimester. The period extending from 24 weeks of gestation until the time of birth is called the perinatal period by embryologists of the central nervous system. The children with autism that have been documented with third trimester insults appear to be mostly affected by infections, such as symptomatic congenital cytomegalovirus infection (Yamashita et al. 2003).

The perinatal and postnatal periods are times when errors established earlier may be expressed or new insults may affect brain function. After the advent of birth, the brain continues to grow, change, and be vulnerable owing to the persistence of some limited neurogenesis, elimination of neurons through apoptosis or programmed cell death, postnatal proliferation and pruning of synapses, and activity-dependent refinement of neuronal connections (Johnston 2004).

Table 1-2   Disease entities in which both neuronal migration and autistic symptoms have been reported

MCA/MR syndrome	Type of neuronal migration disorder
de Lange syndrome	heterotopia
Ehlers-Danlos syndrome	heterotopia
Hypomelanosis of Ito	polymicrogyria, heterotopia
Neurofibromatosis, type 1	polymicrogyria, heterotopia
Rett syndrome	nodular heterotopia
	perisylvian cortical dysplasia
Smith-Lemli-Opitz syndrome	polymicrogyria, rare
Sotos syndrome	neuronal heterotopia
Tuberous sclerosis complex	heterotopia

Reference: Hennekam & Barth (2003)

THE NOSOLOGY OF AUTISM

So in this neurodevelopmental syndrome, the question arises as to how we are going to diagnose children with this core social disorder in the future. One encouraging development is that, in psychiatry and neurology as in all of medicine, nosology is rapidly improving so that diagnosis and treatment can be more individualized. It is now possible to expand the traditional clinicopathological method of general diagnosis into a more comprehensive study of the disease during the lifetime of the individual through chromosomal studies, molecular genetics, brain imaging, electrophysiology, and many other technologies. However, the symptoms of central nervous system disease, showing through an underlying personality structure, remain particularly difficult to interpret. This is especially so in the case of the young child with autistic symptoms.

It has been 60 years since the behavioral syndrome of autism was first described, yet problems of nosology remain. Most physicians working with these patients would agree that current testing instruments to define the symptoms of autism (table 1-3) are clinically useful and appropriate. Autism involves multiple developmental domains; it compromises a wide range of socioemotional, language, and other cognitive skills. However, many patients do not fit exactly into the designated criteria of autism or Asperger, and their condition is called atypical autism or pervasive developmental disorder not otherwise specified (PDD-NOS). Are children with specific language disorders mistakenly being put into a pool with autism? Another unsettled question refers to patients currently classified as having the very rare Childhood Disintegrative Disorder. This is a topic in itself: A family of 2 half-brothers, 1 with autism and 1 with Childhood Disintegrative Disorder, has been described (Zwaigenbaum et al. 2000).

Very important work has been done to recruit populations of children with autism that are as psychiatrically homogeneous as possible for research purposes. Nevertheless, a number of unsolved issues remain in play. These problems are not just academic; they have implications for infant and childhood learning programs, as well as pharmacological approaches.

One persistent nosological challenge is to determine whether Asperger syndrome and autism are variations of the same disease, a question posed by Lot-

Table 1-3   Current instruments that can be used to diagnose or assess the severity of patients with autistic symptoms

Autism Diagnostic Interview–Revised (ADI-R)
Autism Diagnostic Observation Schedule–Generic (ADOS-G)
Childhood Autism Rating Scale (CARS)
Diagnostic Interview for Social and Communication Disorders (DISCO)
Diagnostic and Statistical Manual of Mental Disorders (*DSM–IV*) criteria
The ICD-10 Classification of Mental and Behavioral Disorders (ICD–10) criteria

speich et al. (2004) and others. There is evidence from a number of disciplines including genetics that suggests that the answer is likely to be yes (table 1-4). The same mutations in nuclear DNA (Jamain et al. 2003) and also in mtDNA (Pons et al. 2004) have been found both in patients with autism and in patients with Asperger syndrome. However, an increasingly difficult point is this: Are the criteria for Asperger generally being applied by clinicians too loosely? Where does one draw the line between an eccentric or odd person and a truly sick person; in other words, how broad is the phenotype? Benaron (2003), using the title "Inclusion to the point of dilution," reviewed the topic of diagnosis in autism/Asperger and raised a number of important points. One was that there are no criteria for exclusion, as is seen in so many other syndromes, resulting in increasing dilution.

Another area of debate is the presence of additional brain symptoms. Although it is well accepted that many of the children with autism would be classified on standardized testing as mentally retarded, there is a very significant percentage—up to 40% in some series—who are also prone to other psychiatric conditions, such as mood, attentional, and anxiety disorders. Should there be a neurological or an epilepsy subgroup (chapter 5)? Do mute patients belong in a separate group, since this is a large subgroup (Gillberg & Wahlstrom 1985)? Some of the worse clinical problems with children with autism arise from the so-called secondary symptoms, which are vision and hearing impairments, disturbing forms of self-abuse, sleep disorders that haunt the parents, many types of food faddism, and water fascination with its danger of drowning. Are they found only in certain disease entities or throughout all autism?

Table 1-4   Characteristics shared by autism and Asperger syndrome

Clinical:
   Social impairment
   Nonverbal communication difficulties
   Narrow interests
   Repetitive routines
   Savants or splinter skills
   Predominantly male
Imaging:
   Variability of neural network maps
Neuropathological:
   Diminished Purkinje cells in the cerebellum
   Neuronal migration defects
   Limbic system neuropathology
   Altered minicolumn organization
   Rare neuroepithelial tumors
Genetic:
   Same gene mutations found (e.g., mutations in the X-linked *NLGN3* and *NLGN4* genes, and in mitochondrial DNA)

Before these many questions can be answered, however, the most elementary nosological question that must be addressed is whether autism is one disease or many diseases. A spectrum is the term used to describe continuous clinical variations spread out within the same disease entity. The utility of a spectrum is the ability to assemble a coherent group that is composed of individuals who all share a set of basic underlying pathological traits, such as a genotype, and that thus provides a consistent set of individuals for further research and the development of rational therapies. The implication of the term "autistic spectrum disorders" is that they are, in the end, one underlying disease. Thus, is autism one huge, sprawling, multifaceted spectrum of a disease? Or, perhaps, is autism a syndrome, a final, common phenotype expressed by many different underlying diseases?

Is autism a spectrum or a syndrome? Study of the human genome has led to many changes in medical thinking; one of these changes is that the concepts of "spectrum" and "syndrome" as used in the past have developed extended meanings. For example, mutations of the *ARX* (Aristaless-related homeobox) gene, important in neurodevelopment, have clinical manifestations referred to as the "spectrum of the *ARX* gene" (Kato et al. 2004). Mutations of this gene are associated with the following human phenotypes: (1) hydranencephaly with abnormal genitalia, (2) X-linked lissencephaly with abnormal genitalia, (3) Proud syndrome (X-linked mental retardation, agenesis of the corpus callosum and abnormal genitalia), (4) isolated agenesis of the corpus callosum (in females) (5) X-linked infantile spasms, and (6) nonsyndromic X-linked mental retardation. Other phenotypes include West syndrome, myoclonus, dystonia, spinocerebellar ataxia, and autism. So disease entities that result in very major brain malformations and those that do not cause any detectable malformation of the brain can arise from mutations in this single gene. This is a case of extreme pleiotropy of clinical expression indicating a great allelic heterogeneity; it ranges from the missing cortex of hydranencephaly all the way to the brain apparently without malformations of nonsyndromic mental retardation. The *ARX* gene holds other fascinations as well. The location and types of the mutations inside the *ARX* gene tend to be predictive of the phenotype (Kato et al. 2004). To date, the known *ARX* mutations in humans that do not result in brain malformations are the deletion of exon 5, polyalanine expansions or duplications, and missense mutations. In contrast, truncating mutations, which induce a premature termination of the protein, cause lissencephaly or hydranencephaly. *ARX* was one of the very first genes for which it was noted that there tends to be a consistency of the genotype-phenotype correlation which can be determined by looking inside the gene itself.

Certainly on the face of it, the clinical expression of *ARX* mutations underlies what appears to mimic a syndrome (many separate disease entities) rather than a spectrum (variations of a single disease). However, by some present definitions, all clinically relevant mutations on one gene = one spectrum. So this kind of caveat will be kept in mind during the nosology discussion of autism/Asperger syndrome. At least there is no argument that from the point of view of educational intervention programs, it is often quite useful to consider autism, Asperger syndrome, PDD-NOS, and the other phenotypic variants as part of a rather extensive clinical psychiatric spectrum, using similar individualized approaches to tackle the symptoms.

Based on twin and family studies (Bailey et al. 1995; Pickles et al. 1995) and subsequent genome scans, evidence that more than one gene might be involved in autism began to develop. This led to the conclusion that autism was a complex rather than a monogenic disorder, with the term "oligogenic disorder" used to describe the involvement of multiple loci (Risch et al. 1999; Cook 2001). The assumption was made that, like in other common diseases such as Parkinson disease, multiple genetic and environmental factors would influence the risk of an individual being affected. Susceptibility or protective genes might confer or reduce the risks of developing disease. One strategy, using linkage and association studies, examined the possibility that the responsible genes are not mutated sequences encoding aberrant gene products but apparently normal polymorphisms acting synergistically or even "independently." Investigating the genetics of separate subclinical traits or endophenotypes in relatives of children with autism seemed another constructive way to find susceptibility genes (Leboyer 2003).

After more than 10 years of very hard work on these linkage and association studies by many dedicated investigators, no susceptibility gene for all of autism has yet been identified. In contrast, there is now good and growing information about Parkinson's disease in hand. In Parkinson's disease, genetic studies have found mutations in genes from different families and several susceptibility genes; they affect the misfolding, overexpression, or insufficient disposal or aggregation of brain alpha-synuclein, which has a central role in this disease process (Olanow 2003; Golbe & Mouradian 2004). Researchers are even beginning to understand how damage by toxins such as MPTP to alpha-synuclein might cause clinical Parkinson-like effects similar to those that result from the gene mutations. Although the Parkinson story is not yet over and other genes and alternate mechanisms await discovery, it is currently believed that most gene mutations directly or indirectly lead to a pathogenetic cascade that eventually affects the brain's handling of a central protein, alpha-synuclein.

So now it can be asked if Parkinson's disease is a good pathogenetic model for autism. Will gene mutations be consistently found in autism that eventually lead in most cases to one protein? Or, perhaps, would a more fruitful model be the approach used in studying the mental retardation syndromes in which many, many different factors are involved; in which there are chromosomal duplications, deletions, translocations, and mosaics; and in which where there are genes with different Mendelian patterns of transmission, trinucleotide repeats and maternal inheritance patterns, as well as epigenetic phenomena?

One Disease Entity

The first question is as follows: Is autism, at least as originally described by Kanner, a single disease entity in the great majority of patients? One can make the argument that this is not clear-cut in view of the fact that 2 of his 11 patients developed a seizure disorder, creating 2 subgroups—a seizure group and a non-seizure group—in the very first population of patients (Kanner 1943, 1971). Of course, it is theoretically possible that the same gene, indicating one disease entity, can underlie a phenotype that is similar except that some patients have seizures and others are seizure free. Another theoretical possibility is that classic autism might be caused by epigenetic silencing that can mimic genetic mutation by abolishing the expression of a gene. The mosaicism and nonMendelian inheritance that are characteristic of epigenetic states can produce patterns of disease risk that resemble those of polygenic or complex traits.

But now that genetic screening has begun in large groups of children with autism, different genes have been found in different individuals, and the pleiotropic nature of many genes has become apparent. In the autism literature, there now exists evidence of both locus heterogeneity (mutations in completely different genes causing the same phenotype) and allelic heterogeneity (different mutations in the same gene causing different phenotypes). An example of locus heterogeneity is seen in the tuberous sclerosis complex. In this genetically heterogeneous disorder, approximately 40% of the cases are related to mutations in the *TSC1* gene on chromosome 9 (9q34), while most of the remaining cases are associated with alteration of the *TSC2* gene on chromosome 16 (16p13.3). An example of allelic heterogeneity concerning the *ARX* gene was discussed above; Sherr (2003) lists the autism cases in the *ARX* spectrum.

As the number of genetic loci found by studying children with strictly defined autism has multiplied, investigators have begun to rethink their theories and have begun to wonder if the limited concordance in different genome-wide scans might reflect sample heterogeneity rather than ever more numerous genes of weak effect (Buxbaum et al. 2004). Could it be that autism is more than one disease entity?

Many Disease Entities

That autism might be a syndrome with multiple etiologies has been considered by a number of authors. In 1986, Reiss et al. wrote that autism appears to be a behaviorally defined phenotype that arises from diverse causes of central nervous system damage. Bailey (1993) noted that the genetic factors in autism probably include causative genes, since autism appeared to have one of the highest heritability rates in psychiatry. By 2003, Eigsti and Shapiro were stating that autism is a heterogenous disorder and is likely to have multiple possible etiologies.

Actually, the concept that autism might be a syndrome of more than one disease had already been put forward earlier by neurological, biochemical, stigmata, and family history analyses in a research study of 78 children with autism and their 78 age, sex, parent-income matched controls (Coleman 1976). Virtually everything studied in this early 1976 research project failed to show consistency. The children with autism were not found to be uniform in blood studies: in whole blood serotonin studies, 59% had elevated levels of whole blood serotonin (confirming results from as early as 1961 by Schain and Freedman) and 25% had low levels. Urine studies also lacked uniformity: twenty-two percent of the children had too much uric acid in their urine (hyperuricosuria) and a separate group of 22% had too little calcium (hypocalcinuria). Neurological, stigmata, immunological, autoimmunological, and family history patterns also showed great variability. Although no individual disease entities were identified in this early study, there was a striking lack of homogeneity in the results; hence, the name "the autistic syndromes" was chosen for the study.

Since that study, at least 60 different disease entities have been identified in patients meeting standardized criteria of autism (tables 1-1, 1-5, and 1-6 and the epileptic syndromes in chapter 5). Just as has been seen in the mental retardation syndromes, children with autistic features with chromosomal, genetic, infectious, endocrine, toxic, and space-occupying etiologies have been described. In autism, there are groups of children with no classical neurological signs and there are others with neurological signs such as epilepsy, hypotonia, or tics (see chapter 5). The cranial circumferences are not consistent: they may be normocephalic, macrocephalic, or microcephalic (see chapter 4). All these major variations suggest that autism is not a single disease entity.

If autism in fact is many different diseases, there are a number of implications. One might refer to the study of gender difference in autism. If autism is many diseases, then the underlying factors leading to male predominance in the patients

Table 1-5   Autistic syndromes with subtle or minimal stigmatization

Miles-Hillman subgroup of nonstigmatized phenotypes
Mitochondrial disease subgroups
15q11-q13 duplication syndrome
22q13 deletion syndrome
X-linked neuroligin syndrome
Metabolic disorders (cases are scarce even within these rare diseases):
    Aminoacidurias–phenylketonuria
    GABA metabolism disorders–Succinic semialdehyde dehydrogenase deficiency, pyridoxine-
      dependency syndrome, ?GABA-transaminase deficiency
    Leukodystrophies–metachromatic leukodystrophy
    Mucopolysaccharidoses–Sanfilippo's syndrome
    Organic acidurias–D-glyceric aciduria, (succinic semialdehyde dehydrogenase deficiency)
    Peroxismal disorders–infantile Refsum disease
    Purine disorders–adenylosuccinate lyase deficiency, nucleotidase-associated pervasive
      developmental disorder

Table 1-6 Infectious, endocrine, toxic, and space-occupying disease entities reported in children with autistic symptoms

Infectious
    Congenital encephalopathies: rubella, herpes simplex, cytomegalovirus
    Meningitis
Endocrine–Hypothyroidism
Perinatal toxicity–ROP (retinopathy of prematurity)
Space-occupying lesions
    Arachnoid cysts
    Brain tumors–neuroepithelial tumors
Toxic fetal embryopathies:
    Alcohol, cocaine, lead, thalidomide, valproate

with a normal physical examination and a structurally normal brain by MRI (23 boys to 1 girl) and in the phenotypically abnormal children (1.7 boys to 1 girl) likely have a different origin (Miles & Hillman 2000). As more homogenous populations are identified, pathological studies, functional imaging studies, genetic studies—all research studies—can be more pinpointed and consistent. Another shift might be to move pharmacological research in the direction of tailoring treatment to individual disease entities inside the autistic syndrome.

A look at a few selected chromosomal and genetic aberrations discovered from studying children with autistic features will highlight the great variety of the autistic syndromes.

CHROMOSOMAL DISORDERS

Autism spans the genome. Putting together all the published information on patients who meet the criteria of autism, Asperger syndrome, or PDD-NOS, chromosomal aberrations or genetic mutations have been described in every chromosome (reviewed in Lauritsen et al. 1999; Gillberg & Coleman 2000c). Regarding the pattern seen in the chromosomal aberrations, the autistic syndromes are more likely to be associated with chromosomal deletions than are the mental retardation syndromes, which have more cases of full trisomies. It has been estimated in the past that between 3% and 9% of a population of children with autistic traits have chromosomal aberrations (Gillberg & Wahlstrom 1985; Ritvo et al. 1990; Fombonne et al. 1997; Konstantareas & Homatidis 1999; Wassink et al. 2001). Three examples of chromosomal sites associated with autism will be discussed: regions on chromosome 15, chromosome 22, and the X chromosome.

The 15q11-q13 Cluster

The area on chromosome 15q11-q13, sometimes called the Prader-Willi/Angelman critical region (PWACR), contains a number of imprinted genes. In both the Prader-Willi syndrome and the Angelman syndrome, a large chromosome deletion that spans 4.0 to 4.5 megabases in 15q11.2-q13 has been identified in 60% to 70% of patients. A deletion in the paternally derived chromosome 15 results in Prader-Willi syndrome, while the same deletion in the maternally derived chromosome 15 underlies the Angelman syndrome. These syndromes can also be caused by uniparental disomy (when the two copies of the chromosome are derived from one of the parents); a maternal disomy results in Prader-Willi syndrome, whereas paternal disomy causes Angelman syndrome. Many patients with Angelman syndrome have been reported to have autistic characteristics, but autistic symptoms usually are not described in patients with the Prader-Willi syndrome. However, even here an occasional patient with autistic features has been reported with Prader-Willi (Descheemaker et al. 2002; Veltman et al. 2004).

Patients who do not have clinically apparent Angelman or Prader-Willi syndrome but who definitely have autistic symptoms have been described in association with a number of different aberrations of chromosome 15 that include the PWACR. Most frequently found are duplications, including interstitial ones resulting in trisomic genetic load, or a supernumerary marker chromosome formed by the inverted duplication of proximal chromosome 15, with either a trisomic or tetrasomic genetic load. Translocations, deletions, and microdeletions also are described (for review see Gillberg & Coleman 2000c). The most consistent factor in the aberrations associated with autism is their origin in the maternal chromosome.

Most cases of children with autism and a chromosomal anomaly in the 15q11-13 region appear to have one of the forms of chromosomal duplication. Actually, this area involves probably the most common supernumerary marker chromosome in humans. It should be remembered that not every patient with excessive chromosomal material encompassing 15q11-q13 is autistic (Rineer et al. 1998). If the duplication involves the PWARC, the patients are more likely to have autism or developmental delay; the asymptomatic patients tend to have duplications that fall outside this region (Bolton et al. 2001). Clinically, the presentations in children meeting autistic criteria vary somewhat (Borgatti et al. 2001). Facial stigmata, if present, are usually subtle. Mental retardation is almost always present but ranges from mild to severe. Many but not all children have a seizure disorder. Patients with hypotonia and motor delays have been reported in the literature. Spinal deformities also have been described (Gillberg et al. 1991).

It is not yet known precisely which genes underlie the symptoms of autism in patients with 15q11-13 duplication or deletion in spite of extensive work by excellent laboratories. Of great interest are the three genes encoding GABA$_A$ receptor subunits (GABRB3, GABRA5, GABRG3) located there. In a study of 140 families who had a child with an autistic disorder, Cook et al. (1998) revealed linkage disequilibrium with the GABRB3 gene encoding the beta3 subunit. A GABRB3 polymorphism also was found to be associated with autism in a set of 80 families (Buxbaum et al. 2002). A study of a group of familial cases in which the children had savant skills identified a susceptibility locus within the *GABRB3* gene (Nurmi et al. 2003), while another study using the symptoms of insistence on sameness also found increased linkage to the *GABRB3* gene (Shao et al. 2003). In a study of 226 families with 1 or more children affected with autism, Menold et al. (2001) reported linkage disequilibrium with the *GABRG3* gene. Not all these studies have been duplicated.

Another gene (KIAA0068) that encodes a protein interacting with and modulating the fragile X protein is of interest. The imprinted gene *UBE3A*, involved in Angelman syndrome, is another candidate (Nurmi et al. 2001; Herzing et al. 2002). The gene *ATP10C* exhibits a similar imprinted expression to *UBE3A*, is adjacent to it, and is involved in ion transport (Herzing et al. 2001). And there are still a number of other imprinted genes in the PWACR area.

Probably the most interesting cases to date are those of 2 children with autism and 15q11-q13 inverted duplication, also called isodicentric chromosome 15, who had pronounced mitochondrial proliferation in muscle and partial respiratory chain block most parsimoniously placed at the level of complex III (Filipek et al. 2003). One of these children had no dysmorphic features; the other had dysmorphic features classified as mild. Both had global developmental delay and hypotonia, although it was episodic in one case.

The 22q11 and 22q13 Regions

The chromosomal 22q11 region has been studied by investigators of both schizophrenia and autism; the chromosomal region 22q13 is also under intensive study. These regions are associated with a number of disease entities in which patients have autistic features. There have been several cases of *ring chromosome 22* with autistic disorder (Assumpcao 1998; MacLean et al. 2000), which includes a deletion covering the q11-q13 region. Major malformations are absent in most cases, but it is of note that these children may have the second and third toe syndactyly that is more common in children with autism (Walker 1976).

The 22q11 region is of particular interest because it is the site of the 22q11.2 deletion syndrome, often associated with the *velocardiofacial syndrome*, also known as CATCH 22 (cardiac abnormality, T cell deficit, cleft palate, and hypocalcemia) syndrome. This multiple anomaly syndrome can occur after a de novo mutation or be transmitted as an autosomal dominant trait. Either learning difficulties or mental retardation, as well as problems with speech and language including articulation, are usually present. Common clinical features of this syndrome are cleft palate (velopharyngeal insufficiency), cardiac defects, and a characteristic facial appearance, although there is high phenotypic variability. The patients have a long face, a prominent nose with a bulbous nasal tip and a narrow alar base, almond-shaped or narrow palpebral fissures, malar flattening, malformed ears, and a recessed chin. These facial features are not always apparent in infancy and early childhood. For example, four children with childhood onset schizophrenia and deletions in the chromosome 22q11 region "had subtle cran-iofacial and body dysmorphic characteristics that *had not been noticed previously*" (Sporn et al. 2004).

Neurobehavioral involvement has been reported by many investigators and is thought to be a major feature of the velocardiofacial syndrome (Niklasson et al. 2001), although it has been suggested that it may not be specific but rather related to the level of cognitive development (Feinstein et al. 2002). In 1996, Swillen et al. identified 2 individuals living in residential homes for people with autism as having the velocardiofacial syndrome. A number of children with autism or PDD-NOS have since been reported to have a deletion at 22q11.2 or the velocardiofa-cial syndrome (Kozma 1998; Chudley et al. 1998; Eliez et al. 2000; Niklasson et al. 2001). The velocardiofacial syndrome or the 22q11.2 deletion syndrome also has been described in patients with adult schizophrenia (Coleman & Gillberg 1996) and childhood-onset schizophrenia (Nicolson et al. 1999).

In the velocardiofacial syndrome, the volume of the brain—both grey and white matter but particularly white matter—is decreased (Eliez et al. 2000; Barnea-Goraly et al. 2003b). It is of interest that those patients with a maternal 22q11.2 microdeletion are reported to have a significantly greater loss of grey matter than those with a paternal microdeletion (Eliez et al. 2001a). The velo-cardiofacial syndrome is one of the syndromes in which a diminished size of cerebellar vermal lobules VI-VII and the pons has been demonstrated (Eliez et al. 2001c). Researchers used functional imaging by fMRI to study mathematical reasoning abilities in this patient group and raised the question of aberrant ac-tivation of their brains (Eliez et al. 2001b).

Almost all cases of the velocardiofacial syndrome and two other syndromes—the DiGeorge syndrome and the conotruncal anomaly face syndrome—share a common microdeletion on chromosome 22q11.2. This is one of the most fre-quent interstitial deletions found in humans. A 3-year-old boy with muteness, who met *DSM-IV* criteria for autism, was found to have a 20/22 chromosomal translocation with an interstitial deletion within the 22q11 region; his phenotype was inconsistent with the DiGeorge syndrome. A 99mTc HMPAO brain perfusion SPECT showed a hypoperfusion of the left temporoparietal cortex in this boy (Carratala et al. 1998). Although more than 30 genes have been identified in these deleted segments, neither a single gene nor multiple contiguous genes have yet been identified as responsible for these syndromes (Yamagishi 2002).

The 22q13 region also is involved in disease entities that can occur with au-tism. Adenylosuccinate lyase deficiency is a rare autosomal-recessive disorder of the purine de novo synthesis pathway characterized by developmental delay, hy-potonia, and seizures. The first case report of 3 children with the deficiency indicated that they had infantile autism (Jaeken & Van den Berghe 1984); since then, researchers have identified a number of children who have the deficiency and autistic features (Ciardo et al. 2001). Not all deficient patients are autistic. Adenylosuccinate lyase is an essential enzyme involved in purine biosynthesis; its gene is located at 22q13.1-q13.2. Laboratory investigations have found in the urine and cerebral spinal fluid of patients the presence of succinylpurines, which are normally undetectable in these fluids.

A terminal 22q13 deletion syndrome has been reported in a patient having the autistic syndrome and a de novo cryptic deletion in chromosome 22q13.3 (Goizet et al. 2000); Anderlid et al. (2002) have reported a case with a submicroscopic 22q13 deletion and autistic symptoms. Prasad et al. (2000) described 3 children with the 22q13 deletion syndrome, 1 with autism and 2 with PDD, and suggested that the terminal 22q13 deletion syndrome may represent a recognizable phenotype for genetic evaluation. These authors proposed that children with minor facial stigmata, normal or advanced growth, and significantly delayed speech compared to motor development, combined with deviant behavior, be screened for deletion at 22q13. Macrocrania, a small pointed chin, simple ears, and a high arched palate are other phenotypical features. Disruption of the *ProSAP2* gene, encoding a scaffold protein involved in the postsynaptic density of excitatory synapses and preferentially expressed in the cerebral cortex and cerebellum, has been proposed as the cause of the 22q13 deletion syndrome (Bonaglia et al. 2001). Finally, the meaning is not yet clear regarding a case of Schindler disease (N-acetyl galactosaminidase deficiency) whose gene is located at 22q13→qter; Blanchon et al. (2002) have described a patient with this disease and autistic features.

The X Chromosome

The X chromosome is of particular interest in autism. Compared to the genes on the autosomal chromosomes this chromosome contains a significantly higher number of genes that, when mutated, cause mental impairment (Zechner et al. 2001). Another reason for interest in this chromosome is that the gender ratio favors boys with autism, raising the possibility of increased genetic errors on the X chromosome, which in most known diseases affect males. (For the record, errors on the X chromosome also can be associated with autistic symptoms in subgroups of females; those with Rett syndrome, Turner syndrome, or Xp deletion syndrome [Thomas et al. 1999].) The X chromosome has been studied extensively because of its folate-sensitive fragile sites that have been visualized on the chromosome. These sites are clustered at the Xq27.3-Xq28 region and include the fragile X syndrome and the FRAXE syndrome sites.

The fragile X syndrome is an X-linked disorder that is believed to be the single most common cause of mental retardation, with an incidence estimated at about 1:4000. It is usually caused by an expansion of the trinucleotide repeat (CGG) in the 5'-untranslated region of the *FMR1* gene; however, in a small number of patients, deletions and point mutations of the *FMR1* gene have been identified.

There is perhaps no other developmental disorder in which the pathogenesis from gene to behavioral manifestations is as well described, however imperfectly. Expansion of the number of CGG repeats beyond 230 in the *FMR1* gene usually leads to hypermethylation of this repeat. In addition, a CpG island is formed within the gene which then recruits the transcriptional silencing machinery to the gene, preventing its expression. The *FMR1* gene product, FMRP, is a selective RNA binding protein that shuttles between the nucleus and cytoplasm. FMRP is important in fetal development; the mutated gene is expressed in proliferating and migrating cells (Abitbol et al. 1993), and a fetal brain examined at 23 weeks gestation already had dendritic spine abnormalities (Jenkins et al. 1984). FMRP protein levels have a relationship with functional brain activation during working memory (Menon et al 2000; Kwon et al. 2001), suggesting that these levels are associated with the translational machinery in the dendritic spines. Such regulation of localized protein synthesis is important to the synaptic plasticity that underlies the neural networks of learning and memory. Thus, perhaps it is not unexpected that white matter in the frontostriatal and parietal sensory-motor tracts has been reported to be altered in this syndrome (Barnea-Goraly et al. 2003a).

Facial features of individuals with the fragile X syndrome include a long, narrow face, strabismus, prominent long ears, a thick nasal bridge, dental malocclusion, and a prominent jaw. After puberty, macroorchidism often occurs. Excessive joint laxity, pectus excavatum, kyphoscoliosis, a single palmar crease, and pes planus have been described. The behavioral phenotype of the syndrome includes pronounced gaze aversion (Garrett et al. 2004), language delay and echolalia, perseveration, stereotypies, need for sameness, hypersensitivity to sensory stimuli, preoccupations with constricted interests, and social anxiety, especially with peers or unfamiliar adults.

Although this behavioral phenotype sounds very much like a child with autism, the majority do have emotional relationships with their parents and other familiar adults. They develop strong attachments and concern for others, so they do not have what is considered the core symptom of autism. However, a small percent of patients with the fragile X syndrome do meet full autism criteria; it is not many, but it is higher than can be accounted for by chance (Feinstein & Reiss 1998). Some patients with fragile X appear to be mosaic as judged from their blood cells; there is a trend for autism to be more prevalent in patients with the nonmosaic full mutation. The rate of fragile X among patients with autism is estimated to be about 2–4% (Wassink et al. 2001).

The FRAXE syndrome is also a trinucleotide repeat syndrome, with an expansion of the trinucleotide GCC in the gene *FMR2*. The children are less severely affected and less likely to be stigmatized than those with fragile X. A rare patient with high-functioning autism has been reported (Abrams et al. 1997).

GENES BEING STUDIED IN AUTISM

Genes on the X Chromosome

In addition to the *FMR1* and *FMR2* genes susceptible to excess trinucleotide repeats mentioned above, a number of other genes located on the X chromosome are under investigation in children with permanent or temporary symptoms of autism. Investigators have learned a great deal from the studies of the methyl-CpG-binding protein 2 gene, *MECP2,* located at Xq28. Normally, the function of *MECP2* is to turn off several genes whose promoters have been methylated, an epigenetic phenomenon and many other functions.

Mutations in this gene were first found in girls with Rett syndrome (Amir et al. 1999), a disease that goes through an autistic phase (see chapter 7). A number of variants exist, so the spectrum of diseases is called the Rett Complex. Girls with one of the variants, the Preserved Speech Variant (PSV) of the Rett Complex, have autistic behavior, and most meet *DSM-IV* criteria for autism. The clinical features of PSV include the typical staging of Rett syndrome, but symptoms are milder in that the cranial circumference is often within normal limits, hand washing is more occasional, scoliosis is mild, and body weight may be excessive. Pathogenic mutations of the *MECP2* gene in 55% (10 out of 18) of girls with PSV have been reported; there is a family with two discordant sisters (classic Rett and PSV) bearing a late truncating mutation (Zappella et al. 2001). Investigation of phenotypical variability in the Rett Complex by type of *MECP2* mutation has not shown a consistent pattern, raising the possibility of skewed X-inactivation and/or modifier genes whose products may act in an epistatic matter with MeCP2 protein (De Bona et al. 2000).

A question has been raised about whether girls with autism who apparently do not have a type of the Rett Complex also have mutations in *MECP2*. It sometimes takes in depth background knowledge of both syndromes to distinguish between a Rett variant and autism in a child; Trevathan and Naidu (1988) have listed the differential criteria, and Kammoun et al. (2004) helped pinpoint certain of the criteria. The Rett Complex is much more tightly diagnosed than is autism; it has necessary, supportive, and exclusion criteria, as well as four stages of progression. Two girls with the PSV variant of Rett syndrome were followed closely, and although they had autistic behavior during the first three stages of progression, by early adolescence they lost autistic behavior and reached an IQ close to 45 (Zappella et al. 2003). In addition to differences between the diagnostic criteria, the clinical course often reveals the difference between a girl with a static form of autism and a girl with a Rett Complex variant.

Carney et al. (2003) analyzed 69 girls with autism and found 2 with *MECP2* mutations; neither patient exhibited classic Rett features. Similarly, Lam et al. (2000) screened 21 females with autism and mental retardation and found 1 with a *MECP2* mutation. Shibayama et al. (2004) also identified a mutation and var-

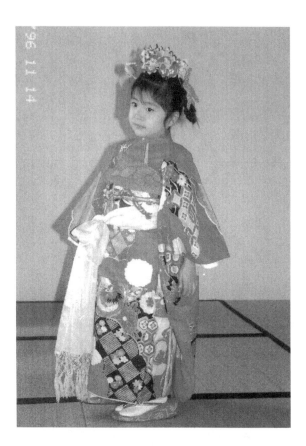

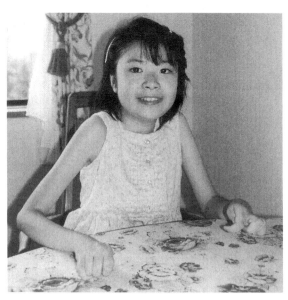

Figures 1.3, 1.4 This Japanese girl, with an A201V mutation of the MeCP2 gene, is seen at 5 and 13 years of age. Dystonic contracture of the hands can be seen at the older age.

iants in children with autism. *MECP2* mutations have also been found in individuals with other brain disorders. These include severe mental retardation, a spastic syndrome in boys, schizophrenia, and bipolar disorder. A previously unknown *MECP2* open reading frame defines a new protein isoform that is different from the previously identified protein; the new isoform is more abundant in the human brain, and this defective form may be the cause of the Rett Complex (Mnatzakanian et al. 2004; Kriaucionis & Bird 2004).

A recent study has shown that 5% (3 out of 63) of Rett girls are carriers of both a *MECP2* mutation and a chromosome 15q11-13 rearrangement (Longo et al. 2004). This is in contrast to the only 1% of patients with autism who have a duplication on chromosome 15q11-q13. Since this study is the first of its kind, the percentage may be due to chance, but the finding itself gives important new information. All three of the girls with the 15q rearrangement were carriers of an *MECP2* mutation at amino-acid R133, a hot spot for mutations in the Rett Complex. Two of the girls with classic Rett had maternally inherited small deletions on 15q11-q13, while the girl with PSV had a paternally inherited small duplication on 15q11-q13.

Another interesting X chromosome gene is *ARX*, a paired-class homeobox gene located at Xp22.13. ARX is specifically expressed in the embryonic forebrain and is involved in the proliferation of neural precursors and differentiation and tangential migration of interneurons. Stromme et al. (2002) have described individuals with autism and mild-to-moderate mental retardation who had *ARX* mutations. Individuals with autism or autistic behavior that had a duplication in this gene have been described by Turner et al. (2002). These authors also found the same duplication in a family with X-linked infantile spasms with hypsarrhythmia, a syndrome that is sometimes associated with the development of later autistic behavior. As discussed above, the phenotypes associated with *ARX* mutations range well beyond autism. Investigators of autism are also interested in another homeobox gene, *EN2,* located at 7q36 (Gharani et al. 2004).

Another important group of genes, those encoding the neuroligins, are also located on the X chromosome. These genes produce proteins that function as cell adhesion molecules during neurodevelopment. Among the proteins involved in the establishment of neural networks (see chapter 2), neuroligins appear to have a central role in the formation of CNS synapses (Chih et al. 2004; Comoletti et al. 2004).

The two neuroligin genes on the X chromosome are *NLGN3*, located at Xq13, and *NLGN4*, located at Xp22.3. Deletions at Xp22.3 that include *NLGN4* have been reported in several individuals with autism (Thomas et al. 1999). Mutations in *NLGN3* and *NLGN4* have now been described in families with autism and Asperger syndrome (Jamain et al. 2003). Researchers have identified an additional family in which the members who have autism, PDD-NOS, or nonsyndromic X-linked mental retardation have a 2-base-pair deletion in *NLGN4* (Laumonnier et al. 2004).

Genes on the Autosomal Chromosomes

Family histories and sibling pairs with autism have enriched the search for candidate genes. In the past 10 years, the combination of identifying gene mutations in individual patients with autistic features and the search for susceptibility genes in strictly defined autism has resulted in a rich harvest of autosomal chromosome sites. Potential sites exist on every chromosome. If autism is, in fact, the cognitive behavioral cousin to the cognitive mental retardation syndromes, then this richness is to be expected, since over 200 monogenetic diseases alone already have been identified for the mental retardation syndromes.

The long lists of potential autosomal gene sites for autism can be found in a number of papers. These include chapter 15 of *The Biology of the Autistic Syndromes* (3rd ed.) (Gillberg & Coleman 2000c) and the two sections on candidate gene analysis and genetic mechanisms in *Autism: Neural Basis and Treatment Possibilities* (Bock & Goode 2003). Data from one genome-wide scan on Asperger syndrome is now available (Ylisaukko-oja et al. 2004). New gene mutations or likely chromosomal sites are constantly being found. While you have been reading this book, it is possible that researchers have found another gene mutation or chromosomal site.

Mitochondrial DNA Studies

The mitochondria are unique among cellular organelles in that they contain their own DNA. Each mitochondrion has 2 to 10 copies of DNA in a circular molecule consisting of 16,569 base pairs. Mitochondrial DNA (mtDNA) differs from DNA in the cell nucleus in that it contains few noncoding sequences (introns), has a slightly different genetic code, and is transmitted almost exclusively from the mother. Over 95% of total brain ATP, the chemical energy of cells, is produced in the mitochondria by the process of oxidative phosphorylation. The regions of the brain that are most functionally active, such as the temporal lobe, are sites of increased mitochondrial activity. Since mitochondria play a pivotal role in cell metabolism, cellular mitochondrial density reflects metabolic activity. Skeletal muscles, as well as neurons, have a high mitochondrial mass, a finding that can be used to detect mitochondrial disease when the mitochondrial function is diminished.

The mutation rate of mtDNA is much higher than that of nuclear DNA. The reason for this higher mutation rate can be ascribed to the absence of a histone coat for mtDNA, a poor repair system for DNA damage, a high turnover rate of mtDNA, exposure to higher oxidative stress, and a high error rate of polymerase gamma, which is responsible for mtDNA replication. This high mutation rate means that even control subjects may sometimes possess mutations, requiring caution in interpreting the complicated literature.

Many mutations in mtDNA have now been associated with human diseases. These are a diverse group of disorders that result from structural, biochemical or genetic derangement of mitochondria. Because mtDNA is inherited almost exclusively through the mother, mtDNA-related defects would be expected to exhibit the maternal inheritance pattern. This is indeed seen, but to date most cases are sporadic. This maternal inheritance pattern of mtDNA does represent a well-recognized non-Mendelian genetic system. However, to make things more complicated, it is necessary to consider that some of the mitochondrial diseases affecting the respiratory chain can also be due to mutations of genes in the nuclear genome, resulting in Mendelian patterns of inheritance. Thus, the family history of a child with a mitochondrial disease may be characterized by a disease that is sporadic, has a maternal inheritance pattern, or has a classical Mendelian pattern. Other genetic characteristics—heteroplasmy, mitotic segregation, and threshold effects—can be seen.

This background detail about mitochondrial diseases has been offered because evidence is mounting that a significant number of children with autism may belong to the mitochondrial subgroup. In fact, the first population-based epidemiological study of mitochondrial disease in autism, completed in Portugal, has arrived at an estimate of 7.2% or more of children with autism (Oliveira et al. 2005). If confirmed, this is the largest subgroup of patients with autism yet described. Furthermore, some of the children reported with mtDNA abnormalities in the literature did not appear to be different from children with "primary autistic spectrum disorders" (Pons et al. 2004).

Speculation that children with autism might have mitochondrial diseases began after it was discovered that some children with autism had high lactate levels (Coleman & Blass 1985), raising the possibility of mitochondrial oxidative phosphorylation dysfunction (Lombard 1998). The impairment of mitochondrial energy metabolism has been documented in individuals with autism and Asperger syndrome (Minshew et al. 1993, Laszlo et al. 1994; Chugani et al. 1999). Thus, it is no surprise that cases of autism and mitochondrial disease are now being reported; the reported cases have a variety of mitochondrial defects. In some children, there are mutations in mtDNA itself (Graf et al. 2000; Pons et al. 2004), as well as deletion (Fillano et al. 2002) and depletion of mtDNA (Pons et al. 2004). In other children, there is alteration of mitochondrial function likely secondary to duplication of the maternally derived chromosome 15q11-q13 region (Filipek et al. 2003).

A growing body of evidence indicates that certain children with autism might be evaluated for mitochondrial cytopathies. This includes those who have lactic acidosis, although it may not be always detectable, and those who have a family pattern of maternal inheritance. Other possible indications include the presence of major neurological signs including seizures, if other known etiologies have been ruled out, and a family history of depression.

Table 1-7   Examples of children with clinical nonsyndromic autism who have a genetic error

Diagnosis	Genetic error	Reference
Autism	24 bp duplication in exon 2 of *ARX* gene (Xp22.13)	Turner et al. 2002
Autism and Asperger	frameshift mutation (1-bp insertion in exon 5) in gene encoding neuroligin *NLGN4* (Xp22.3)	Jamain et al. 2003
Autism and PDD-NOS	2-bp deletion in exon 5 of the *NLGN4* gene (Xp22.3)	Laumonnier et al. 2004
Autism and Asperger	C→T transition (R451C) in gene encoding neuroligin *NLGN3* (Xq13)	Jamain et al. 2003
Autistic spectrum disorder	A3243 mtDNA mutation	Pons et al. 2004
Autism	1-bp deletion in exon 5 (c.183delT) of the CDKL5/STK9 gene (Xp22.1), resulting in a frameshift and premature truncation	Weaving et al. 2004

Genes in Nonsyndromic Autism

Genetic diagnosis has recently become possible in a few patients with nonsyndromic autism and Asperger syndrome. The literature now describes children who clinically present with these disorders and have genetic mutations (table 1-7). However, genetic diagnosis in the majority of such children still eludes us as of the writing of this book.

GENETIC COUNSELING IN AUTISM

That autism is a disorder with a major genetic component is no longer in doubt (see Cook 2001, for a summary of the evidence). Furthermore, variations such as Asperger syndrome and PDD-NOS breed true in some families (Micali et al. 2004). One group of patients have what are called single-gene diseases; this concept of mutations in a single gene as an essential minimum for such genetic diseases is a clinically useful tool, in spite of its scientific limitations. Other members of the family of these patients sometimes have subclinical traits; these traits are called the broader autism phenotype, or endophenotypes, encompassing both psychological and biological data.

Genetic counseling for a disease entity needs to be based on valid information about the family risk of recurrence. In the disease entities listed in tables 1-1, 1-4, and 1-5, informed sources of such information often are available. Although many cases of autism are sporadic, there are some patients within each disease entity in which family patterns can be discerned. For example, genetic patterns of autosomal recessive (adenylosuccinate lyase deficiency), autosomal dominant (tuberous sclerosis complex), X-linked (mutations in the X-linked neuroligins), trinucleotide repeat (fragile X), and mitochondrial (A3243G mtDNA mutations) inheritance can be used to counsel a family.

Unfortunately, for the majority of children with autistic features, often with nonsyndromic autism, such information is not available or may not be relevant. Here, the information gathered from studies of families of children with autism put together as a single disease entity can at least be a guideline. Family studies have shown that the risk of another sibling born with autism to parents who have already had a child with autism may be 4.5% (Jorde et al. 1991). Another way of saying this is that, based on current prevalence estimates, the risk of reoccurrence among siblings appears to be 6 times more frequent than it is in the population as a whole (Micali et al. 2004), a much higher recurrence rate than the prevalence rate in the general population. However, it should be noted that this rate is much lower than is found in single-gene diseases. In the case of autism, there is a high concordance of monozygotic twins, first reported by Rimland (1964) and later confirmed by many studies. When twins are studied using a broader spectrum of autism including related cognitive and social abnormalities, 92% of monozygotic twins were concordant versus only 10% of dizygotic twins (Bailey et al. 1995).

Neurogenetic Diseases

The sequencing of the human genome has turned out to be a necessary first step in a yet unfolding journey; sometimes the answers appear to be much more complex than mere DNA sequence. In patients with autism and their families, discovery of a genetic mutation is a most important but not necessarily full picture of what leads to the disease process.

Inactivating mutations that result in loss of protein function can occur. The unstable trinucleotide repeat, a common type of mutation frequently found in diseases of the brain, has a different genetic mechanism, toxic gain-of-function. For example, when abnormally long polyglutamine stretches are present, cascades of sequential genes often occur, so that a mutation in the first gene in a series results in low expression of others that follow; it may be difficult to determine whether a detected underexpression of a later gene is primary or secondary. Genes sequences may be shuffled and create different proteins with alternate functions when being expressed in different organs (Mnatzakanian et al. 2004), making it harder to anticipate brain function or dysfunction from the study of a gene taken from the blood. This finding in Rett syndrome has received special attention because of its clinical implications; the concept of alternative splicing, in which a gene produces different versions of a protein, is well established.

Another genetic factor to consider in autism, especially in the mitochondrial diseases, is the amount of heteroplasmy (a mixture of wild-type and mutant mtDNA) present in living patients (DiMauro & Moraes 1993). This helps account for tremendous clinical variation inside the same family. In addition, new information may arise from epigenetics. These are modifications that help control gene activity by acting like switches. The best known epigenetic signal is DNA methylation, which is generally associated with silencing of gene expression; DNA methylation patterns tend to be stable over time in postmitotic cells. Growing evidence indicates that imprinted genes are probably involved in autism, and epigenetics may help disentangle future diagnoses. Finally, in regard to laboratory studies, evolutionary research into both genes expressed in the brain and established neural circuits in animals shows that sometimes earlier systems have been changed when recruited for specific "human" functions, placing limitations on animal studies that simulate a human genetic disease of the brain. A great deal of work lies ahead.

SUMMARY

This chapter can be summarized as follows: It asserts the principle that, although we can not yet define many of them, autistic symptoms reflect a great variety of underlying disease entities, each perhaps with a somewhat different neuropathological mechanism. Autism/Asperger is a big syndrome. Now it is time, in the next chapter, to explore how so many different diseases can all lead to the same symptom complex of autism by modifying, interrupting, or redirecting the neural pathways of behavior.

REFERENCES

Abitbol M, Menini C, Delezoide AL, Rhyner T, Vekemans M, Mallet J (1993) Nucleus basalis magnocellularis and hippocampus are the major sites of *FMR-1* expression in the human fetal brain. *Nature Genetics* 4:147–153.

Abrams MT, Doheny KF, Mazzocco MM, Knight SJ, Baumgardner TL, Freund LS, Davies KE, Reiss AL (1997) Cognitive, behavioral, and neuroanatomical assessment of two unrelated male children expressing *FRAXE*. *American Journal of Medical Genetics* 74:73–81.

Amir RE, Van den Veyver IB, Wan M, Tran CO, Franke U, Zoghi HY (1999) Rett syndrome is caused by mutations in X-linked *MECP2*, encoding methyl-CpG-binding protein 2. *Nature Genetics* 23:185–188.

Anderlid BM, Schoumans J, Anneren G, Tapia-Paez I, Dumanski J, Blennow E, Nordenskjold M (2002) FISH-mapping of a 100-kb terminal 22q13 deletion. *Human Genetics* 110:439–443.

Assumpcao FB Jr. (1998) Brief report: a case of chromosome 22 alteration associated with autistic syndrome. *Journal of Autism and Developmental Disorders* 28:253–256.

Bailey AJ (1993) The biology of autism. *Psychological Medicine* 23:7–11.

Bailey A, Le Couteur A, Gottesman I, Bolton P, Simonoff E, Yuzda E, Rutter M (1995)

Autism as a strongly genetic disorder: evidence from a British twin study. *Psychological Medicine* 25:63–77.

Barnea-Goraly N, Eliez S, Hedeus M, Menon V, White CD, Moseley M, Reiss AL (2003a) White matter tract alterations in fragile X syndrome: preliminary evidence from diffusion tensor imaging. *American Journal of Medical Genetics* 118B:81–88.

Barnea-Goraly N, Menon V, Krasnow B, Ko A, Reiss A, Eliez S (2003b) Investigation of white matter structure in velocardiofacial syndrome: a diffusion tensor imaging study. *American Journal of Psychiatry* 160:1863–1869.

Benaron LD (2003) Inclusion to the point of dilution. *Journal of Autism and Developmental Disorders* 33:355–359.

Blanchon YC, Gay C, Gibert G, Lauras B (2002) A case of N-acetyl galactosaminidase deficiency (Schindler disease) associated with autism. *Journal of Autism and Developmental Disorders* 32:145–146.

Bock G, Goode J (2003) *Autism: Neural Basis and Treatment Possibilities.* Chichester, UK: Wiley.

Bolton PF, Dennis NR, Browne CE, Thomas NS, Veltman MW, Thompson RJ, Jacobs P (2001) The phenotypic manifestations of interstitial duplications of proximal 15q with special reference to the autistic spectrum disorders. *American Journal of Medical Genetics* 105:675–685.

Bonaglia MC, Giorda R, Borgatti R, Felisari G, Gagliardi C, Selicorni A, Zuffardi O (2001) Disruption of the *ProSAP2* gene in a t(12;22)(q24.1;q13.3) is associated with the 22q13.3 deletion syndrome. *American Journal of Human Genetics* 69:261–268.

Borgatti R, Piccinelli P, Passoni D, Dalpra L, Miozzo M, Micheli R, Gagliardi C, Balottin U (2001) Relationship between clinical and genetic features in "inverted duplicated chromosome 15" patients. *Pediatric Neurology* 24:111–116.

Bryson SE, Clark BS, Smith IM (1988) First report of a Canadian epidemiological study of autistic syndromes. *Journal of Child Psychology and Psychiatry* 29:433–445.

Buxbaum JD, Silverman J, Keddache M, Smith CJ, Hollander E, Ramoz N, Reichert JG (2004) Linkage analysis for autism in a subset of families with obsessive-compulsive behaviors: evidence for an autism susceptibility gene on chromosome 1 and further support for susceptibility genes on chromosome 6 and 19. *Molecular Psychiatry* 9: 144–150.

Buxbaum JD, Silverman JM, Smith CJ, Greenberg DA, Kilifarski M, Reichert J, Cook EH Jr, Fang Y, Song CY, Vitale R (2002) Association between a *GABRB3* polymorphism and autism. *Molecular Psychiatry* 7:311–316.

Campbell M, Geller B, Small AM, Petti TA, Ferris SH (1978) Minor physical anomalies in young psychotic children. *American Journal of Psychiatry* 135:573–575.

Carney RM, Wolpert CM, Ravan SA, Shahbazian M, Ashley-Koch A, Cuccaro ML, Vance JM, Pericak-Vance MA (2003) Identification of *MECP2* mutations in a series of females with autistic disorder. *Pediatric Neurology* 28:205–211.

Carratala F, Galan F, Moya M, Estivill X, Pritchard MA, Llevadot R, Nadal M, Gratacos M (1998) A patient with autistic disorder and a 20/22 chromosomal translocation. *Developmental Medicine and Child Neurology* 40:492–495.

Chess S (1977) Follow-up report on autism in congenital rubella. *Journal of Autism and Childhood Schizophrenia* 7:68–81.

Chih B, Afridi SK, Clark L, Scheiffele P (2004) Disorder-associated mutations lead to functional inactivation of neuroligins. *Human Molecular Genetics* 13:1471–1477.

Chudley AE, Gutierrez E, Jocelyn LJ, Chodirker BN (1998) Outcomes of genetic evaluation in children with pervasive developmental disorder. *Journal of Developmental and Behavioral Pediatrics* 19:321–325.

Chugani DC, Chugani HT, Muzik O, Shah JR, Shah AK, Canady A, Mangner TJ, Chakraborty PK (1998) Imaging epileptogenic tubers in children with tuberous sclerosis complex using alpha-[11C]methyl-L-tryptophan positron emission tomography. *Annals of Neurology* 44:858–866.

Chugani DC, Sundram BS, Behen M, Lee ML, Moore GJ (1999) Evidence of altered energy metabolism in autistic children. *Progress in Neuropsychopharmacology and Biological Psychiatry* 23:635–641.

Ciardo F, Salerno C, Curatolo P (2001) Neurologic aspects of adenylosuccinate lyase deficiency. *Journal of Child Neurology* 16:301–308.

Coleman M (Ed) (1976) *The Autistic Syndromes.* Amsterdam: North-Holland Publishing Company.

Coleman M (1994) Second trimester of gestation: a time of risk for classical autism? *Developmental Brain Dysfunction* 7:104–109.

Coleman M, Blass JP (1985) Autism and lactic acidosis. *Journal of Autism and Developmental Disorders* 15:1–8.

Coleman M, Gillberg C (1996) *The Schizophrenias.* New York: Springer.

Comoletti D, De Jaco A, Jennings LL, Flynn RE, Gaietta G, Tsigelny I, Ellisman MH, Taylor P (2004) The Arg451Cys-neuroligin-3 mutation associated with autism reveals a defect in protein processing. *Journal of Neuroscience* 24:4889–4893.

Cook EH Jr (2001) Genetics of autism. *Child and Adolescent Psychiatric Clinics of North America* 10:333–350.

Cook EH Jr, Courchesne RY, Cox NJ, Lord C, Gonen D, Guter SJ, Lincoln A, Nix K, Haas R, Leventhal BL, Courchesne E (1998) Linkage-equilibrium mapping of autistic disorder, with 15q11-q13 markers. *American Journal of Human Genetics* 62:1077–1083.

Croen LA, Grether JK, Yoshida CK, Odouli R, Van de Water J (2005) Maternal authoimmune diseases, asthma and allergies, and childhood autism spectrum disorders: a case-control study. *Arch Pediatratric Adolescence Medicine* 159:151–157.

De Bona C, Zappella M, Hayek G, Meloni I, Vitelli F, Bruttini M, Cusano R, Loffredo P, Longo I, Renieri A (2000) Preserved speech variant is allelic of classic Rett syndrome. *European Journal of Human Genetics* 8:325–330.

Descheemaeker MJ, Vogels A, Govers V, Borghgraef M, Willekens D, Swillen A, Verhoeven W, Fryns JP (2002) Prader-Willi syndrome: new insights in the behavioural and psychiatric spectrum. *Journal of Intellectual Disability Research* 46:41–50.

DiMauro S, Moraes CT (1993) Mitochondrial encephalomyopathies. *Archives of Neurology* 50:1197–1208.

Down JLH (1866) Observations on the ethnic classification of idiots. *Clinical Lectures and Reports by the Medical and Surgical Staff of the London Hospital* 3:259–262.

Eigsti IM, Shapiro T (2003) A systems neuroscience approach to autism: biological, cognitive and clinical perspectives. *Mental Retardation and Developmental Disabilities Research Reviews* 9:205–215.

Eliez S, Antonarakis SE, Morris MA, Dahoun SP, Reiss AL (2001a) Parental origin of the deletion 22q11.2 and brain development in velocardiofacial syndrome: a preliminary study. *Archives of General Psychiatry* 58:64–68.

Eliez S, Blasey CM, Menon V, White CD, Schmitt JE, Reiss AL (2001b) Functional brain imaging study of mathematical reasoning abilities in velocardiofacial syndrome (del22q11.2) *Genetic Medicine* 3:49–55.

Eliez S, Schmitt JE, White CD, Reiss AL (2000) Children and adolescents with velocardiofacial syndrome: a volumetric MRI study. *American Journal of Psychiatry* 157:409–415.

Eliez S, Schmitt JE, White CD, Wellis VG, Reiss Al (2001c) A quantitative MRI study of posterior fossa development in velocardiofacial syndrome. *Biological Psychiatry* 49:540–546.

Feinstein C, Eliez S, Blasey C, Reiss AL (2002) Psychiatric disorders and behavioral problems in children with velocardiofacial syndrome: usefulness as phenotypic indicators of schizophrenia risk. *Biological Psychiatry* 15:312–318.

Feinstein C, Reiss AL (1998) Autism: the point of view from fragile X studies. *Journal of Autism and Developmental Disorders* 28:393–405.

Filipek PA, Juranek J, Smith M, Mays LZ, Ramos ER, Bocian M, Masser-Frye D, Laulhere TM, Modahl C, Spence MA, Gargas JJ (2003) Mitochondrial dysfunction in autistic patients with 15q inverted duplication. *Annals of Neurology* 53:801–804.

Fillano JJ, Goldenthal MJ, Rhodes CH, Marin-Garcia J (2002) Mitochondrial dysfunction in patients with hypotonia, epilepsy, autism and developmental delay: HEADD syndrome. *Journal of Child Neurology* 17:435–439.

Folstein SE, Rosen-Sheidley B (2001) Genetics of autism: complex aetiology for a heterogeneous disorder. *Nature Reviews Genetics* 2:943–955.

Fombonne E, Du Mazaubrun C, Cans C, Grandjean H (1997) Autism and associated medical disorders in a French epidemiological survey. *Journal of the American Academy of Child and Adolescent Psychiatry* 36:1561–1569.

Garrett AS, Menon V, MacKenzie K, Reiss AL (2004) Here's looking at you, kid: neural systems underlying face and gaze processing in fragile X syndrome. *Archives of General Psychiatry* 61:281–288.

Gharani N, Benayed R, Mancuso V, Brzustowicz LM, Millonig JH (2004) Association of the homeobox transcription factor, ENGRAILED 2,3, with autism spectrum disorder. *Molecular Psychiatry* 9:474–484.

Gillberg C, Coleman M (2000) *The Biology of the Autistic Syndromes*. London: Cambridge University Press. a: chapter 12. Epilepsy and electrophysiology; b: chapter 9. Neuropsychology in autism and spectrum disorders. c: chapter 15. The genetics of autism.

Gillberg C, Steffenburg S, Wahlstrom J, Gillberg IC, Sjöstedt A, Martinsson T, Liedgren S, Eeg-Olofsson O (1991) Autism associated with marker chromosome. *Journal of the American Academy of Child and Adolescent Psychiatry* 30:489–494.

Gillberg C, Wahlstrom J (1985) Chromosomal abnormalities in infantile autism and other childhood psychoses: a population study of 66 cases. *Developmental Medicine and Child Neurology* 27:293–304.

Goizet C, Excoffier E, Taine L, Taupiac E, El Moneim AA, Arveiler B, Bouvard M, Lacombe D (2000) Case with autistic syndrome and chromosome 22q13.3 deletion detected by FISH. *American Journal of Medical Genetics* 96:839–844.

Golbe LI, Mouradian MM (2004) Alpha-synuclein in Parkinson's disease: light from two new angles. *Annals of Neurology* 55:153–156.

Graf WD, Marin-Garcia J, Gao HG, Pizzo S, Naviaux RK, Markusic D, Barshop BA,

Courchesne E, Haas RH (2000) Autism associated with the mitochondrial DNA G8363A transfer RNA (Lys) mutation. *Journal of Child Neurology* 15:357–361.

Harrison JE, Bolton PF (1997) Annotation: tuberous sclerosis. *Journal of Child Psychology and Psychiatry* 38:603–614.

Hennekam RCM, Barth PG (2003) Syndromic cortical dysplasias: a review. In Barth PG (Ed) *Disorders of Neuronal Migration* London: Mac Keith Press.

Herzing LB, Cook EH Jr, Ledbetter DH (2002) Allele-specific expression analysis by RNA-FISH demonstrates preferential maternal expression of *UBE3A* and imprint maintenance within 15q11-q13 duplications. *Human Molecular Genetics* 11:1707–1718.

Herzing LB, Kim S, Cook EH Jr, Ledbetter D (2001) The human aminophospholipid-transporting ATPase gene *ATP10C* maps adjacent to *UBE3A* and exhibits similar imprinted expression. *American Journal of Human Genetics* 68:1501–1505.

Humphrey A, Higgins JN, Yates JR, Bolton PF (2004) Monozygotic twins with tuberous sclerosis discordant for the severity of developmental deficits. *Neurology* 9:795–798.

Ivarsson SA, Bjerre I, Vegfors P, Ahlfors K (1990) Autism is one of several disabilities in two children with congenital cytomegalovirus infection. *Neuropediatrics* 21:102–103.

Jacobson JW, Janicki MP (1983) Observed prevalence of multiple developmental disabilities. *Mental Retardation* 21:87–94.

Jaeken J, Van den Berghe G (1984) An infantile autistic syndrome characterised by the presence of succinylpurines in body fluids. *Lancet* 2:1058–1061.

Jamain S, Quach H, Betancur C, Rastam M, Colineaux C, Gillberg IC, Soderstrom H, Giros B, Leboyer M, Gillberg C, Bourgeron T, Paris Autism Research International Sibpair Study (2003) Mutations of the X-linked genes encoding neuroligins *NLGN3* and *NLGN4* are associated with autism. *Nature Genetics* 34:27–29.

Jenkins EC, Brown WT, Brooks J, Duncan CJ, Rudelli RD, Wisniewski HM (1984) Experience with prenatal fragile X detection. *American Journal of Medical Genetics* 17:215–239.

Johnston MV (2004) Clinical disorders of brain plasticity. *Brain Development* 26:73–80.

Jorde LB, Hasstedt SJ, Ritvo ER, Mason-Brothers A, Freeman BJ, Pingree C, McMahon WM, Petersen B, Jenson WR, Mo A (1991) Complex segregation analysis of autism. *American Journal of Human Genetics* 49:932–938.

Kammoun F, de Roux N, Boespflug-Tanguy O, Vallee L, Seng R, Tardieu M, Landrieu P (2004) Screening of *MECP2* coding sequence in patients with phenotypes of decreasing likelihood for Rett syndrome: a cohort of 171 cases. *Journal of Medical Genetics* 41:e85.

Kanner L (1943) Autistic disturbances of affective contact. *Nervous Child* 2:217–250.

Kanner L (1971) Follow-up study of eleven children originally reported in 1943. *Journal of Autism and Childhood Schizophrenia* 1:119–145.

Kato M, Das S, Petras K, Kitamura K, Morohashi K, Abuelo DN et al. (2004) Mutations of ARX are associated with striking pleiotropy and consistent genotype-phenotype correlation. *Human Mutations* 23:147–159.

Kielinen M, Rantala H, Timonen E, Linna S-L, Moilanen I (2004) Associated medical disorders and disabilities in children with autistic disorder: a population-based study. *Autism* 8:49–60.

Konstantareas MM, Homatidis S (1999) Chromosomal abnormalities in a series of children with autistic disorder. *Journal of Autism and Developmental Disorders* 29:275–285.

Kozma C (1998) On cognitive variability in velocardiofacial syndrome: profound mental retardation and autism. *American Journal of Medical Genetics* 81:269–270.

Kriaucionis S, Bird A (2004) The major form of *MECP2* has a novel N-terminus generated by alternative splicing. *Nucleic Acids Research* 32:1818–1823.

Kwon H, Menon V, Eliez S, Warsofsky IS, White CD, Dyer-Friedman J, Taylor AK, Glover GH, Reiss AL (2001) Functional neuroanatomy of visuospatial working memory in fragile X syndrome: relation to behavioral and molecular measures. *American Journal of Psychiatry* 158:1040–1051.

Lam CW, Yeung WL, Ko CH, Poon PM, Tong SF, Chan KY, Lo IF, Chan LY, Hui J, Wong V, Pang CP, Lo YM, Fok TF (2000) Spectrum of mutations in the *MECP2* gene in patients with infantile autism and Rett syndrome. *Journal of Medical Genetics* 37:E41.

Laszlo A, Horvath E, Eck E, Feket M (1994) Serum serotonin, lactate and pyruvate levels in infantile autistic children. *Clinical Chimica Acta* 229:205–207.

Laumonnier F, Bonnet-Brilhault F, Gomot M, Blanc R, David A, Moizard MP, Raynaud M, Ronce N, Lemonnier E, Calvas P, Laudier B, Chelly J, Fryns JP, Ropers HH, Hamel BC, Andres C, Barthelemy C, Moraine C, Briault S (2004) X-linked mental retardation and autism are associated with mutation in the *NLGN4* gene, a member of the neuroligin family. *American Journal of Human Genetics* 74:552–557.

Lauritsen M, Mors O, Mortensen PB, Ewald H (1999) Infantile autism and associated autosomal chromosome abnormalities: a register-based study and a literature survey. *Journal of Child Psychology and Psychiatry* 40:335–345.

Leboyer M (2003) Searching for alternative phenotypes in psychiatric genetics. In Leboyer M, Bellivier F (Eds) *Psychiatric Genetics: methods and reviews*. Totowa, New Jersey: Humana Press.

Links PS, Stockwell M, Abichandani F, Simeon J (1980) Minor physical anomalies in childhood autism. I. Their relationship to pre- and perinatal complications. *Journal of Autism and Developmental Disorders* 10:273–285.

Lombard J (1998) Autism: a mitochondrial disorder? *Medical Hypotheses* 50:497–500.

Longo I, Russo L, Meloni I, Ricci I, Ariani F, Pescucci C, Giordano C, Canitano R, Hayek G, Zappella M, Neri G, Renieri A, Gurrieri F (2004) Three Rett patients with both *MECP2* mutation and 15q11-q13 rearrangements. *European Journal of Human Genetics* 12:682–685.

Lotspeich LJ, Kwon H, Schumann CM, Fryer SL, Goodlin-Jones BL, Buonocore MH, Lammers CR, Amaral DG, Reiss AL (2004) Investigation of neuroanatomical differences between autism and Asperger syndrome. *Archives of General Psychiatry* 61:291–298.

MacLean JE, Teshima IE, Szatmari P, Nowaczyk MJ (2000) Ring chromosome 22 and autism: report and review. *American Journal of Medical Genetics* 90:382–385.

Menold MM, Shao Y, Wolpert CM, Donnelly SL, Raiford KL, Martin ER, Ravan SA, Abramson RK, Wright HH, DeLong GR, Cuccaro ML, Pericak-Vance MA, Gilbert JR (2001) Association analysis of chromosome 15 GABA$_A$ receptor subunit of genes in autistic disorder. *Journal of Neurogenetics* 15:245–259.

Menon V, Kwon H, Eliez S, Taylor AK, Reiss AL (2000) Functional brain activation during cognition is related to *FMR1* gene expression. *Brain Research* 877:367–370.

Micali N, Chakrabarti S, Fombonne E (2004) The broad autism phenotype: findings from an epidemiological study. *Autism* 8:21–37.

Miles JH, Hillman RE (2000) Value of a clinical morphology examination in autism. *American Journal of Medical Genetics* 91:245–253.

Minshew NJ (1996) Brief report: Brain mechanism in autism: functional and structural abnormalities. *Journal of Autism and Developmental Disorders* 26:205–209.

Minshew NJ, Goldstein G, Dombrowski SM, Panchalingam K, Pettegrew JW (1993) A preliminary 31P MRS study of autism: evidence for undersynthesis and increased degradation of brain membranes. *Biological Psychiatry* 33:762–773.

Mnatzakanian GN, Lohi H, Munteanu J, Alfred SE, Yamada T, MacLeod PJM, Jones JR, Scherer SW, Schanen NC, Friez MJ, Vincent JB, Minassian BA (2004) A previously unidentified *MECP2* open reading frame defines a new protein isoform relevant to Rett syndrome. *Nature Genetics* 36:339–341.

Nelson KB, Grether JK, Croen LA, Dambrosia JM, Dickens BF, Jelliffe LL, Hansen RL, Phillips TM (2001) Neuropeptides and neurotrophins in neonatal blood of children with autism or mental retardation. *Annals of Neurology* 49:597–606.

Nicolson R, Giedd JN, Lenane M, Hamburger S, Singaracharlu S, Bedwell J, Fernandez T, Thaker GK, Malaspina D, Rapoport JL (1999) Clinical and neurobiological correlates of cytogenetic abnormalities in childhood-onset schizophrenia. *American Journal of Psychiatry* 156:1575–1579.

Niklasson L, Rasmussen P, Oskarsdottir S, Gillberg C (2001) Neuropsychiatric disorders in the 22q11 deletion syndrome. *Genetic Medicine* 3:79–84.

Nokelainen P, Flint J (2002) Genetic effects on human cognition: lessons from the study of mental retardation syndromes. *Journal of Neurology Neurosurgery and Psychiatry* 72:287–296.

Nurmi EL, Bradford Y, Chen Y, Hall J, Arnone B, Gardiner MB, Hutcheson HB, Gilbert JR, Pericak-Vance MA, Copeland-Yates SA, Michaelis RC, Wassink TH, Santangelo SL, Sheffield VC, Piven J, Folstein SE, Haines JL, Sutcliffe JS (2001) Linkage disequilibrium at the Angelman syndrome gene *UBE3A* in autism families. *Genomics* 77:105–113.

Nurmi EL, Dowd M, Tadevosyan-Leyfer O, Haines JL, Folstein SE, Sutcliffe JS (2003) Exploratory subsetting of autism families based on savant skills improves evidence of linkage to 15q11-q13. *Journal of the American Academy of Child and Adolescent Psychiatry* 42:856–863.

Olanow CW (Ed) (2003) Neurodegeneration and prospects for neuroprotection and rescue in Parkinson's disease. *Annals of Neurology*, Supplement 3:S1–S170.

Oliveira G, Diogo L, Grazina M, Garcia P, Ataide A, Marques C, Miguel T, Borges L, Vicente AM, Oliveira CR (2005) Mitochondrial dysfunction in autism spectrum disorders: evidence for the association of a mitochondrial respiratory chain functional abnormality with autism. *Developmental Medicine and Child Neurology*, 47: 185–189.

Orstavik KH, Stromme P, Ek J, Torvik A, Skjeldal OH (1997) Macrocephaly, epilepsy, autism, dysmorphic features, and mental retardation in two sisters: a new autosomal recessive syndrome? *Journal of Medical Genetics* 34:849–851.

Pickles A, Bolton P, Macdonald H, Bailey A, Le Couteur A, Sim CH, Rutter M (1995) Latent-class analysis of recurrence risk for complex phenotypes with selection and measurement error: twin and family history of autism. *American Journal of Human Genetics* 57:717–726.

Pons R, Andreu AL, Checcarelli N, Vila MR, Englestad K, Sue CM, Shungu D, Haggerty R, De Vivo DC, DiMauro S (2004) Mitochondrial DNA abnormalities and autistic spectrum disorders. *The Journal of Pediatrics* 144:81–85.

Prasad C, Prasad AN, Chodirker BN, Lee C, Dawson A, Jocelyn LJ, Chudley A (2000) Genetic evaluation of pervasive developmental disorders: the terminal 22q13 deletion syndrome may represent a recognizable phenotype. *Clinical Genetics* 57:103–109.

Reiss AL, Feinstein C, Rosenbaum KN (1986) Autism and genetic disorders. *Schizophrenia Bulletin* 12:724–738.

Rice D, Barone S Jr (2000) Critical periods of vulnerability for the developing nervous system: evidence from humans and animal models. *Environmental Health Perspectives* 108:511–533.

Rimland B (1964) *Infantile Autism: The Syndrome and Its Implication for a Neural Theory of Behavior.* Englewood Clifts, NJ: Prentice Hall.

Rineer S, Finucane B, Simon EW (1998) Autistic symptoms among children and young adults with isodicentric chromosome 15. *American Journal of Medical Genetics* 81: 428–433.

Risch N, Spiker D, Lotspeich L, Nouri N, Hinds D, Hallmayer J, Kalaydjieva L, McCague P, Dimiceli S, Pitts T, Nguyen L, Yang J, Harper C, Thorpe D, Vermeer S, Young H, Hebert J, Lin A, Ferguson J, Chiotti C, Wiese-Slater S, Rogers T, Salmon B, Nicholas P, Petersen PB, Pingree C, McMahon W, Wong DL, Cavalli-Sforza LL, Kramer HC, Myers RM (1999) A genomic screen of autism: evidence for a multi-locus etiology. *American Journal of Human Genetics* 65: 493–507.

Ritvo ER, Mason-Brothers A, Freeman BJ, Pingree C, Jenson WR, McMahon WM, Petersen PB, Jorde LB, Mo A, Ritvo A (1990) The UCLA-University of Utah epidemiologic survey of autism: the etiologic role of rare diseases. *American Journal of Psychiatry* 147:1614–1621.

Rodier PM, Bryson SE, Welch JP (1997a) Minor malformations and physical measurements in autism: data from Nova Scotia. *Teratology* 55:319–325.

Rodier PM, Ingram JL, Tisdale B, Croog VJ (1997b) Linking etiologies in humans and animal models: studies of autism. *Reproductive Toxicology* 11:417–422.

Rodier PM, Ingram JL, Tisdale B, Nelson S, Romano J (1996) Embryological origin for autism: developmental anomalies of the cranial nerve motor nuclei. *Journal of Comparative Neurology* 370:247–261.

Schain R, Freedman DX (1961) Studies on 5-hydroxyindole metabolism in autistic and other mentally retarded children. *Journal of Pediatrics* 58:315–320.

Shao Y, Cuccaro ML, Hauser ER, Raiford KL, Menold MM, Wolpert CM, Ravan SA, Elston L, Decena K, Donnelly SL, Abramson RK, Wright HH, DeLong GR, Gilbert JR, Pericak-Vance MA (2003) Fine mapping of autistic disorder to chromosome 15q11-q13 by use of phenotypic subtypes. *American Journal of Human Genetics* 72:539–548.

Sherr EH (2003) The *ARX* story (epilepsy, mental retardation, autism and cerebral malformations): one gene leads to many phenotypes. *Current Opinion in Pediatrics* 15: 567–571.

Shibayama A, Cook EH Jr, Feng J, Glanzmann C, Yan J, Craddock N, Jones IR, Goldman

D, Heston LL, Sommer SS (2004) MECP2 structural and 3'-UTR variants in schizo-phrenia, autism, and other pyschiatric diseases: a possible association with autism. *American Journal of Medical Genetics* 128B:50–53.

Smalley SL (1998) Autism and tuberous sclerosis. *Journal of Autism and Developmental Disorders* 28:407–414.

Splawski I, Timothy KW, Sharpe LM, Decher N, Kumar P, Bloise R, Napolitano C, Schwartz PJ, Joseph RM, Condouris K, Tager-Flusberg H, Priori SG, Sanguinetti MC, Keating MT (2004) Ca(V)1.2 calcium channel dysfunction causes a multisys-tem disorder including arrhythmia and autism. *Cell* 119:19–31.

Sporn A, Addington A, Reiss AL, Dean M, Gogtay N, Potocnik U, Greenstein D, Hallmayer J, Gochman P, Lenane M, Baker N, Tossell J, Rapoport JL (2004) 22q11 deletion syndrome in childhood onset schizophrenia: an update. *Molecular Psychiatry* 9:225–226.

Steg JP, Rapoport JL (1975) Minor physical anomalies in normal, neurotic, learning dis-abled, and severely disturbed children. *Journal of Autism and Childhood Schizophre-nia* 5:299–307.

Stromme P, Mangelsdorf ME, Scheffer IE, Gecz J (2002) Infantile spasms, dystonia and other X-linked phenotypes caused by mutation in Aristaless related homeobox gene, ARX. *Brain Development* 24:266–268.

Swillen A, Hellemans H, Steyaert J, Fryns JP (1996) Autism and genetics: high incidence of specific genetic syndromes in 21 autistic adolescents and adults living in two residential homes in Belgium. *American Journal of Medical Genetics* 67:315–316.

Thomas NS, Sharp AJ, Browne CE, Skuse D, Hardie C, Dennis NR (1999) Xp deletions associated with autism in three females. *Human Genetics* 104:43–48.

Titomanlio L, Marzano MG, Rossi E, D'Armiento M, De Brasi D, Vega GR, Andreucci MV, Orsini AV, Santoro L, Sebastio G (2001) Case of Myhre syndrome with autism and peculiar skin histological findings. *American Journal of Medical Genetics* 103: 163–165.

Torrey EF, Hersh SP, McCabe KD (1975) Early childhood psychosis and bleeding during pregnancy. A prospective study of gravid women and their offspring. *Journal of Autism and Childhood Schizophrenia* 5:287–297.

Trevathan E, Naidu S (1988) The clinical recognition and differential diagnosis of Rett syndrome. *Journal of Child Neurology* 3(Suppl): S6–S16.

Turner G, Partington M, Kerr B, Mangelsdorf M, Gecz J (2002) Variable expression of mental retardation, autism, seizures, and dystonic hand movements in two families with an identical *ARX* gene mutation. *American Journal of Medical Genetics* 112: 405–411.

Van Karnebeek CD, van Gelderen I, Nijhof GJ, Abeling NG, Vreken P, Redeker EJ, van Eeghen AM, Hoovers JM, Hennekam RC (2002) An aetiological study of 25 mentally retarded adults with autism. *Journal of Medical Genetics* 39:205–213.

Veltman MW, Thompson RJ, Roberts SE, Thomas NS, Whittington J, Bolton PF (2004) Prader-Willi syndrome—a study comparing deletion and uniparental disomy cases with reference to autism spectrum disorders. *European Child and Adolescent Psy-chiatry* 13:42–50.

Walker HA (1976) Incidence of minor physical anomalies in autistic patients. In Coleman M (Ed) *The Autistic Syndromes*. Amsterdam: North-Holland Publishing Co.

Wassink TH, Piven J, Patil SR (2001) Chromosomal abnormalities in a clinic sample of individuals with autistic disorder. *Psychiatric Genetics* 11:57–63.

Weaving LS, Christodoulou J, Williamson SL, Friend KL, McKenzie OL, Archer H, Evans J, Clarke A, Pelka GJ, Tam PP, Watson C, Lahooti H, Ellaway CJ, Bennetts B, Leonard H, Gecz J (2004) Mutations of CDKL5 cause a severe neurodevelopmental disorder with infantile spasms and mental retardation. *American Journal of Human Genetics* 75:1079–1093.

Wing L, Leekam SR, Libby SJ, Gould J, Larcombe M (2002) The diagnostic interview for social and communication disorders: background, inter-rater reliability and clinical use. *Journal of Child Psychology and Psychiatry* 43:307–325.

Yamagishi H (2002) The 22q11.2 deletion syndrome. *Keio Journal of Medicine* 51:77–88.

Yamashita Y, Fujimoto C, Nakajima E, Isagai T, Matsuishi T (2003) Possible association between congenital cytomegalovirus infection and autistic disorder. *Journal of Autism and Developmental Disorders* 33:455–459.

Ylisaukko-oja T, Nieminen-von Wendt T, Kempas E, Sarenius S, Varilo T, von Wendt L, Peltonen L, Jarvela I (2004) Genome-wide scan for loci of Asperger syndrome. *Molecular Psychiatry* 9:161–168.

Zappella M, Meloni I, Longo I, Canitano R, Hayek G, Rosaia L, Mari F, Renieri A (2003) Study of *MECP2* gene in Rett syndrome variants and autistic girls. *American Journal of Medical Genetics* 119B:102–107.

Zappella M, Meloni I, Longo I, Hayek G, Renieri A (2001) Preserved speech variants of the Rett syndrome: molecular and clinical analysis. *American Journal of Medical Genetics* 104:14–22.

Zechner U, Wilda M, Kehrer-Sawatzki H, Vogel W, Fundele R, Hameister H (2001) A high density of X-linked genes for general cognitive ability: a run-away process of shaping human evolution? *Trends in Genetics* 17:697–701.

Zwaigenbaum L, Szatmari P, Mahoney W, Bryson S, Bartolucci G, MacLean J (2000) High functioning autism and childhood disintegrative disorder in half brothers. *Journal of Autism and Developmental Disorders* 30:121–126.

Chapter 2

A Neurological Framework

Mary Coleman

Autism is the result of a neurodevelopmental disease process; where in the brain it is localized is under intense study. Our present thinking on the cortical organization of primate memory is undergoing a Copernican change, from a neuropsychology that localizes different memories in different areas to one that views memory as a distributed property of cortical systems (Fuster 1997). And these systems are almost beyond imagination: 30 billion neurons of 200 different types with 1 million billion connections between them. Recently, the distribution was observed via infrared mapping of the brain; it was found to be consistent with distributed and complex functional representation of the cerebral cortex (Gorbach et al. 2003), rather than the traditional concepts of discrete functional loci as demonstrated by brief cortical stimulation or by noninvasive functional imaging techniques. As Bachevalier (1996) has suggested, it is unlikely that the symptoms of autism are going to be explained by the older lesion paradigms. A neurodevelopmental disease has a much different origin at an earlier stage of formation than a disease process attacking an already intact brain.

In the twentieth century, a brilliant behavioral neurologist, Norman Geschwind, introduced the concept of the cerebral disconnection syndromes as central to the classical syndromes of behavioral neurology (Geschwind 1965). For example, the signature syndromes of the brain, such a Wernicke's aphasia or Broca's aphasia, were originally based on reports of the effect of lesions in a localized brain area. Mesulam (1990) has proposed that the complex behavioral domains are coordinated by large-scale distributed networks, and damage to any network component can impair behavior in the relevant domain. Focal brain lesions that interfere with these processing streams lead to Geschwind's disconnection syndromes, such as apraxia, prosopagnosia, color anomia, amnesia, etc.

Mega and Cummings (2001) agreed that neuropsychiatric symptoms undoubtedly reflect the dysfunction of 1 or more neural circuits that pass through several different areas of the brain. In the case of autism, decreased functional connections within the cerebral cortex and between the cortex and subcortical regions were suggested in 1988 by Horwitz et al. Zilbovicius et al. (1995) proposed the existence of poor connections due to delayed maturation of the circuitry of the frontal lobe in autism.

NEURAL NETWORK MODELS OF AUTISM

These connections, these large-scale distributed networks in the brain, are called the neural networks. Neural networks are believed to have "emergent properties," that is, new properties not explicitly programmed into them from the onset. Since it has been found that more than 90% of children with autism appear to have a genetic component to their disease, interest in the early neurodevelopment of these networks in autism and their constraints has increased. In 2001, Batshaw and Towbin stated it plainly: The findings suggest that autism involves the abnormal development of a distributed neural network involving a number of regions of the brain. Many now consider autism a disorder of neural information processing of cognition and behavior (Belmonte et al. 2004), likely based on neural networks (McClelland 2000). Neural network models of autism have been suggested by Cohen (1994, 1998, 2004), Gustafsson (1997), and Casanova et al. (2003) using computer models and neurobiological data. An attempt at a one-paragraph comment on each theory, which can not even begin to touch the complexity of these brilliant publications, follows.

Cohen (1994, 1998, 2004) has proposed a neural network model of autism in which too many connections are established during development, perhaps owing to inadequate pruning of irrelevant connections. Thus, while too few neurons may not be able to solve a problem to begin with, having too many may impair generalization and produce rigidity and resistance to change. Among many other predictions, Cohen's model explains savant skills.

According to Gustafsson's 1997 model of the autistic brain, inhibitory lateral feedback synaptic connection strengths of Kohonen-type neural networks are excessive. This results in networks that attend to a restricted set of features in a stimulus configuration (i.e., too much discrimination.) Excessive inhibition is the primary culprit. Gustafsson and Paplinki (2004) used their neural network model to test assumptions about attention shift impairments and familiarity preference in autism.

Casanova et al. (2002, 2003) have reported that the minicolumns in the brains of autistic subjects are narrower, with less peripheral neurophil space. This leads to a neural network model in which autism could result from an imbalance between the process of excitation and inhibition toward too little inhibition. Casanova's theory has been challenged by a regional brain chemistry study that disputes the hypothesis of diffuse increased neuronal packing density (Friedman et al. 2003).

All three neural network models are, in one sense, conceptually similar. They all focus on a neurodevelopmental impairment in the neural networks that leads to the concept that connectivity constraints are responsible for the attention to the restricted range of details. They differ only in the types of constraints that produce these problems (Cohen 2004).

In these neural network models, the brain in autism becomes impaired during early neurodevelopment. That the connectivity of the networks is formed, at least in part, in an unusual and aberrant fashion has been suggested by a variety of studies of patients with high-functioning autism and Asperger syndrome that raise the question of abnormal variability and scatter of functional maps in autism (Muller et al. 2001). Evidence suggests that when standard circuits are inadequate for a task, other circuits from other regions may be recruited for to perform that task (Hazlett et al. 2004).

Another hypothesis that attempts to explain impairment during neurodevelopment in autism is that the usual networks form but are underdeveloped with underconnectivity (Tsatsanis et al. 2003; Just et al. 2004). A rather different possibility is the hypothesis that overconnected neural systems prone to noise and crosstalk result in hyperarousal and reduced selectivity (Belmont & Yurgelun-Todd 2003). There also is a theory that networks are formed in a standard pattern in the first place, but a later impinging on these tracts causes diminution of function or the actual uncoupling of a disconnection syndrome (as might be seen, for example, with neuroepithelial tumors). Many factors may slow or disconnect conduction in any neural network. Neural circuits can transverse through a number of different brain regions and involve neurotransmitters, receptor subtypes, and second messengers. In many disease entities presenting with autism, it is still unclear exactly which circuits and where in those circuits the slowing or interruption occurred, an essential first step in deciding which mechanism caused the dysfunction.

Minshew et al. (1997) described a recurring profile in autism of dissociation between intact or enhanced simple abilities with impaired higher order abilities across cognitive and neurological domains; the investigators described a pattern effecting memory, motor, language, abstract reasoning, and probably also sensory domains. Further work by this group has led to their theory of underconnectivity (Just et al. 2004). A related theory based on similar clinical observations is Frith's (1989) theory of weak central coherence. The Frith theory notes that higher level processes impose coherence on lower level processes and that these components may be normal except for weak coherence between them, which is expressed in reduced connectivity and synchrony resulting in a bottleneck in the interaction between higher order and lower order perceptual processes (Castelli et al. 2002). The underconnectivity theory of Just et al. (2004) is somewhat different in that it treats coherence as an emergent property of the collaboration among cortical centers that may be or become abnormal because of their development without adequate collaboration.

It is too early to know at this time whether any or all of the network scenarios can explain the symptoms of autism. In fact, if autism has many different etiologies, it is even possible that some or all of these models are correct in at least some individuals. Much of this theoretical work has arisen from the study of speaking, high-functioning individuals with autism or Asperger syndrome. The next frontier is investigation of the large group of low-functioning children with autism, including those who are mute. This work might combine the information already gleaned from studies of individuals with high-functioning autism combined with those of individuals who are lower functioning.

In reality, our ignorance about how the brain creates normal behavior patterns, much less the dysfunctional behavior seen in children with autism, is abysmal. Even with the best of methodological rigor, questions remain. In autism, evidence suggests that both temporal and spatial maldevelopment or interruption of behavioral circuits occur. Like the mental retardation syndromes, autism probably represents selected delays or dysmaturation in the central nervous system. An example showing that even high-functioning children are not spared major delays is the evidence of abnormal brain lateralization in high-functioning autism, which probably signals maturational disturbances in establishing lateral preference (Escalante-Mead et al. 2003).

Nevertheless, the scaffolding in which to begin to build blocks of enduring information about autism may now be in place. The available sources of data include those from the disciplines of neuropsychology, neuropathology, molecular biology, biochemistry, electrophysiology, a number of different types of neuroimaging, and infrared mapping. In particular, the powerful tools of imaging studies have raised many fascinating questions. However, these new imaging studies have their limitations; the relationship between neural activity and blood flow, which these methods often measure, is still uncertain; there also are limitations on spatial and temporal resolution of the image and difficulties establishing statistical criteria of neural activation. Studies are now emerging that caution against using functional imaging as the sole method of establishing cognitive neuroanatomy (Bird et al. 2004).

The way stations of neurocircuitry for social cooperation (Rilling et al. 2002) and empathy (Carr et al. 2003) in the human brain are under intense investigation. In the case of autism, the task is complimentary to the task of studying the way stations in the neurocircuits impaired in the mental retardation syndromes. Since so many individuals with autism function in the mental retardation range, much overlapping useful information is being developed.

CENTRAL NERVOUS SYSTEM ONTOLOGY

A genetic plan for the development of the entire observable structure of the cortex clearly exists (Fuster 2003). Events of central nervous system ontogeny have their specific timetables that dictate when the genes for neuronal development and their enabling factors express themselves. Each has its critical period, a time window when the particular set of enabling factors is essential for normal development. This is the time when genetic errors or extraneous factors can most readily derail or arrest this development. Thus, early neurodevelopmental pathogenesis in autism can directly affect or alter the emerging functional maps. The plasticity of the human brain is greatest during the early developmental periods, which might explain the utilization of alternative, but often less than fully satisfactory, circuitry when essential neural pathways fail to develop or are blocked. In the case of autism, a small literature showing utilization of several alternative circuits in different individuals with autism already exists (Schultz et al. 2000; Pierce et al. 2001; Muller et al. 2001, 2003; Nishitani et al. 2004). Thus, the autistic syndrome is likely to be a disease entity affecting certain final common circuits whose symptoms reflect inadequate, interrupted, or alternative function of connecting pathways, beginning in the fetal period with clinical expression in early childhood.

DNA, discussed in the previous chapter, is the first step of a long just-beginning-to-be-deciphered process from gene to behavior. This complex process involves the expression of protein patterns at particular sites and at particular times affecting the biological function groups of cytoskeleton arrangement, chromatin modeling, energy metabolism, and cell signaling, each with distinct neurodevelopmental consequences. It is hard to be sure at this time which neurodevelopmental processes are specifically affected in autism. One process that has drawn attention recently in autism studies is that of a possible diminution of programmed cell death, apoptosis, that might account for the increased grey matter identified in some studies (Waiter et al. 2004).

A number of factors known to affect neurodevelopment have been identified as abnormal in children with autism. In neonatal blood samples, Nelson et al. (2001) identified abnormal levels of two proteins of the mammalian neurotrophin family, BDNF and NGF, which were originally identified as neuronal survival factors. Perry et al. (2001) found increased levels of BDNF in postmortem brain tissue taken from patients with autism. BDNF is also thought to be involved in regulation of synaptic transmission, synaptogenesis in the CNS, and possibly as an intercellular synaptic messenger in long-term potentiation in the hippocampus (Lessmann et al. 2003). BDNF is the clearest example of a growth factor with neurotropic properties whose concentration in venous blood increases with increasing gestation age (Kaukola et al. 2004). Many factors such as maternal infection regulate the expression of BDNF; the first evidence of abrogation of BDNF-induced expression of synaptic vesicle proteins by a virus has been found (Hans et al. 2004) and it may be the crucial end-product of the protein-synthesis-dependent step in L-LTP. However, the neurotrophins and neuropeptides found in the study by Nelson et al. (2001) to be abnormal are not specific to autism; they also are abnormal in children who become mentally retarded without autism.

Identified genetic mutations appear to play a primary role during the neurodevelopment of some children with autism. There are many examples: the tuberous sclerosis complex, caused by mutations in the gene, is the most frequent diagnosis of a MCA/MR syndrome in a child with autism. Other known examples of how early genetic mutations can cause primary aberrations in cell lineages are the dysembryoplastic neuroepithelial tumors and the Hypomelanosis of Ito, rare disease entities with autistic subgroups.

Cortical neurons are first formed in specialized proliferative regions with neuronogenesis complete at 15 weeks of gestation. Then they migrate often as far as a 1,000 cell-body lengths. There appear to be three different modes of neuronal migration, including 2 forms of radial migration (somal translocation and glia-guided locomotion), as well as tangential or nonradial migration. The third form, tangential migration, is used by GABAergic neurons, a major class of inhibitory neurons. Disorders of neuronal migration have been described in nonsyndromic autism, as well as in a number of the MCA/MR syndromes in which a subgroup of patients with autism exist (table 1-2). One of the initial MRI studies of carefully selected children with nonsyndromic autism compared to controls found evidence of UBOs, which are small white matter lesions of uncertain etiology now usually interpreted as heterotopias (Nowell et al. 1990). The pathology study by Bailey et al. (1998) showed neuronal heterotopias, focally increased numbers of single neurons in the white matter, and neuronal disorganization. Most types of neuronal migration appear to have a primary genetic basis, but this is not necessarily true when migration fails. The type of neuronal heterotopias described in autistic brains probably are due to genetic misinformation in most cases, but they also may be caused by focal infarction of subcortical white matter during fetal life. These infarctions destroy radial glial fibers that guide the migrating neuroblasts and gliablasts to the cortical plate; disruption of their monorail transport system leaves neuroblasts arrested in the middle course of migration, short of their destination, where they mature as heterotopic cells but are unable to establish their intended synaptic relations (Sarnat & Flores-Sarnat 2004). Neuronal migration ends around the 20th week of gestation.

It is already known that whatever is going wrong in the young autistic brain is unlikely to be uniform in its effect; marked variation across the cerebral regions can occur. Certain abilities are preserved in most children with autism, suggesting that those circuits remain intact; these abilities include visual-spatial perception (Ozonoff et al. 1991) and noncerebellar motor function (Haas et al. 1996). Other regions may experience the positive or negative effects of postulated abnormal feedback systems; for example, Carper and Courchesne (2000) found in their patients a significant inverse correlation between smaller, more abnormal cerebellar regions VI-VII and larger, more abnormal frontal lobe volumes.

There also appear to be both general and regional issues of neurodevelopmental timing which appear to be factors; idiosyncratic patterns of growth have been described. A very interesting study of children with predominantly high-functioning autism revealed early hyperplasia of cerebral cortex and cerebral

Table 2-1   Shared symptoms of frontotemporal dementia and autism

---

Marked male predominance
Impairment of social interaction
    lack of social awareness
    theory of mind impairment
    absence (or loss of) empathy
    difficulty learning or indifference to rules
Impairment in communication
    speech abnormalities
Repetitive and stereotyped patterns of behavior
    repetitive compulsive behaviors
    perseveration
Lack of imagination
    pathologically rigid personality
Eating disorders
Evidence of savant skills

References for symptoms of frontotemporal dementia: Gregory et al. 2002; Miller et al. 2003)

white matter in the 2- and 3- year-old age groups, followed by slowed growth in later ages (Courchesne et al. 2001; Carper et al. 2002).

Finally, before moving on from central nervous system ontology and its apparently critical role in the genesis of the symptoms of autism in most affected children, it helps to remember the limitations on how to interpret even the most reasonable of hypotheses. At the other end of life there is a neurological disease called frontotemporal dementia. In table 2-1, it can be seen that this disease of old age mimics infantile autism in a number of ways. It is a surprise to see so many shared symptoms, such as language problems, impairment of theory of mind (ToM) and stereotyped behaviors in these older adult patients (Miller et al. 2003). It is actually startling to note that adults with frontotemporal dementia sometimes acquire gifted artistic drawing and colorist abilities even if they previously had no particular interest in art; these individuals are described by some as at the same level of visual creativity observed in autistic savants!

CANDIDATE REGIONS IN AUTISM

A complex neurocircuitry in the brain handles social relationships with others through visual social clues, vocal social clues, communication by language, gesture, body language, affiliative behavior, etc. These social cognition circuits are in process of being mapped in human volunteers by studying the way stations of the social neurocircuitry. These centers, these waystations, also can be evaluated neuroanatomically by imaging techniques in patients with behavioral disorders. However, the problem of neuroanatomical correlates with specific behaviors is particularly difficult when dealing with neurodevelopmental diseases that begin in utero. In adult neurology, the cortical anatomy of particular gyri is likely to be fairly consistent from 1 patient to the next. For example, modern technical advances (preoperative fMRI and extraoperative ECS mapping with placement of subdural electrodes combined with intraoperative iECS mapping and sensory evoked potential monitoring) help neurosurgeons pinpoint precise function of gyri where they are planning to operate. However, in the case of children in general with their potential for neural plasticity, and particularly in children with a neurodevelopmental disease such as autism, exact neuroanatomical diagnosis is a much greater challenge in both neurology and neurosurgery.

The information about social, language, and behavioral circuits in autism has been gathered mostly from the large group of nonsyndromic patients. It remains difficult to unjumble the various underlying disease entities and subgroups in the autistic populations used in these studies. The functional imaging information that requires active participation is mostly based on a set of adult men with Asperger syndrome or those with what is known as high-functioning/able autism. This omits the majority of the population of individuals with autism, those who test as mentally retarded. Based on the information reported, it seems likely that individuals who have autism with ventriculomegaly or microcephaly have rarely been tested. The not unreasonable rationale appears to be that, since the high-functioning children with autism may have domains of superior functioning yet still have autism, only certain selected networks can be involved in all patients for autistic symptoms in general.

The candidate regions for autistic dysfunction being studied included many of the major neural centers found on neural networks in the central nervous system. These circuits are thought to be widely distributed and functionally diverse. They are being located by 2 different paradigms: hypothesis-driven and non–hypothesis driven approaches. The hypothesis-driven approach was to try to find the brain location of specific symptoms of autism by analogy with behavioral information from neurological cases or adult psychiatric cases. The non–hypothesis (or less–hypothesis) driven approach was to study the brains of individuals with autism, usually by looking at the whole brain. Selected examples of these studies are as follows:

The frontal lobes: The frontal lobes are the last to mature in the human brain, as is seen in the frontal circuits with their executive function over other brain areas. Their full expression may not be seen until the end of adolescence, so they seemed unlikely to be involved in a disease like autism that begins so early in brain development. Nevertheless, the relationship between brain maturation and cognitive development during infancy includes a number of functions that appear to be strengthened by the maturation of frontal and prefrontal cortices (Diamond et al. 1989). Higher order cognitive processes such as spatial working memory are subserved by a distributed neural network in which prefrontal cortex plays a primary role. The orbitofrontal cortex, located right above the eyes, is thought to process rewards and set up impulse control. The lateral orbitofrontal cortex processes both the visual and vocal social cues that make it possible to recognize the emotions of others and allows its integration into contextually appropriate behavioral responses. The frontal region is important in the fundamental job of executive function, processing and directing the development of socially appropriate behavior that is slowly coming "online" throughout childhood.

Many different types of studies completed in children and adults with autism/Asperger syndrome show dysfunction in the frontal region. The most common site of localized spikes in paroxysmal EEGs in children with autism and seizures are at the Fz and Cz electrodes in the frontal region on both sides of the midline, although not that specific (Hashimoto et al. 2001). Salmond et al. (2003) looked at 14 children with autism individually using MRI and VBM and found an orbitofrontal cortex abnormality in all but 1. The dorsolateral prefrontal cortex had decreased activation during a spatial working memory task in non–mentally retarded people with autism (Luna et al. 2002). However, during a different verbal memory task, patients had lower glucose metabolism in medial/cingulate regions but not in lateral regions of the frontal area (Hazlett et al. 2004).

The effects of orbitofrontal lesions in nonhuman primates are said to provide parallels to the emotional and affiliative dysfunction seen in Asperger syndrome (Zald & Kim 2001). A PMRS study in Asperger syndrome found abnormalities in the medial prefrontal lobe that were related to the severity of clinical symptoms of autism (Murphy et al. 2002). The SPECT study by Ohnishi et al. (2000) found hypoperfusion in the left prefrontal cortices. Higher metabolic rates of the right anterior cingulate gyrus at baseline have been reported to predict response to the serotonin-reuptake inhibitor drug fluoxetine in adults with autism, a similar pattern of predictability to that found in depression (Buchsbaum et al. 2001). Focal regions of decreased uptake of alpha[11C]methyl-L-tryptophan, interpreted as serotonin, have been shown in the frontal cortex of boys with autism (Chugani et al. 1999). Wilcox et al. (2002) reported that the abnormal findings in the prefrontal area are more prominent with age.

The temporal lobes: The temporal lobes were one of the first areas of the brain that fell under suspicion by autistic investigators owing to their clinical involvement although their involvement is hard to establish (Hazlett et al. 2004). The temporal lobes were found to be damaged in diseases with significant subgroups of patients with autistic symptoms, such as tuberous sclerosis and herpes encephalitis; tumors in both temporal lobes have been found in patients with autism. Bilateral involvement of the temporal lobes in autism has been reported by several imaging studies (Boddaert et al. 2002; Ohnishi et al. 2000), while bilateral temporal hypometabolism in early infancy even has been used to predict DSM-IV autism (Chugani et al. 1996).

The superior temporal gyrus has become an area of focus of many autism studies; it is marked in its posterior aspect by the presence of horizontal convolutions (the transverse temporal gyri) known as Heschl's convolutions. The superior temporal gyrus appears to be specialized for perception and comprehension of spoken words, although the degree of laterality is still somewhat controversial. This gyrus is where the N1c/Tb wave of late auditory evoked potentials are generated. In the study by Bruneau et al. (2003) utilizing such potentials, a stronger intensity on the right side was seen in children with autism instead on the left side as was seen in the matched control children. A PET study by Boddaert et al. (2003) also confirmed greater right temporal activation to speech sounds in autism.

Processing the human face is at the focal point of most social interactions. The fascination of the infant with the mother's face starts up that social learning process as early as the neonatal period. From birth, human infants prefer to look at faces that engage them in mutual gaze; from an early age, healthy babies show enhanced neural processing during a direct gaze. This exceptionally early sensitivity to mutual gaze in human babies is arguably a major foundation for the development of social skills (Farroni et al. 2002). Face processing goes through identified visual pathways, parts of which appear deficient in autism (Deruelle et al. 2004). A study using differential event-related potentials found that the specific potential usually used for processing faces was larger for furniture than faces in adolescents and adults with autism (McPartland et al. 2001).

The fusiform gyrus in particular has a region in its lateral aspect that is more engaged by human faces than any other category of image; it is known as the fusiform face area (FFA). Functional MRI has shown that typical children consistently activate several neural areas, especially the FFA, when performing a face perception test. Hypoactivation of the fusiform gyrus has been reported in children with autism (Critchley et al. 2001). However, the hypoactivation reported in autism probably should be interpreted not as caused by a simple dysfunction of the FFA, but rather due to more complex anomalies in the distributed network of brain areas involved in social perception and cognition (Schultz et al. 2003; Hadjikhani et al. 2004). It should be noted that some children with autism, however, "see" faces utilizing their own aberrant and individual-specific neural sites outside FFA (Pierce et al. 2001). Each child may have his or her own unique and compensatory neural circuitry, often omitting the FFA site. Dysfunction of the fusiform gyrus, however, is not unique to autism; the volume of the fusiform gyrus is bilaterally reduced in first-episode patients with schizophrenia (Lee et al. 2002a).

The insula: Another area of interest is the insula, where a SPECT study by Ohnishi et al. (2000) found hypoperfusion bilaterally in autism. The insula is believed to play a fundamental role in a mechanism of action representation that allows for empathy and modulates our emotional content (Carr et al. 2003).

The limbic system: The limbic system seemed like an obvious choice for pathology because of the nature of autistic symptoms. When Bauman and Kemper (1985, 1994) began neuropathological studies of autism, they found small, densely distributed neurons there, especially in fields CA1 and CA4. Brothers (1990) and Baron-Cohen et al. (1999) have proposed that the amygdala is the most likely site of damage to the impaired neural network in autism. Based on nonautistic neurological cases with focal bilateral amygdala damage, Adolphs et al. (2001) hypothesized that, in autism, the poor recognition of emotional and social information from faces might be due to bilateral amygdala dysfunction. By directly comparing test results from neurological cases, these authors found some parallels since the 8 subjects with autism made abnormal social judgments regarding the trustworthiness of faces. However, other studies of both patients with bilateral damage to the amygdala (Amaral et al. 2003) and with autism (Salmond et al. 2003) do not support the hypothesis that impairment of the amygdala is always an underlying component of autistic symptoms. Regarding its size, the amygdala has been reported to be both decreased (Aylward et al. 1999) and increased (Sparks et al. 2002) in autism.

Other areas within the limbic system, such as the area dentata, have been reported to be significantly smaller in young children with autism (Saitoh et al. 2001).

If one turns from areas of underperformance to areas of overperformance in autism, at least part of the limbic system appears quite intact. The most functional sensory system of many children with autism is the olfactory system, which is part of the limbic pathways. Children who are savants might use some aspect of a memory circuit that includes the amygdala.

The corpus callosum: Studies, including an MRI study in which enlarged cortical lobes were found, have suggested that the corpus callosum is diminished in size (Piven et al. 1997); however, later studies dispute this (Herbert et al. 2004). Whether anterior or posterior subregions may be abnormal is another point of contention.

The thalamus: The thalamus is a vital part of sensory pathways. There is evidence of focal areas of decreased uptake (Ryu et al. 1999). Researchers have found reduced thalamic volume (Tsatsanis et al. 2003; Waiter et al. 2004). Alteration of the circuits through the thalamus may account for some of the perceptual peculiarities so noticeable in individuals with autism.

The brainstem: The brainstem was first identified as possibly abnormal in autism by Rimland (1964) who targeted its reticular formation. Piven et al. (1992) found the size of the pons did not differ between autistic subjects and controls and Hardan et al. (2001) reported that the brain stem had a normal volume. However, Rodier et al. (1996), Hashimoto et al. (1993) and others have shown neuropathological shortening of the brainstem and abnormal inferior olive in some cases. Evidence from other neurological forms of mutism in children suggests that brainstem malfunction might be a factor underlying autistic mutism (chapter 5). A brain stem location in some forms of autism also is suggested by the common group of anomalies noted in the Möbius sequence, a congenital palsy of the 6th and 7th cranial nerves, as well as thalidomide embryopathy; these

2 syndromes contain a subgroup of children who meet autistic criteria (Miller et al. 1998).

The cerebellum: Abnormalities in the cerebellum have been identified by a number of different disciplines. This was the first location in which abnormalities were consistently found by the early pathological studies (Ritvo et al. 1986; Kemper & Bauman 1998) and many subsequent studies of autism. The finding of hypoplasia of neocerebellar vermal lobules VI-VII appeared at first to be an important key to autism (Courchesne et al. 1988), as these regions give rise to output pathways that eventually connect the cerebellum with the cerebral cortex. It is likely that this finding remains relevant to individuals with autism who have such vermal hypoplasia. But it is not abnormal in all patients with autism, nor is such hypoplasia specific to autism since it can be found in nonautistic disease entities. McAlonan et al. (2002) also report significantly less grey matter in the cerebellum. Reduced Purkinje cell size and specific receptor abnormalities in cerebellar cortex are now being described (Lee et al. 2002b; Fatemi et al. 2002a, 2002b). Yet studies by Abell et al. (1999) and Hardan et al. (2001) found increased grey matter volume in regions of the cerebellum, while Waiter et al. (2004) reported no significant changes in grey matter volume. A monozygotic twin study found clinical discordance was echoed in discordance of grey and white matter volume of the cerebellum only (Kates et al. 2004). Behavioral studies have found evidence for a cerebellar role in the symptoms of reduced exploration and stereotyped behavior in autism (Pierce & Courchesne 2001). See chapter 3 for in-depth information about the cerebellum in autism, including the effect of cerebellar lesions on affective control and executive functioning circuits.

Summary of candidate regions: Regarding the ability to evaluate these attempts of brain localization, there are limitations to questions of homogeneity of the populations studied and to technical, attentional, and age-dependent problems (Wilcox et al. 2002). But one thing does seem clear: the totality of all the information just discussed suggests that there can not be just a single anatomical location, one specific regional pathology, whose abnormality underlies the symptoms of autism in all patients. To quote Salmond et al. (2003) "Autism is unlikely to be associated with abnormality in one particular location alone. Instead the autistic phenotype may reflect abnormalities within a particular neural system or, indeed, multiple systems."

The neuronal centers being studied are part of a massively connected brain, yet a developmentally dysregulated brain. Earlier attempts to localize the symptoms of autism in a single brain region are being replaced by models that postulate a disruption and/or modification of parallel distributed or dynamic circuits with evidence of aberrant connectivity. The variety of anatomical locations involved in these circuits reflects early developmental changes and early neuromodulary discrepancies. With so many different disease entities associated with autistic symptoms, it is possible that the social circuitry of the brain is affected at a number of different sites and by a number of different means. Just as there is no one genetic error, there likely is no one neuroanatomical site of circuit disruption. To look at the many factors involved, evidence available about synaptogenesis, the neurotransmitters at the synapse, the circuits of the neural networks themselves, and the myelin that covers them must be reviewed. These pathological processes may continue to play out throughout gestation and the perinatal period and into early childhood.

TROUBLE AT THE CELLULAR LEVEL: SYNAPTOGENESIS

The formation of synaptic contacts in human cerebral cortex in auditory cortex (Herschl's gyrus) and the prefrontal cortex begin before gestational age 27 weeks, before the beginning of the third trimester (Huttenlocher & Dabholkar 1997). The phase of net synapse elimination occurs late in childhood, earlier in auditory cortex where it has ended by age 12 years, than in prefrontal cortex where it extends to midadolescence. As examples of problems with synaptogenesis in a brain in which autistic symptoms have been demonstrated, there will be 2 examples, 1 from syndromic and 1 from nonsyndromic autism.

Probably the best studied MCA/MR disease with autistic features is the fragile X syndrome, although only a small minority of children have the complete autistic syndrome. It has been demonstrated that people with the fragile X syndrome show immature dendritic spine morphology (Irwin et al. 2000), and it now is known that the fragile X protein made from the gene is synthesized in dendrites (Govek et al. 2004). Since there is evidence that this neurotransmitter-evoked protein synthesis is reduced in vivo (Greenough et al. 2001), the intriguing question is whether one role of the FMR protein in normal brains could be to regulate the translational response to synaptic stimulation, a prerequisite for synaptic plasticity. (Plasticity is of course necessary for modification of learning and is the opposite of rigid thinking, a characteristic of the autistic symptom of "need for sameness.")

In nonsyndromic patients with autism/Asperger, mutations have been found in the 2 X-linked genes encoding neuroligins NL6N3 and NL6N4 (Jamain et al. 2003) (Laumonnier et al. 2004). Deletions at Xp22.3 that include NL6N4 had previously been reported in several autistic individuals (Thomas et al. 1999). Neuroligins are part of the machinery employed during the formation and remodeling of CNS synapses (Scheiffele et al. 2000). Among the various proteins involved in the establishment of neural networks, cell-adhesion molecules are essential factors for the identification of the appropriate partner cell and the formation of the functional synapse. NL6N3 and NL6N4 encode cell-adhesion molecules present at the postsynaptic side of the synapse.

TROUBLE WITH THE NEUROTRANSMITTERS

Abnormal levels of body fluids that might implicate biochemical pathways important for brain function have been found in children with autism; imaging studies have added even more data. In fact, the more scientific questions that are posed, the greater the number of neurotransmitters that appear to be involved. However, the interpretation of these findings is far from clear. Although some investigators believe that these abnormal levels may signal a primary defect, others believe that the biochemical abnormalities of these systems in almost all cases appear to be nonspecific, with what apparently could be interpreted as secondary or compensatory roles. Different sets of cousin neurotransmitter pathways have been identified in a number of studies in individuals with autistic traits: one set is the tryptophan/tyrosine systems and another is the purine/pyrimidine systems. Other neurotransmitter systems also are of interest. The glutamate/GABA neurotransmitter system has been studied because of the frequency of epilepsy in autism and because subunits of the $GABA_A$ receptors cluster within the region of chromosome 15q11-q13. Another neurotransmitter under investigation is acetylcholine (Lee et al. 2002b; Martin-Ruiz et al. 2004); an early study reported that the symptoms of irritability and hyperactivity in children with autism respond to an acetylcholinesterase inhibitor, donezipil (Hardan & Hardan 2002).

The tryptophan/tyrosine system

The very first biochemical abnormality found in a group of children with autism was a high level of serotonin in the whole blood of 6 of 23 patients (38%) (Schain & Freedman 1961). Serotonin is a neurotransmitter in the tryptophan pathway, and this finding has stood the test of time. A number of studies have confirmed that approximately 40% of children with autistic features have a high level of serotonin in their platelets as measured by the whole blood method, while a small number, less than 5%, have a low level. Besides being a neurotransmitter, serotonin also plays a role in neurogenesis, neuronal differentiation, neuropil formation, axon myelination, and synaptogenesis (Whitaker-Azmitia 2001). An early low level of serotonin causes narrow neural columns in animals. A rat model of autism, created by treating fetal rats with the serotonin agonist 5-methoxytryptamine, is said to partially mimic both clinical and imaging findings found in children with autism (Kahne et al. 2002). During childhood, serotonin synthesis capacity in the brain of children with autism has been shown to start to increase at a later age and persist longer than the increase seen in normal children, but still never reach the top capacity of the controls and these abnormalities may be specific to clinical subgroups (Chugani et al. 1999; Behen et al. 2004).

A number of studies of genes related to serotonin in children with autism have been performed, so far without clear-cut results. In spite of the questions raised by studies of serotonin transporter genes (Coutinho et al. 2004), another study did not find a significant relationship between serotonin blood levels and serotonin transporter gene polymorphisms in children with autism (Betancur et al. 2002), nor did a study of the serotonin transporter locus in an autistic phenotypic subset of families with compulsive behaviors and rigidity (McCauley et al. 2004). Serotonin type 2A receptors are now under study.

Table 2-2 Disease entities with abnormal levels of serotonin in syndromic autism

High levels of serotonin	Low levels of serotonin
Congenital hypothyroidism	de Lange syndrome
Maternal rubella	Phenylketonuria
Tuberous sclerosis	West syndrome
Williams syndrome	

At this time, one explanation of the abnormalities found in the serotonin system of children with autism appears to be that they are nonspecific and secondary to other biochemical abnormalities. Abnormal levels of serotonin in blood have been found in certain diseases that have a subgroup of patients with autistic features (table 2-2), as well as many other diseases. It is of historical interest that the serotonin level in the blood of children who may have diseases with a subgroup of autism has been brought toward or into the normal range by correcting the underlying disease biochemistry. Examples of this correction phenomenon are bringing down into the normal range the high whole-blood serotonin levels in patients with congenital hypothyroidism by the administration of the thyroid hormone (Coleman 1970), and bringing the low level of serotonin up into the normal range in children with phenylketonuria by placing them on the low phenylalanine diet (McKean 1971).

In the tyrosine pathway, the first enzyme in the pathway, phenylalanine hydroxylase, is involved in PKU autism. Dopamine-beta-hydroxylase (DBH), the enzyme responsible for the final step in norepinephrine biosynthesis, has neen shown to be statistically lower in children with autism (Goldstein et al. 1976).

Both the tryptophan and tyrosine pathways utilize monoamine oxidase at the catabolic end of the pathway. Although there were 7 negative studies of monoamine oxidase in the platelets, plasma, and fibroblasts of children with autism from 1976 to 1980 (summarized in Coleman & Gillberg 1985), a relationship has now been described between severe autistic behavior and low IQ with a functional polymorphism (a low-activity MAOA allele) in the monoamine oxidase promoter region (Cohen et al. 2003).

The purine/pyrimidine system

Hyperuricosuria, the presence of excessive amounts of uric acid in the urine in children with autism, appears to be a phenomenon of childhood only; it was found in more than 25% of the children under the age of 12 years (Coleman et al. 1976). The uric acid in the urine is the final endproduct of all the purine pathways. With the onset of adolescence, however, the hyperuricosuria tapers off or disappears in almost all cases. This creates the rule that if a child loses hyperuricosuria after puberty, a diligent search for a purine enzyme error is unlikely to be rewarded.

However, a few children with autism do have established metabolic errors of the purine metabolic pathway. One such disease is adenylosuccinate lyase deficiency (ADSL), which is based on genetic errors in the enzyme that catalyzes 2 different steps in the purine pathway. The error is usually due to a point mutation in the gene, although a deletion in the gene also has been reported (Kohler et al. 1999). In the original paper by Jaeken and Van den Berghe (1984), describing the abnormal biochemistry of succinyl purine compounds, 3 children with autism were described. There are now many more reported ADSL cases with autism, although not all children with this disease meet autistic criteria. Another metabolic error results in nucleotidase-associated pervasive developmental disorder (NAPDD) (Page et al. 1997). In this very rare disease entity, 5' nucleotidase, an enzyme that cleaves purines and pyrimidines equally well, is elevated.

Virtually all the children who have hyperuricosuria during childhood do not have an established disease entity of purine metabolism; the reason for the hyperuricosuria is not known. A remote possibility is that these children might be showing during their childhood years only a secondary effect of the overproduction of purines that are part of the response to their genetic makeup, as suggested by elevated mRNA levels (Purcell et al. 2001), or of other indirect genetic effects.

The GABA/glutamate system

The GABA/glutamate system in autism is under increasing scrutiny. In the case of GABA, diminution of benzodiazepine binding sites (Blatt et al. 2001) and alterations in plasma, platelets and urine have been reported. Patients with autism have been described in succinic semialdehyde dehydrogenase deficiency and the pyridozine-dependency syndrome, disorders which involve GABA (see table 1-5). There is evidence pointing toward autism risk alleles in the $GABA_A$ receptors (McCauley et al. 2004) and the reelin gene. A question has been raised about levels of GABAergic interneurons. Regarding glutamate, it has been proposed that autism may be a hypoglutamingeric disorder. Subjects with autism may have abnormalities in glutamatte receptors (Jamain et al. 2002) and transporters (Purcell et al. 2001).

TROUBLE WITH CIRCUITRY IN AUTISM

The effect of the neurotransmitters is translated postsynaptically into electrical impulses of the neural circuits. According to the distributed cortical network theory of brain function, all thoughts and actions are believed to be encoded in patterns of neuronal electrical activity, and the circuits of nerve cells connected by synapses are dedicated to processing the information in these patterns. However, the question of exactly which are the candidate circuits that might be impaired in autism is difficult to study at this time for a number of reasons. A major problem at present is that the dysfunctional circuits identified in children with the social cognition problems of autism appear to be involved in other disease entities as well and do not appear to be unique to autism. Another major problem is that, like some individuals with the multiple cognitive dysfunctions of mental retardation, a number of individuals with autism may have developed somewhat unusual circuitry. In mental retardation research, the pathways of shared cognitive pathogenesis show defects in synapses, axon maintenance, and trafficking (Nokelainen & Flint 2002).

ToM refers to the ability to attribute mental states to self and others, and to predict and understand other people's behavior on the basis of their mental states. Clinical deficiencies of ToM are well documented in children with autism and can be one of their most devastating clinical handicaps. In control subjects, the ToM task is performed in a network consisting of the amygdala (Fine et al. 2001), the medial prefrontal cortex (Shallice 2001), the cingulate cortex, the extrastriate cortex, and the temporoparietal junction. However, the same clinical deficiency of ToM can be found in other disease entities such as paranoid delusional schizophrenia and frontotemporal dementia (table 2-1). Interestingly, Gregory et al. (2002) found a striking correlation between the magnitude of impairment on ToM testing and the degree of frontal atrophy in patients with frontotemporal dementia; this helped reinforce the supposition that functioning frontal lobes are an essential part of the circuit for ToM processing (Stuss 2001).

A number of studies show that individuals with autism have aberrant activation in the regions associated with ToM, including the medial prefrontal cortex (Castelli et al. 2002), while performing ToM tasks and "mentalizing" (Happe et al. 1996; Baron-Cohen et al. 1999). However, such a circuit is far from certain; a recent stroke patient with extensive damage to medial frontal lobes thought to be critical for ToM did not have significant ToM impairment (Bird et al. 2004). Corticocingulate circuitry was also implicated during an oculomotor spatial working memory task; there was evidence of decreased activation of the dorsolateral prefrontal and posterior cingulate circuitry (Luna et al. 2002). Whether ToM is domain specific, with its own dedicated neural circuit, or whether it is processed by domain-general cognitive functions is not yet established. In fact, the neural systems implicated in ToM and in responding to the emotional expression of others appear to be the same neural systems involved in working memory, impulse control, and decision-making (Bechara 2002).

In 1997, Chugani et al. studied boys with autism and proposed that the connectivity of a dentato-thalamo-cortico pathway might be disrupted during development, causing decreased serotonin synthesis in the cerebral cortex, which has developmental implications including sensory integration and concomitant language impairment. A study of adults with autism also reported atypical functional impairment of the dentato-thalamo-cortical pathway for language activation (Muller et al. 1998). Hardan et al. (2001) also noted a cerebellothalamocortical circuit involved in information reception and processing in adolescents and adults with autism. In addition, Townsend et al. (2001) interpreted their event-related potential study of spatial attention as evidence of impaired cerebellofrontal circuits. The dentato-thalamo-cortical tract is an interesting circuit that can be surgically injured resulting in cerebellar mutism (Wang et al. 2002), yet the phenomenon of diaschisis may occur. Diaschisis produces a disruption of cerebral oxygen metabolism, glucose metabolism, and blood flow in the secondarily affected cortical area (Meyer et al. 1993), and in the case of diaschisis, function partially or completely returns in that remote, temporarily deactivated region as the primary cerebellar lesion heals.

Regarding circuits that might be involved in Asperger's syndrome, McAlonan et al. (2002) have suggested that abnormalities in the frontal-striatal circuits result in defective sensory-motor gating with consequently characteristic difficulties inhibiting repetitive thoughts, speech, and actions. Frontal-parietal circuits may be involved in some patients, as exemplified by the circuits involved in catatonia, the orbitofrontal/prefrontal-parietal/cortical circuits.

What is already known is that different circuits may be involved in different disorders. Networks impaired in bipolar disorder might also be involved in the infantile autistic bipolar disorder (frontotemporal, ventral and medial prefrontal, and amygdalar) (Blumberg et al. 2002). Networks under siege in Tourette's syndrome may also be involved in the Zappella dysmaturational syndrome of children with autism and tics, such as the cortico-striatal-thalamo-cortical circuits.

But, although we can make educated guesses, we do not yet know which networks are involved in most children with autism. It is important to acknowledge what is not known.

TROUBLE WITH MYELINATION OF THE NEURAL NETWORKS

Myelin plays an essential but largely under appreciated role in human brain structure and function. Myelin is a vital part of any neural network. Its importance in increasing axonal transmission, reducing action potential time, and improving synchrony of brain function is well established. Myelination is inextricably associated with the speed of human brain cognitive processing; there is early evidence that processing speed has a genetically influenced association with white matter volume (Posthuma et al. 2003). The process of myelination is regionally and temporally heterochronologic; females have a faster developmental trajectory, reaching peak myelination levels earlier than males in multiple regions. One possible extrapolation of that data might explain why girls tend to have a faster trajectory of language acquisition (Karrass et al. 2002). According to the model developed by Bartzokis (2004), the promyelinating effects of female gender may help protect from the developmental vulnerabilities of the myelination process. He speculates that dysregulation of the uniquely vulnerable developmental trajectory of myelination in humans might interfere with special human functions such as language and higher executive function.

In 1986, a hypothesis was proposed that a potential etiological factor in autism was abnormal brain development resulting from dysfunctional myclination (Rciss et al. 1986) White matter pathways of the limbic and paralimbic circuits have been found significantly different in socially deprived orphans. To examine this question, first there will be a look at a few of the established diseases with syndromic autism in which there is relevant data and then review more recent data on nonsyndromic autism. It is known that each disease entity has its own mechanism of harming the myelin; some are characterized by dysmyelination (abnormal development of myelin because of a metabolic error preventing the normal sequence of events) and others by demyelination (the loss of previously acquired normal myelin through some superimposed neuropathologic process).

Phenylketonuria (PKU) is an aminoaciduria whose symptoms occur as a consequence of mutations in the PAH gene, leading to the underperformance of phenylalanine-4-hydroxlase, a critical enzyme for the catecholamine pathway of dopamine and norepinephrine. The high level of the amino acid phenylalanine and its metabolites backed-up behind the poorly functioning enzyme also interfere with related metabolic pathways, such as the serotonin pathway. Phenylalanine-4-hydroxlase fails to function either because the enzyme itself is genetically diminished or the amount of its cofactor tetrahydrobiopterin (BH4) is inadequate owing to a metabolic defect in the synthesis or regeneration of BH4. A percentage of patients with phenylketonuria have been diagnosed as having autism in the past; fortunately, PKU autism is becoming a rare disease in countries where children undergo newborn screening (Baieli et al. 2003). Neuropathological studies have shown that myelin is primarily affected in phenylketonuria. Evidence indicates that high levels of phenylalanine may induce oligodendrocytes, the brain cells that make myelin, to adopt a nonmyelinating phenotype (Dyer et al. 1996). In untreated PKU patients, findings that suggest the process of dysmyelination is delayed myelination, fibrillary gliosis, excess white matter water, and low concentration of myelin components such as cerebrosides, sulfatides, and cholesterol (Martin & Schlote 1972). However, in this complex disease, myelin is only one of several brain tissues injured by the blockage of phenylalanine-4-hydroxylase.

Congenital rubella is also primarily a disease of the past. It is responsible for very few children with autism since vaccination against rubella has been instituted, (although a few rubella cases are resurfacing in segments of modern societies in which families refuse rubella vacations for their children). After the last big epidemic in the United States in 1964, many cases of children with rubella autism were published. One rubella birth defect evaluation project in New York identified 10 children with autism and 8 more with limited autistic symptoms (Chess et al. 1971). It is interesting that a longitudinal study of these 18 cases found that 7 had improved or recovered with respect to autistic symptoms (Chess 1977). Neuropathological studies of congenital rubella show extensive involvement of cerebral blood vessels. The most frequently affected are the penetrating vessels in the deep white matter and the basal ganglia. This is believed to lead to foci of inflammation or eventual necrosis in the white matter, ischemic sequelae of periarterial and pericapillary degeneration that is a direct effect of the rubella virus on the blood vessels (Lane 1996). In this disease entity, there appears to be demyelination secondarily to cerebral vascular pathology.

A number of the phakomatoses, or neurocutaneous syndromes, are best known for their propensity to produce benign and malignant tumors. In recent years, MRI and various neuropathological studies have brought to light a number of abnormalities of the cerebral white matter in these entities. In the case of tuberous sclerosis complex (see chapter 5), despite the name of the disease being derived from the tubers, most of the other lesions are found in the white matter (Filley 2001). The white matter lesions are usually found in the frontal cortex. Tuberous sclerosis complex affects a significant number of children who present with autism: in a population of all children with autism, 1% to 4% have tuberous sclerosis complex. Another neurocutaneous syndrome, neurofibromatosis, results in 2 kinds of lesions in the white matter. In the subcortical white matter high signal changes are seen on MRI and thought to represent dysmyelination, hamartoma, heterotopias, or even edema. Also, increased cerebral white matter volume has been observed, both in the cerebrum as a whole and in the corpus callosum. A number of children with neurofibromatosis have been described with autistic symptoms. Hypomelanosis of Ito, with hypopigmentation and neurological features, is associated with a number of peculiar white matter findings. These include periventricular white matter hyperintensity and absent delineation between cortical gray and white matter. Up to 10% of children with this disease show autistic features.

Only a small number of patients (summarized in Gillberg & Coleman 2000) have been described with autism and one of the mucopolysaccharidoses, a group of lysosomal storage diseases. Although many brain tissues are involved (Zafeiriou et al. 2001), diffusely delayed myelination has been reported (Johnson et al. 1984). More commonly, cribiform (sieve-like or multicystic) changes occur in the white matter and may even mimic a leukodystrophy (Barone et al. 2002).

The leukodystrophies are the classic disorders of white matter in childhood, but autism is almost never found among them. There is only 1 patient in the literature with autism and adrenomyeloneuropathy (Swillen et al. 1996) and 10 PDD children with a nonspecific pseudodeficiency of the enzyme arylsulfatase A that underlies metachromatic leukodystrophy (Alessandri et al. 2002). This virtual absence of reports in the leukodystrophies could be interpreted to suggest that autistic symptoms are related to myelin, they must arrive from alterations with selective myelinated pathways rather than a direct problem in myelin itself.

Moving on to the subject of nonsyndromic autism, such possible selective pathways have been described by Barnea-Goraly et al. (2004). They examined the white matter in 7 male children and adolescents with autism and compared them to matched controls. Diminished white matter tracts were found adjacent to a number of cortical centers, as well as in the occipitotemporal tracts and the corpus callosum; Bigler et al. (2003) found a trend toward smaller white matter stem volume of the temporal lobe. McAlonan et al. (2002) also had found widespread differences in white matter, as they also reported less gray matter in the frontostriatal and cerebellar regions.

It can be confusing to note that another set of research papers report a somewhat opposite phenomenon: an abnormally large white matter volume in autism. Studies of high-functioning individuals with nonsyndromic autism or Asperger syndrome have often shown enlargement of both global brain volumes and specific neural structures. In some cases, white matter volume increase appeared to be the major factor in increased brain volume, although there may have been a selected increase in gray matter, too. Herbert et al. (2004) report that the increase in white matter is limited to the radiate outer white matter, which is myelinated later or during a longer time interval. In the Courchesne et al. (2001; 2003) papers, the brain volume increase occurred postnatally so that, by 2 to 3 years of age, up to 37% of high-functioning children had become macrocephalic. In the series by Carper et al. (2002), 2- and 3-year-old children had a white matter and gray matter hyperplasia with an anterior to posterior gradient, while older children had neither gray nor white matter differences.

In syndromic autism, both decreased cerebral cortex (Kagawa et al. 2004) or postnatal forms of brain enlargement or actual macrocephaly developing throughout infancy been described as in Sotos syndrome (see chapter 4). In some studies on syndromic autism, these changes can be due to gray rather than white matter. Total gray matter was greater in high-functioning individuals with autism of the average age of 16 years than it was in controls (Waiter et al. 2004). The increased gray matter volume was primarily in the right posterior and left anterior cerebral hemispheres; in this paper, a decrease of global white matter volume did not reach significance. A paper by Abell et al. (1999) that used similar voxel-based morphology to study individuals with autism of the average age of 28 years found less extensive differences, with decreases in gray matter in anterior and increases in posterior parts of the system.

The failure of so many of the various papers mentioned throughout this chapter to confirm each others' findings does not necessarily discredit these often carefully done studies. The contradictions and confusions seen in the literature reflect technical differences, as well as our lack of diagnostic knowledge regarding nonsyndromic autism. In spite of rigorous standards of psychiatric diagnosis, homogeneity in the populations chosen for investigation is likely lacking.

HOW THE INFORMATION IN THIS CHAPTER MIGHT RELATE TO CLINICAL FINDINGS IN THE AUTISTIC SYNDROME

In spite of the amount of information detailed in this chapter, our understanding of the neural substrate of the symptoms of autism/Asperger is largely unknown. A review of the clinical symptoms themselves shows only islets of knowledge.

Children with autistic syndromes have impaired social interaction and lack empathy

Social perception in typical control subjects causes activation of a network that performs face recognition (right fusiform gyrus), perception of eye gaze (superior temporal gyrus), and ToM (anterior cingulate and superior temporal sulcus). In studies in autism, the information is confusing and inadequate. Selected deficits of components of the social network have been demonstrated in the ToM studies, face perception tests, and other related studies, yet both increases and decreases in gray matter also have been reported in the same areas. Another postulated circuit involved in autism is the cerebellothalamocortical circuit. In truth, it is not known exactly which or how many circuits are involved in autism symptoms. Some children with autism appear to function with aberrant and individual-specific circuits.

The word "empathy" appears to refer to 2 different and separate phenomena generated by 2 different neural circuits (Eslinger 1998). Evidence suggests that the empathy deficit in autism/Asperger may be due to the inability to integrate the cognitive and affective facets of another person's life (Shamay-Tsoory et al. 2002). In a recently developed Empathy Quotient, adults with high-functioning autism or Asperger syndrome scored significantly lower than did age, sex-matched peers (Baron-Cohen & Wheelwright 2004).

Children with autistic syndromes have a disabling need for sameness

Insistence on sameness is a primary symptom of autism that can be extremely troubling to family life. Dysfunction of the right medial temporal lobe has been implicated in the insistence on sameness in autism. Preliminary molecular genetic analysis of this phenotypical trait has shown linkage to the chromosomal 15q11-q13 region at the GABRB3 genetic locus (Shao et al. 2003).

Children with autistic syndromes exhibit repetitive and stereotyped patterns of behavior

The repetitive and stereotyped patterns of behavior in autism have been compared to obsessive-compulsive disorder in older patients, but this can be misleading. Obsessive-compulsive behavior has been associated with hypermetabolism of the orbitofrontal cortex both at rest and when confronted with triggering stimuli; also, successful pharmacological treatment of this behavior is associated with significant reductions in orbitofrontal metabolism (Zaid & Kim 2001). There is reason to think that this may not always be the same circuits involved in the repetitive behavior in autism, where subcortical circuits must be considered. For example, in patients with autism secondary to the tuberous sclerosis complex, stereotypical repetitive behaviors and impaired social interaction were associated with an imbalance in circuits including glucose hypermetabolism in the deep cerebellar nuclei and increased uptake of tryptophan in the caudate nuclei (Asano et al. 2001).

Speaking children with autism begin to talk at unusually late ages and have a qualitative impairment in communication

Many studies show abnormal metabolism in the temporal and frontal language sites in children with autism. Also, both the frontal and temporal language-related association cortices appear in studies of brain perfusion in autism to become more abnormal with age (Wilcox 2002). There is a reversed asymmetry in language sites in many boys with autism compared to controls (Muller et al. 1999; Herbert et al. 2002; Boddaert et al. 2003) but the Broca's area neural asymmetry is related more to language impairment than specifically to autism (DeFosse et al. 2004).

A significant minority of children with autism may be mute

Based on the known neuroanatomy of speech, the mutism of autism is likely to involve bilateral dysfunction of the language circuits. The brainstem is a primary candidate area, although networks involving prefrontal, temporal, and cerebellar areas are also at risk (see chapter 5).

Part of the social communication problem in children with autism is a failure to comprehend human mime and gesture

Social imitation is lacking or deficient in children with autism. The fact that limb gestural skills mature before the verbal route in normally developing children (Zoia et al. 2002) is relevant to the early presentation of the communication problem in autism.

The level of development at 5 years of age is a milestone that has some predictive value in children with autism

This may have something to do with the regional localization and strong lateralization of auditory language processing that is attained by 5 years of age.

Some children with autism smell other people to identify them

Olfaction usually is intact in children with autism, even those that are mute (Soussignan et al. 1995). The olfactory pathway is the sensory system that is not processed through the thalamus, the grey matter substation processing the other major sensory pathways of audition, vision, and touch.

What is the meaning of the extensive literature on immunological and autoimmunological abnormalities in children with autism? Is there neuroinflamation of the brain?

It is unknown at this time.

Is autism unique?

In the end, autistic symptoms appear to be due the very young developmental age at which the central nervous system is first impaired, resulting in selective impairments of particular neural networks of behavior and cognition. But these clinical patterns apparently are not unique to autism. The same network impairments can become clinically evident at the other end of life, producing somewhat similar symptoms as described in frontotemporal dementia, a complex syndrome with overlapping pathology with other forms of dementia.

SUMMARY

The autistic syndromes might be considered as one extensive set of impaired final common circuits presenting with dysfunctional information processing of behavior and cognition in very young children. Deficits in pragmatics, linguistic abilities, mindreading, executive functions, episodic memory, self-awareness, central coherence, and affective processing have been documented. These deficits are caused by many disease entities whose shared symptoms likely occur owing to malfunction of certain distributed neural networks. This malfunction in most cases is likely due to aberrant neurodevelopment, leading either to (1) abnormally varied neural circuits or to (2) abnormality in network components of more standard neural pathways. In fact, it is now apparent that autism/Asperger is not a final diagnosis in itself; it is a descriptive set of syndromes due to the result of fetal or early childhood dysfunction in certain common pathways in the brain caused by many different diseases. It is hypothesized that each of the disease entities underlying the autistic syndromes will eventually be identified and found to have its own distinctive variation of clinical symptoms and its own specific neuropathology.

REFERENCES

Abell F, Krams M, Ashburner J, Passingham R, Friston K, Frackowiaki R, Happe F, Frith C, Frith U (1999) The neuroanatomy of autism; a voxel-based whole brain analysis of structural scans. *Neuroreport* 10:1647–1651.

Adolphs R, Sears L, Piven J (2001) Abnormal processing of social information from faces in autism. *Journal of Cognitive Neuroscience* 13:232–240.

Alessandri MG, De Vito G, Fornai F (2002) Increased prevalence of pervasive developmental disorders in children with slight arylsulfatase A deficiency. *Brain and Development* 24:688–692.

Amaral DG, Bauman MD, Schumann CM (2003) The amygdala and autism: implications from non-human primate studies. *Genes, Brain and Behavior* 2:295–302.

Asano E, Chugani DC, Muzik O, Behen M, Janisse J, Rothermel R, Manger TJ, Chakraborty PK, Chugani HT (2001) Autism in tuberous sclerosis complex is related to both cortical and subcortical dysfunction. *Neurology* 57:1269–1277.

Aylward EH, Minshew NJ, Goldstein G, Honeycutt NA, Augustine AM, Yates KO, Barta PE, Pearlson GD (1999) MRI volumes of amygdala and hippocampus in non–mentally retarded autistic adolescents and adults. *Neurology* 53:2145–2150.

Bachevalier J (1996) Brief report: medial temporal lobe and autism: a putative animal model in primates. *Journal of Autism and Developmental Disorders* 26:217–220.

Baieli S, Pavone L, Meli C, Fiumara A, Coleman M (2003) Autism and phenylketonuria. *Journal of Autism and Developmental Disorders* 33:201–204.

Bailey A, Luthert P, Dean A, Harding B, Janota I, Montgomery M, Rutter M, Lantos P (1998) A clinicopathological study of autism. *Brain* 121:889–905.

Barnea-Goraly N, Kwon H, Menon V, Eliez S, Lotspeich L, Reiss AL (2004) White matter structure in autism: preliminary evidence from diffusion tensor imaging. *Biological Psychiatry* 55:323–326.

Baron-Cohen S, Ring HA, Wheelwright S, Bullmore ET, Ashweii C, Williams SC (1999) The amygdala theory of autism. *Neuroscience Biobehavioral Review* 24:355–364.

Baron-Cohen S, Wheelwright S (2004) The empathy quotient: An investigation of adults with Asperger syndrome or high-functioning autism, and normal sex differences. *Journal of Autism and Developmental Disorders* 34:163–175.

Barone R, Parano E, Trifiletti RR, Fiumara A, Pavone P (2002) White matter changes mimicking a leukodystrophy in a patient with mucopolysaccharidoses; characterization by MRI. *Journal of Neurological Science* 195:171–175.

Bartzokis G (2004) Quadratic trajectories of brain myelin content: unifying construct for neuropsychiatric disorders. *Neurobiology of Aging* 25:49–62.

Batshaw ML, Towbin KE (2001) Research news: the origins of autism. *Pediatric Research* 50:1–2.

Bauman M, Kemper TL (1985) Histoanatomic observations of the brain in early infantile autism. *Neurology* 35:866–874.

Bauman M, Kemper TL (1994) *The Neurobiology of Autism*. Baltimore: Johns Hopkins University Press.

Bechara A (2002) The neurology of social cognition. *Brain* 125:1673–1675.

Behen ME, Chandana SR, Rothermel R, Muzik O, Juhasz C, Chugani HT, Chugani DC (2004) Lateralized cortical serotonergic abnormalities in autistic children are associated with social subtypes. *Annals of Neurology* 56(8):S95. (abstract)

Belmonte MK, Cook EH, Anderson GM, Rubenstein JL, Greenough WP, Beckel-Mitchener A, Courchesne E, Boulanger LM, Powell SB, Levitt P, Perry EK, Kiang YH, DeLorey TM, Tierney E (2004) Autism as a disorder of neural information processing: directions for research and targets for therapy (1). *Molecular Psychiatry* 9:646–663.

Belmonte MK, Yurgelun-Todd DA (2003) Functional anatomy of impaired selective attention and compensatory processing in autism. *Brain Research and Cognition Brain Research* 17:651–664.

Betancur C, Corbex M, Spielewoy C, Phillippe A, Laplanche JL, Launay JM, Gillberg C,

Mouren-Simeoni MC, Hamon M, Giros B, Nosten-Bertrand M, Leboyer M (2002) Serotonin transporter gene polymorphisms and hyperserotonemia in autistic disorder. *Molecular Psychiatry* 7:67–71.

Bigler ED, Tate DF, Neeley ES, Wolfson LJ, Miller MJ, Rice SA, Cleavinger H, Anderson C, Coon H, Ozonoff S, Johnson M, Dinh E, Lu J, Mc Mahon W, Lainhart JE (2003) Temporal lobe, autism, and macrocephaly. *American Journal of Neuroradiology* 24: 2066–2076.

Bird CM, Castelli F, Malik O, Frith U, Husain M (2004) The impact of extensive medial frontal lobe damage on 'Theory of Mind' and cognition. *Brain* 127:914–928.

Blatt GJ, Fitzgerald CM, Guptill JT, Booker AB, Kemper TL, Bauman ML (2001) Density and distribution of hippocampal neurotransmitter receptors in autism; an autoradiographic study. *Journal of Autism and Developmental Disorders* 31:537–543.

Blumberg HP, Charney DS, Krystal JH (2002) Frontotemporal neural systems in bipolar disorder. *Seminars in Clinical Neuropsychiatry* 7:243–254.

Boddaert N, Belin P, Chabane N, Poline JB, Barthelemy C, Mouren-Simeoni MC, Brunelle F, Samson Y, Zilbovicius M (2003) Perception of complex sounds: abnormal pattern of activation in autism. *American Journal of Psychiatry* 160:2057–2060.

Boddaert N, Chabane N, Barthelemy C, Bourgeois M, Poline JB, Brunel F, Samson Y, Zilbovicius M (2002) Bitemporal lobe dysfunction in infantile autism: a positron emission tomography study. *Journal of Radiology* 83:1829–1833.

Brothers L (1990) *Concepts in Neuroscience* 1:27–51.

Bruneau N, Bonnet-Brilhault F, Gomot M, Adrien JL, Barthelemy C (2003) Cortical auditory processing and communication in children with autism: electrophysiological/ behavioral relations. *International Journal of Psychophysiology* 51:17–23.

Buchsbaum MS, Hollander E, Haznedar MM, Tang C, Spiegel-Cohen TC, Solimando A, Buchsbaum BR, Robins D, Bienstock C, Cartwright Mosovich S (2001) Effect of fluoxetine on regional cerebral metabolism in autistic spectrum disorders: a pilot study. *International Journal of Neuropsychopharmacology* 4:119–125.

Carper RA, Courchesne E (2000) Inverse correlation between frontal lobe and cerebellum sizes in autism. *Brain* 123:836–844.

Carper RA, Moses P, Tigue ZD, Courchesne E (2002) Cerebral lobes in autism: early hyperplasia and abnormal age effects. *Neuroimage* 16:1038–1051.

Carr L, Iacoboni M, Dubeau MC, Mazziotta JC, Lenzi GL (2003) Neural mechanisms of empathy in humans: a relay from neural systems for imitation to limbic areas. *Proceedings of the National Academy of Science USA* 100:5497–5502.

Casanova MF, Buxhoeveden D, and Gomez J (2003) Disruption in the inhibitory architecture of the cell minicolumn: implications for autism. *The Neuroscientist* 9:496–507.

Casanova MF, Buxhoeveden DP, Switala AE, Roy E (2002) Minicolumnar pathology in autism. *Neurology* 58:428–32.

Castelli F, Frith C, Happe F, Frith U (2002) Autism, Asperger's syndrome and brain mechanism for the attribution of mental state to animated shapes. *Brain* 125:1839–1849.

Chess S (1977) Follow-up report on autism in congenital rubella. *Journal of Autism and Childhood Schizophrenia* 7:69–81.

Chess S, Korn SJ, Fernandez PB (1971) *Psychiatric disorders of children with congenital rubella.* New York: Brunner/Mazel.

Chugani HT, Da Silva El, Chugani DC (1996) Infantile spasms III: prognostic implications of bitemporal hypometabolism on positron emission tomography. *Annals of Neurology* 39:643–649.

Chugani DC, Muzik O, Behen M, Rothermel R, Janisse JJ, Lee J, Chugani HT (1999) Developmental changes in brain serotonin synthesis capacity in autistic and non-autistic children. *Annals of Neurology* 45:287–295.

Chugani DC, Muzik O, Rothermel R, Behen M, Chakraborty P, Mang de Silva EA, Chugani HT (1997) Altered serotonin synthesis in the dentatothalamocortical pathway in autistic boys. *Annals of Neurology* 42:666–669.

Cohen IL (1994) An artificial neural network analogue of learning in autism. *Biological Psychiatry* 36:5–20.

Cohen IL (2004) A neural network model of autism: implications for theory and treatment. In Mareschal D, Sirois S, Westermann G, and Johnson MH (Eds) *Neuroconstructivism. Vol. 2: Perspectives and Prospects.* Oxford, UK: Oxford University Press.

Cohen IL (1998) Neural network analysis of learning in autism. In Stein DJ and Ludik J (Eds) *Neural Networks and Psychopathology.* New York: Cambridge University Press.

Cohen IL, Liu X, Schutz C, White BN, Jenkins EC, Brown WT, Holden JJ (2003) Association of autism severity with a monoamine oxidase. A functional polymorphism. *Clinical Genetics* 64:190–197.

Coleman M (1970) Serotonin levels in infant hypothyroidism. *Lancet* 2:235.

Coleman M, Gillberg C (1985) *The Biology of the Autistic Syndromes.* New York: Praeger Scientific.

Coleman M, Landgrebe MA, Landgrebe AR (1976) Purine autism: hyperuricosuria in autistic children: does this identify a subgroup of autism? In Coleman M (Ed) *The Autistic Syndromes.* Amsterdam: North Holland Publishing Co.

Courchesne E, Carper R, Akshoomoff N (2003) Evidence of brain overgrowth in the first year of life in autism. *JAMA* 290:337–344.

Courchesne E, Karns C, Davis HR, Ziccardi R, Carper RA, Tigue ZD, Chisum HJ, Moses P, Pierce K, Lord C, Lincoln AJ, Pizzo S, Schreibum L, Haas RH, Akshoomoff NA, Courchesne RY (2001) Unusual brain growth patterns in early life in patients with autistic disorder: an MRI study. *Neurology* 57:2345–2254.

Courchesne E, Yeung-Courchesne R, Press G, Hesselink J, Jernigan T (1988) Hypoplasia of cerebellar vermal lobules 6 and 7 in autism. *New England Journal of Medicine* 318:1349–1354.

Coutinho AM, Oliveira G, Morgadinho T, Fesel C, Macedo TR, Bento C, Marques C, Ataíde A, Miguel T, Borges L, Vicente AM (2004) Variants of the serotonin transporter gene (SLC6A4) significantly contribute to hyperserotonemia in autism. *Molecular Psychiatry* 9:264–271.

Critchley HD, Daly EM, Bullmore ET, Williams SC, Van Amelsvoort T, Robertson DM, Rowe A, Phillips M, McAlonan G, Howlin P, Murphy DG (2001) The functional neuroanatomy of social behavior; changes in cerebral blood flow when people with autistic disorder process facial expressions. *Brain* 124:2059.

Diamond A, Zola-Morgan S, Squire LR (1989) Successful performance by monkeys with lesions of the hippocampal formation on AB and object retrieval, two tasks that mark developmental changes in human infants. *Behavioral Neuroscience* 103:526–537.

De Fosse L, Hodge SM, Makris N, Kennedy DN, Caviness VS Jr, McGrath L, Steele S, Ziegler DA, Herbert MR, Frazier JA, Tager-Flusberg H, Harris GJ (2004) Language-association cortex asymmetry in autism and specific language impairment. *Annals of Neurology* 56:757–766.

Deruelle C, Rondan C, Gepner B, Tardif C (2004) Spatial frequency and face processing in children with autism and Asperger syndrome. *Journal of Autism and Developmental Disorders* 34:199–210.

Dyer CA, Kendler A, Philibotte T, Gardiner P, Cruz J, Levy HL (1996) Evidence for central nervous system glial cell plasticity in phenylketonuria. *Journal of Neuropathology and Experimental Neurology* 55:795–814.

Escalante-Mead PR, Minshew NJ, Sweeney JA (2003) Abnormal brain lateralization in high-functioning autism. *Journal of Autism and Developmental Disorder* 33:539–543.

Eslinger PJ (1998) Neurological and neuropsychological bases of empathy. *European Neurology* 39:193–199.

Farroni T, Csibra G, Simion F, Johnson MH (2002) Eye contact detection in humans from birth. *Proceedings of the National Academy of Science USA* 99:9602–9605.

Fatemi SH, Halt AR, Realmuto G, Earle J, Kist DA, Thuras P, Merz A (2002a) Purkinje cell size is reduced in the cerebellum of patients with autism. *Cell and Molecular Neurobiology* 22:171–175.

Fatemi SH, Halt AR, Stary JM, Kanodia R, Schulz SC, Realmuto GR (2002b) Glutamic acid decarboxylase 65 and 67 kDa proteins are reduced in autistic parietal and cerebellar cortices. *Biological Psychiatry* 52:805–810.

Filley CM (2001) *The Behavioral Neurology of White Matter*. New York: Oxford University Press.

Fine C, Lumsden J, Blair RJR (2001) Dissociation between "theory of mind" and executive functions in a patient with early left amygdala damage. *Brain* 124:287–298.

Friedman SD, Shaw DW, Artru AA, Richards TL, Gardner J, Dawson S, Dager SR (2003) Regional brain chemical alterations in young children with autistic spectrum disorder. *Neurology* 60:100–107.

Frith U (1989) *Autism: explaining the enigma*. Oxford, England: Blackwell.

Fuster JM (2003) *Cortex and Mind: Unifying Cognition*. Oxford, England: Oxford University Press.

Fuster JM (1997) Network memory. *Trends in Neuroscience* 20:451–459.

Geschwind N (1965) Disconnection syndromes in animals and man. *Brain* 88:237–294, 585–644.

Gillberg C, Coleman M (2000) *The Biology of the Autistic Syndromes*. London: Mac Keith Press. Chapter 11. Double Syndromes.

Goldstein M, Mahanand D, Lee J, Coleman M (1976) In Coleman M (Ed) *The Autistic Syndromes*. Amsterdam: North-Holland Publishing Co.

Gorbach AM, Heiss J, Jufta C, Sata S, Fedio P, Kammerer WA, Solomon J, Oldfield EH (2003) Intraoperative infrared functional imaging of the human brain. *Annals of Neurology* 54:297–309.

Govek E-E, Newey SE, Akerman CJ, Cross JR, van der Veken L, van Aeist L (2004) The X-linked oligophrenin-1 is required for dendritic spine morphogenesis. *Nature Neuroscience* 7:364–372.

Greenough WT, Klintsova AY, Irwin SA, Galvez R, Bates KE, Weiler IJ (2001) Synaptic regulation of protein synthesis and the fragile X protein. *Proceedings of the National Academy of Science USA* 98:7101–7106.

Gregory C, Lough S, Stone V, Erzinclioglu S, Martin L, Baron-Cohen S, Hodges JR (2002)

Theory of mind in patients with frontal variant frontotemporal dementia and Alzheimer's disease: theoretical and practical implications. *Brain* 125:752–764.

Gustafsson L (1997) Inadequate cortical feature maps: a neural circuit theory of autism. *Biological Psychiatry* 42:1138–1147.

Gustafsson L, Paplinski AP (2004) Self-organization of an artificial neural network subjected to attention shift impairments and familiarity preference, characteristics studied in autism. *Journal of Autism and Developmental Disorders* 34:189–198.

Haas RH, Townsend J, Courchesne E, Lincoln AJ, Schreibman L, Yeung CR (1996) Neurologic abnormalities in infantile autism. *Journal of Child Neurology* 11:84–92.

Hadjikhani N, Joseph RM, Synder J, Chabris CF, Clark J, Steele S, McGrath L, Vangel M, Aharon I, Feczko E, Harris GJ, Tager-Flusberg H (2004) Activation of the fusiform gyrus when individuals with autism spectrum disorder view faces. *Neuroimage* 22: 1141–1150.

Hans A, Bajramovic JJ, Syan S, Perret E, Dunia I, Brahic M, Gonzalez-Dunia D (2004) Persistent, non-cytolytic infectin of neurons by Borna disease virus interferes with ERK ½ signaling and abrogates BDNF-induced synaptogenesis. *FASEB Journal* 18: 863–865.

Happe F, Ehlers P, Fletcher P, Frith U, Johansson M, Gillberg C, Dolan R, Frackowiak R, Frith C (1996) "Theory of mind" in the brain. Evidence from a PET scan study of Asperger syndrome. *Neuroreport* 8:197–201.

Hardan AY, Hardan BL (2002) A retrospective open trial of adjunctive donepezil in children and adolescents with autistic disorder. *Journal of Child and Adolescent Psychopharmacology* 12:237–241.

Hardan AY, Minshew NJ, Harenski K, Keshaven MS (2001) Posterior fossa magnetic resonance imaging in autism. *Journal of the American Academy of Child and Adolescent Psychiatry* 40:666–672.

Hashimoto T, Sasaki M, Sugai K, Hanaoka S, Fukumizu M, Kato T (2001) Paroxysmal discharges on EEG in young autistic patients are frequent in the frontal regions. *Journal of Medical Investigations* 48:175–180.

Hashimoto T, Tayama M, Miyazaki M, Murakawa K, Kuroda Y (1993) Brainstem and cerebellar vermis involvement in autistic children. *Journal of Child Neurology* 8:149–153.

Hazlett EA, Buchsbaum MS, Hsieh P, Hazxnedar MM, Platholi J, LiCalzi EM, Cartwright C, Hollander E (2004) Regional glucose metabolism within cortical Brodmann areas in healthy individuals and autistic patients. *Neuropsychobiology* 49:115–125.

Herbert MR, Harris GJ, Adrien KT (2002) Abnormal asymmetry in language association in autism. *Annals of Neurology* 52:588–596.

Herbert MR, Ziegler DA, Makris N, Filipek PA, Kemper TL, Normandin JJ, Sanders HA, Kennedy DN, Caviness VS Jr. (2004) Localization of white matter volume increase in autism and developmental disorder. *Annals of Neurology* 55:530–540.

Horwitz B, Rumsey JM, Grady CL, Rapoport SI (1988) The cerebral metabolic landscape in autism: intercorrelations of regional glucose metabolism. *Archives of Neurology* 45:749–755.

Huttenlocher PR, Dabholkar AS (1997) Regional differences in synaptogenesis in human cerebral cortex. *Journal of Comparative Neurology* 387:167–178.

Irwin SA, Galvez R, Greenough WT (2000) Dendritic spine structural anomalies in fragile-X mental retardation syndrome. *Cerebral Cortex* 10:1039–1044.

Jaeken J, Van den Berghe G (1984) An infantile autistic syndrome characterized by the presence of succinylpurines in body fluid. *Lancet* 2:1058–1061.

Jamain S, Betancur C, Quach H, Philippe A, Fellous M, Giros B, Gillberg C, Leboyer M, Bourgeron T; Paris Autism Research International Sibpair (PARIS) Study (2002) Linkage and association of the glutamate receptor 6 gene with autism. *Molecular Psychiatry* 7:302–310.

Jamain S, Quach H, Betancur C, Rastam M, Colineaux C, Gillberg IC, Soderstrom H, Giros B, Leboyer M, Gillberg C, Bourgeron T, Paris Autism Research International Sibpair Study (2003) Mutations of the X-linked genes encoding neuroligins and are associated with autism. *Nature Genetics* 27–29.

Johnson MA, Desai S, Hugh-Jones K, Starer F (1984) Magnetic resonance imaging of the brain in Hurler syndrome. *American Journal of Neuroradiology* 5:816–819.

Just MA, Cherkassy VL, Keller TA, Minshew NJ (in press) Cortical activation and synchronization during sentence comprehension in high-functioning autism.

Kagawa K, Chugani DC, Behen M, Chandana SR, Juhasz C, Muzik O, Chugani HT (2004) Altered brain growth in children with tuberous sclerosis complex and autism. *Annals of Neurology* 56(8):S93. (abstract)

Kahne D, Tudorica A, Borella A, Shapiro L, Johnstone F, Huang W, Whitaker-Azmitia PM (2002) Behavioral and magnetic resonance spectroscopic studies in the hyperserotonemic model of autism. *Physiological Behavior* 75:403–410.

Kates WR, Burnette CP, Eliez S, Strunge LA, Kaplan D, Landa R, Reiss AL, Pearlson GD (2004) Neuroanatomic variation in monozygotic twin pairs discordant for the narrow phenotype of autism. *American Journal of Psychiatry* 161:539–546.

Karrass J, Braungart-Rieker JM, Mullins J, Lefever JB (2002) Processes in language acquistion: the roles of gender, attention, and maternal encouragement of attention over time. *Journal of Child Language* 29:519–543.

Kaukola T, Satyraj E, Patel DD, Tchernev VT, Grimwade BG, Kingsmore SF, Kosekela P, Tammela O, Vainionpaa L, Pinko H, Aarimaa T, Hallman M (2004) Cerebral palsy is characterized by protein mediators in cord serum. *Annals of Neurology* 55:186–194.

Kemper TL, Bauman M (1998) Neuropathology of infantile autism. 1998 Jul;57(7):645–652.

Kohler M, Assmann B, Brautigam C, Storm W, Marie S, Vincent MF, Van den Berghe G, Simmonds HA, Hoffmann GF (1999) Adenylosuccinase deficiency; possibly underdiagnosed encephalopathy with variable clinical features. *European Journal of Paediatric Neurology* 3:3–6.

Lane B, Sullivan EV, Lim KO, Beal M, Harvey RL, Myers T, Faustman WO, Pfefferbaum A (1996) White matter MR hyperintensities in adult patients with congenital rubella. *American Journal of Neuroradiology* 17:99–103.

Laumonnier F, Bonnet-Brilhault F, Gomot M, Blanc R, David A, Moizard MP, Raynaud M, Ronce N, Lemonnier E, Calvas P, Laudier B, Chelly J, Fryns JP, Ropers HH, Hamel BC, Andres C, Barthelemy C, Moraine C, Briault S (2004) X-linked mental retardation and autism are associated with a mutation in the NLGN4 gene, a member of the neuroligin family. *American Journal of Human Genetics* 74:552–557.

Lee CU, Shenton ME, Salisbury DF, Kasia K, Onitsuka T, Dickey CC, Yurgelun-Todd D, Kikinis R, Jolesz FA, McCarley RW (2002a) Fusiform gyrus volume reduction in first-episode schizophrenia: a magnetic imaging study. *Archives of General Psychiatry* 59:775–781.

Lee M, Martin-Ruiz C, Graham A, Court J, Jaros E, Perry R, Iversen P, Bauman M, Perry E (2002b) Nicotinic receptor abnormalities in the cerebellar cortex in autism *Brain* 125:1483–1495.

Lessmann V, Gottmann K, Malcangio M (2003) Neurotrophin secretion: current facts and future prospects. *Progress in Neurobiology* 69:341–374.

Luna B, Minshew NJ, Garver KE, Lazar NA, Thulborn KR, Eddy WF, Sweeney JA (2002) Neocortical system abnormalities in autism: an fMRI study of spatial working memory. *Neurology* 59:834–840.

Martin JJ, Schlote W (1972) Central nervous system lesions in disorders of amino-acid metabolism. A neuropathological study. *Journal of Neurological Science* 15:49–76.

Martin-Ruiz CM, Lee M, Perry RH, Bauman M, Court JA, Perry EK (2004) Molecular analysis of nicotinic receptor expression in autism. *Brain Research & Molecular Brain Research* 123:81–90.

McAlonan GM, Daly E, Kumari V, Critchley HD, van Amelsvoort T, Suckling J, Simmons A, Sigmundsson T, Greenwood K, Russell A, Schmitz N, Happe F, Howlin P, Murphy DG (2002) Brain anatomy and sensorimotor gating in Asperger's syndrome. *Brain* 125:1594–1606.

McCauley JL, Olson LM, Delahanty R, Amin T, Nurmi EL, Organ EL, Jacobs MM, Folstein SE, Haines JL, Sutcliffe JS (2004) A linkage disequilibrium map of the 1-Mb 15q12 GABA(A) receptor subunit cluster and association to autism. 131B(1):51–59.

McCauley JL, Olson LM, Dowd M, Amin T, Steele A, Blakely RD, Folstein SE, Haines JL, Sutcliffe JS (2004) Linkage and association analysis at the serotonin transporter (SLC6A4) locus in a rigid-compulsive subset of autism. *American Journal of Medical Genetics* 127:104–112.

McClelland JL (2000) The basis of hyperspecifity in autism: a preliminary suggestion based on properties of neural nets. *Journal of Autism and Developmental Disorders* 97:359–372.

McKean CM (1971) Effects of a totally synthetic, low phenylalanine diet on adolescent phenylketonuria patients. *Archives of the Diseases of Childhood* 46:608.

McPartland J, Dawson G, Webb SJ, Panagiotides H, Carver LJ (2004) Event-related brain potentials reveal anomalies in temporal processing of faces in autism spectrum disorder. *Journal of Child Psychology and Psychiatry* 45:1235–1245.

Mega MS, Cummings LJ (2001) Frontal subcortical circuits: Anatomy and function. In Salloway SP, Malloy PF, Duffy JD (Eds) *The Frontal Lobes and Neuropsychiatric Illness*. Washington DC: American Psychiatric Publishing, Inc.

Mesulam MM (1990) Large-scale neurocognitive networks and distributed processing for attention, language, and memory. *Annals of Neurology* 28:597–613.

Meyer JS, Obara K, Muramatsu K (1993) Diaschisis. *Neurological Research* 15:362–366.

Miller BL, Diehl J, Freedman M, Kertesz A, Mendez M, Rascovsky K (2003) International approaches to frontotemporal dementia diagnosis: from social cognition to neuropsychology. *Annals of Neurology* 54(Suppl 5) S7–S10.

Miller MT, Stromland K, Gillberg C, Johansson M, Nilsson EW (1998) The puzzle of autism: an ophthalmologic contribution. *Transactions of the American Ophthalmological Society* 96:369–385. Discussion 385–387.

Minshew NJ, Goldstein G, Siegel D (1997) Neuropsychologic functioning in autism: profile of a complex information processing disorder. *Journal of the International Neuropsychological Society* 3:303–316.

Muller RA, Behen ME, Rothermel RD, Chugani DC, Muzik O, Magner TJ, Chugani HT (1999) Brain mapping of language and auditory perception in high-functioning autistic adults: a PET study. *Journal of Autism and Developmental Disorders* 29:19–31.

Muller RA, Chugani DC, Behen ME, Rothermel RD, Muzik O, Chakraborty PK, Chugani HT (1998) Impairment of dentato-thalamo-cortical pathway in autistic men: language activation data from positron emission tomography. *Neuroscience Letters* 245:1–4.

Muller RA, Kleinhans N, Kemmotsu N, Pierce K, Courchesne E (2003) Abnormal variability of functional maps in autism: an fMRI study of visuomotor learning. *American Journal of Psychiatry* 160:1847–1862.

Muller RA, Pierce K, Ambrose JB, Allen G, Courchesne E (2001) Atypical patterns of cerebral motor activation in autism: a functional magnetic resonance imaging study. *Biological Psychiatry* 49:665–676.

Murphy DG, Critchley HD, Schmitz N, McAlonan G, Van Amesvoort T, Robertson D, Daly E, Rowe A, Russell A, Simmons A, Murphy KC, Howlin P (2002) Asperger syndrome: a proton magnetic resonance spectroscopy study of the brain. *Archives of General Psychiatry* 59:885–891.

Nelson KB, Grether JK, Croen LA, Dambrosia JM, Dickens BF, Jellife LL, Hansen RL, Phillips TM (2001) Neuropeptides and neurotrophins in neonatal blood of children with autism or mental retardation. *Annals of Neurology* 49:597–606.

Nishitani N, Avikinen S, Hari R (2004) Abnormal imitation-related cortical activation sequences in Asperger's syndrome. *American Neurological Association* 55:558–562.

Nokelainen P, Flint J (2002) Genetic effects on human cognition: lessons from the study of mental retardation syndromes. *Journal of Neurology, Neurosurgery and Psychiatry* 72:287–290.

Nowell MA, Hackney DB, Muraki AS, Coleman M (1990) Varied MR appearance of autism: fifty-three pediatric patients having the full autistic syndrome. *Magnetic Resonance Imaging* 8:811–816.

Ohnishi T, Matsuda H, Hashimoto T, Kunihiro T, Nishikawa M, Uema T, Sasaki M (2000) Abnormal regional cerebral blood flow in childhood autism. *Brain* 123:1838–1844.

Ozonoff S, Pennington BF, Rogers SJ (1991) Executive function deficits in high-functioning autistic individuals: relationship to theory of mind. *Journal of Child Psychology and Psychiatry and Allied Disciplines* 32:1081–1105.

Page T, Yu A, Fontane J, Nyhan WL (1997) Developmental disorder associated with increased cellular nucleotidase activity. *Proceedings of the National Academy of Sciences* 94:11601–11606.

Perry EK, Lee ML, Martin-Ruiz CM, Court JA, Volsen SG, Merrit J, Folly E, Iversen PE, Bauman ML, Perry RH, Wenk GL (2001) Cholinergic activity in autism; abnormalities in the cerebral cortex and basal forebrain. *American Journal of Psychiatry* 158:1058–1066.

Pierce K, Courchesne E (2001) Evidence for a cerebellar role in reduced exploration and stereotyped behavior in autism. *Biological Psychiatry* 49:655–664.

Pierce K, Muller RA, Ambrose J, Allen G, Courchesne E (2001) Face processing occurs outside the fusiform "face area" in autism: evidence from functional MRI. *Brain* 124:2059–2073.

Piven J, Bailey J, Ranson BJ, Arndt S (1997) An MRI study of the corpus callosum in autism. *American Journal of Psychiatry* 154:1051–1056.

Piven J, Nelune E, Simon J, Barta P, Pearlson G, Falstein SE (1992) Magnetic resonance imagery in autism: measurement of the cerebellum, pores, and fourth ventricle. *Biological Psychiatry* 31:491–504.

Posthuma D, Baare WF, Hulshoff Pol HE, Kahn RS, Boomsma DI, De Geus EJ (2003) Genetic correlations between brain volumes and the wais-iii dimensions of verbal comprehension, working memory, perceptual organization, and processing speed. *Twin Research* 6:131–139.

Purcell AE, Jeon OH, Zimmerman AW, Blue ME, Pevsner J (2001) Postmortem brain abnormalities of the glutamate neurotransmitter system in autism. *Neurology* 57: 1618–1628.

Reiss AL, Feinstein C, Rosenbaum KN (1986) Autism and genetic disorders. *Schizophrenia Bulletin* 12:724–738.

Rilling J, Gutman D, Zeh T, Pagnoni G, Berns G, Kilts C (2002) A neural basis for social cooperation. *Neuron* 35:395–405.

Rimland B (1964) *Infantile Autism: The Syndrome and Its Implications for a Neural Theory of Behavior*. Englewood Cliffs, N.J.: Prentice-Hall, Inc.

Ritvo ER, Freeman BJ, Scheibel AB, Duong T, Robinson H, Guthrie D, Ritvo A (1986) Lower Purkinje cell counts in the cerebella of four autistic subjects: initial findings of the UCLA-NSAC Autopsy Research Report. *American Journal of Psychiatry* 143: 862–866.

Rodier PM, Ingram JL, Tisdale B, Nelson S, Romano J (1996) Embryological origin for autism: developmental anomalies of the cranial nerve motor nuclei. *Journal of Comparative Neurology* 370:247–261.

Ryu YH, Lee JD, Yoon PH, Kim DI, Lee HB, Shin YJ (1999) Perfusion impairments in infantile autism on technetium-99m ethyl cysteinate dimer brain single-photon emission tomography; comparison with findings on magnetic resonance imaging. *European Journal of Nuclear Medicine* 26:253–259.

Saitoh O, Karns CM, Courchesne E (2001) Development of the hippocampal formation from 2 to 42 years: MRI evidence of smaller area dentata in autism. *Brain* 124:317–324.

Salmond CH, de Haan M, Friston KJ, Gadian DG, Vargha-Khadem F (2003) Investigating individual differences in brain abnormalities in autism. *Philosophical Transactions of the Royal Society London B* 358:405–413.

Sarnat HB, Flores-Sarnat L (2004) Integrative classification of morphology and molecular genetics in central nervous system malformations. *American Journal of Medical Genetics* 126A:386–392.

Schain R, Freedman DX (1961) Studies of 5-hydroxyindole metabolism in autistic and other mentally ill children. *Journal of Pediatrics* 58:315–320.

Scheiffle P, Fan J, Choih J, Fetter R, Serfini T (2000) Neuroligin expressed in nonneuronal cells triggers presynaptic development in contacting axons. *Cell* 101:657–659.

Schultz TR, Gauthier I, Klin A, Fulbright RK, Anderson AW, Volkmar F, Skudlarski P,

Lacadie C, Cohen DJ, Gore JC (2000) Abnormal ventral temporal cortical activity during face discrimination among individuals with autism and Asperger syndrome. *Archives of General Psychiatry* 57:331–340.

Schultz TR, Grelotti DJ, Klin A, Kleinman J, Van der Gaag C, Marois R, Skudlaski P (2003) The role of the fusiform face area in social cognition: implications for the pathobiology of autism. *Philosophical Transactions Royal Society of London B: Biological Science* 358:415–427.

Shallice T (2001) "Theory of Mind" and the prefrontal cortex. *Brain* 124:247–248.

Shamay-Tsoory SG, Tomer R, Yaniv S, Aharon-Peretz J (2002) Empathy deficits in Asperger syndrome: a cognitive profile. *Neurocase* 8:245–252

Shao Y, Cuccaro ML, Hauser ER, Raiford KL, Monold MM, Wolpert CM, Ravan SA, Elston L, Decena K, Donnelly SL, Abramson RK, Wrigley HH, DeLong GR, Gilbert JR, Pericak-Vance MA (2003) Fine mapping of autistic disorder to chromosome 15q11-q13 by use of phenotypic subtypes. *American Journal of Human Genetics* 72:539–548.

Soussignan R, Schaal B, Schmidt G, Nadel J (1995) Facial responsiveness to odours in normal and pervasively developmentally disordered children. *Chemical Senses* 20:47–59.

Sparks BF, Friedman SD, Shaw DW, Aylward EH, Echelard D, Artru AA, Maravilla KR, Gield JN, Munson J, Dawson G, Dager SR (2002) Brain structural abnormalities in young children with autism. *Neurology* 59:184–192.

Stuss DT, Gallup GG Jr, Alexander MP (2001) The frontal lobes are necessary for "theory of mind." *Brain* 124:279–286.

Swillen A, Hellemans H, Steyaert J, Fryns J-P (1996) Autism and genetics: high incidence of specific genetic syndromes in 21 autistic adolescents and adults living in 2 residential homes in Belgium. *American Journal of Medical Genetics* (Neuropsychiatric Genetics) 67:315–316.

Thomas NS, Sharp AJ, Browne CE, Skuse D, Hardie C, Dennis NR (1999) Xp deletions associated with autism in three females. *Human Genetics* 104:43–48.

Townsend J, Westerfield M, Leaver E, Makeig S, Jung T, Pierce K, Courchesne E (2001) Event-related brain response abnormalities in autism: evidence of impaired cerebello-frontal spatial attention networks. *Brain Research–Cognitive Brain Research* 11:127–145.

Tsatsanis KD, Rouke BP, Klin A, Volkmar FR, Cicchetti D, Schultz RT (2003) Reduced thalamic volume in high-functioning individuals with autism. *Biological Psychiatry* 53:121–129.

Waiter GD, Williams JHG, Murray AD, Gilchrist A, Perrett DI, Whiten A (2004) A voxel-based investigation of brain structure in male adolescents with autistic spectrum disorder. *NeuroImage* 22:619–625.

Wang MC, Winston KR, Breeze RE (2002) Cerebellar mutism associated with a midbrain cavernous malformation. Case report and review of the literature. *Journal of Neurosurgery* 96:607–610.

Whitaker-Azmitia P (2001) Serotonin and brain development: role in human developmental disease. *Brain Research Bulletin* 56:479–485.

Wilcox J, Tsuang MT, Ledger E, Alego J, Schnurr T (2002) Brain perfusion with autism varies with age. *Neuropsychobiology* 46:13–16.

Zafeiriou DI, Savvopoulou-Augoustidou PA, Sewell A, Papadopoulou F, Badouraki M,

Vargiami E, Gombakis NP, Katzos GS (2001) Serial magnetic resonance imaging findings in mucopolysaccharidoses IIIB (Sanfilippo's syndrome B). *Brain Development* 23:385–389.

Zaid DH, Kim SW (2001) The Orbitofrontal cortex. In Salloway SP, Malloy PF, Duffy JD (Eds). *The Frontal Lobes and Neuropsychiatric Illness.* Washington, DC: American Psychiatric Publishing, Inc.

Zilbovicius M, Garreau B, Samson Y, Remy P, Barthelemy C, Syrota A, Lelord G (1995) Delayed maturation of the frontal cortex in childhood autism. *American Journal of Psychiatry* 152:248–252.

Zoia S, Pelamatti G, Cuttini M, Casotto V, Scabar A (2002) Performance of gesture in children with and without DCD: effects of sensory input modalities. *Developmental Medicine and Child Neurology* 44:699–705.

Chapter 3

The Cerebellum in Autism

G. Robert DeLong

At one time, the cerebellum—thought to be primarily involved in motor control—seemed to be the least likely area of the brain to be implicated in autism. That view was clearly wrong. It is probably accurate to say the that study of patients with autism has contributed much to our general understanding of cerebellar function in at least two ways: it has focused interest on the consequences of cerebellar disease in early life, and it has helped elucidate the extensive influence of the cerebellum on cerebral hemisphere functions, including cognition. Here we will attempt to review what has been learned about the role of the cerebellum in autism, and how that has expanded our understanding of cerebellar function.

CEREBELLAR PATHOLOGY IN AUTISM

Cerebellar pathology has been confirmed in autism, both by evidence from MRI studies and, more convincingly, by pathological studies. The latter have shown a decrease in numbers of Purkinje cells, greatest in posterior cerebellar vermis and hemispheres. Neuron loss is seen in the fastigial nucleus, the output pathway for the vermis; no neuron loss occurs in interpositus or dentate nucleus, the output pathways for the hemispheres. The neuron loss is not accompanied by gliosis, a finding that suggests a prenatal event. Kemper and Bauman (2002) also found that the number of Purkinje cells appears to decrease the older the patient, suggesting a progressive degenerative process.

Neuropathology in Autism

Kemper and Bauman's (2002) careful examinations of nine autistic brains, painstakingly compared with age- and sex-matched controls, have revealed consistent findings of a curtailment of maturation in the forebrain limbic system, abnormalities in the cerebellar circuits, and an unusual pattern of change of postnatal brain size. Many components of the limbic system showed unusually small neurons that were more closely packed together than those of the controls. This pattern is similar to that seen at an earlier stage of brain development. The areas most consistently involved were the amygdala, hippocampal formation, entorhinal cortex, and the mammillary body. In the nucleus of the diagonal band of Broca, a part of the septum, younger individuals had a normal number of unusually large neurons, while in older individuals (more that 21 years of age), the neurons were unusually small and decreased in number. In occasional specimens, Kemper and Bauman (2002) found malformations of neocortex, but these were inconspicuous and uncommon; otherwise the neocortex showed no abnormality.

The cerebellar neuropathology was different. The number of Purkinje cells in all the autistic brains had decreased, a finding that was similar at all ages. (In a separate study, Purkinje cell size was small; the cells of 2 of 5 autistic subjects were 50% smaller than those of controls [Fatemi et al. 2002a].) In the deep cerebellar nuclei, into which the Purkinje cells project, the neurons in the younger brains were abnormally large, whereas in the older brains, these neurons were abnormally small and, in some nuclei, decreased in number. A similar pattern of change in cell size was noted in the inferior olive in the brain stem but without evidence of neuronal loss. Changes in the inferior olive were most evident in the part of the inferior olive that projects to the area of the cerebellar cortex, with the most marked decrease in Purkinje cells being in the posterior-lateral part of the lateral lobes of the cerebellum. The postnatal changes in cell size (from unusually large to small) and number (reduced) in the deep cerebellar nuclei, inferior olives, and septal nuclei, represented an obscure kind of neuropathology, indicating an active and progressive pathological process. Atrophy of the cerebellar vermis, a much studied observation, was inconsistent in this series. Kemper and Bauman noted that a clinical correlate of these cerebellar abnormalities was not readily apparent.

Cerebellar Neurochemical Abnormalities in Autism

The neuropathology in autism has rapidly progressed to the study of neurochemical components. In a study of autistic and normal control cerebellar cortices matched for age, sex, and postmortem interval, characteristics of a number of the proteins related to synaptic growth and neurotransmitter function were altered (Fatemi et al. 2001). In autistic cerebellum, reelin expression was reduced by 44%; Bcl-2 levels were decreased by 34% to 51%; and beta-actin expression did not differ between groups (Fatemi et al 2001). Glutamic acid decarboxylase 65 kDa and 67 kDa protein expression was reduced by 51% in autistic parietal and cerebellar cortices (Fatemi et al. 2002b). Purcell et al. (2001) studied the expression of genes associated with glutamate neurotransmission in autistic cerebellums. The mRNA levels of several genes, including those encoding the excitatory amino acid transporter 1 and glutamate receptor AMPA 1, were significantly increased in autism. AMPA-type glutamate receptor density was significantly decreased in the cerebellum of individuals with autism. Other investigators have reported abnormalities of nicotinic receptors in the cerebellar cortex in autism (Lee et al. 2002). These authors found a 40–50% decrease in the high-affinity nicotinic receptor in the granule cell, Purkinje, and molecular layers in the autistic group; and an opposite 3-fold increase in the low-affinity nicotinic receptor. Overall results indicated a loss of the cerebellar nicotinic alpha4 receptor subunit in autism, possibly related to the loss of Purkinje cells, and a compensatory increase in the alpha7 subunit.

It is too early to put this puzzle together. Some or all of these changes may be secondary to the presently unknown primary abnormality. Particular interest has focused on reelin as a factor predisposing individuals to autistic disorder. Genetic analyses yielded a significant association between autistic disorder and a polymorphic triplet repeat in the 5' untranslated region of the *RELN* gene (Persico et al. 2001), a result not confirmed in a second study (Zhang et al. 2002). Studies of blood levels of reelin (Fatemi et al. 2002) have shown remarkable (70%) reductions in unprocessed reelin in blood from autistic twins, their parents, and their normal siblings versus controls. It is not clear how to interpret these changes, particularly in phenotypically normal first-order relatives. Most striking have been findings of decreased reelin in prefrontal cortex in brains from autistic subjects, which is associated with reduced levels of BDNF; the latter is related to synaptic function and plasticity (Fatemi 2002). Serotonin synthesis is decreased in the frontal lobes in autism, but is increased in the right dentate nucleus of cerebellum (Chugani et al. 1997).

Cerebellar Size in Autism

Measurement of cerebellar size in autistic patients by MR imaging has been the subject of much controversy, with differing findings and interpretations. Not surprisingly, this data has been less useful than that from autopsy. It is not necessary to review the imaging controversies here. Over time, measurement techniques have improved and something like a consensus reached. Sparks et al. (2002) examined brain morphometric features in a large sample of carefully diagnosed 3- to 4-year-old children with autism spectrum disorder and compared them to age-matched control groups of typically developing and developmentally delayed children. Children with autism spectrum disorder had significantly higher cerebral volumes than did the other groups, and cerebellar volume was increased in proportion to overall increases in cerebral volume. The developmentally delayed group had smaller cerebellar volume than did both of the other groups. These appear to be the most reliable results to date.

Kates et al. (1998) investigated the neuroanatomical similarities and differences between a pair of monozygotic, 7.5-year-old twin boys discordant for autism. The unaffected twin, while not fulfilling the traditional diagnostic criteria for autism, displayed constrictions in social interaction and play consistent with a broader phenotype for autism. MRI scans were obtained for each brother and compared with scans of 5 age- and sex-matched unaffected peers. Quantitative analysis of brain anatomy using MRI revealed that the affected twin had markedly smaller caudate, amygdaloid, and hippocampal volumes, and small cerebellar vermis lobules VI and VII, than did brother. Both twins showed disproportionately reduced volumes of the superior temporal gyrus and the frontal lobe relative to the comparison sample. The authors suggested the dysfunction of two separate but overlapping neuroanatomical pathways; that is, one subcortical network (the caudate, amygdala, hippocampus, and cerebellar lobules VI and VII), differentiating the twins from each other, that may underlie the traditional neurobehavioral phenotype for strictly defined autism, and a second cortical network, (the superior temporal gyrus and the frontal lobe) differentiating the twins from the comparison sample, that may lead to the broader phenotype for autism.

DelBello et al. (1999), long interested in putative relationships between bipolar illness and autism, noted an MR morphometry study comparing 30 bipolar patients hospitalized with a manic episode (16 with a first episode and 14 with prior manic episodes) to 15 normal volunteers matched for age, sex, race, and education. Regions of interest were right and left cerebellar hemisphere volumes and the vermal areas 6 (lobules 1–5), V2 (lobules 6–7), and V3 (lobules 8–10). The V3 area only was significantly smaller in multiple-episode patients than in first-episode patients or healthy volunteers. Such results need confirmation but bear watching.

CEREBELLAR DEVELOPMENT AND CONNECTIONS IN AUTISM: THE ROLE OF SEROTONIN

Serotonin has an important role in brain development (reviewed by Chugani 2002). Evidence from both pharmacological and knock-out experiments demonstrates that serotonin plays a role in modulation of synaptogenesis. As an example, the serotonergic innervation of thalamocortical axons controls the tangential arborization and branching of these axons, resulting in altered thalamocortical connectivity. Decreased or increased brain serotonin during this period of development results in disruption of synaptic connectivity in sensory cortices; similarly, in the hippocampus, depletion of serotonin in neonatal rat pups resulted in large decreases in the number of dendritic spines of hippocampal neurons. While there are many serotonin receptors, the 5HT1A receptor plays important roles in brain regions showing abnormalities in autism. In the first 2 postnatal weeks in rat pups, the cerebellum contained high concentrations of 5HT1A receptors. In the cerebellum, immunolabelling of 5HT1A receptors was localized to the soma and dendrites of Purkinje cell. This localization is important in light of consistent reports of decreased numbers of Purkinje cells in brains from autistic individuals. The enrichment of 5HT1A receptors is most pronounced in the cerebellar vermis lobules VI and VII (an area found in two recent studies to be significantly small in high-functioning autistic patients (Kaufman et al. 2003). As noted above, this area is smaller in bipolar patients who have had repeated episodes of mania, but not in patients with a first episode of mania (DelBello et al. 1999); this is interesting in light of the putative association between bipolar affective disorder and autism. In developing human cerebellum, the highest expression of 5HT1A mRNA was measured in neonatal cerebellar samples.

Research indicates that serotonin regulates several aspects of brain development, including cell division, differentiation, neurite outgrowth as described above, and synaptogenesis (reviewed in Chugani 2002). Evidence supports serotonergic modulation of synaptic development in the lateral superior olive in gerbils and of segregation of retinal projections in MAO-A knock-out mice. There is evidence that one mechanism by which serotonin has trophic effects during brain development is through the regulation of trophic factors, such as the 5HT1A mediated release of S100 and brain derived neurotrophic factor (BDNF). This latter factor is particularly intriguing because of evidence indicating that BDNF is required for antidepressants (such as fluoxetine, which makes more serotonin available in the synapse by inhibiting reuptake) to relieve depression (Saarelainen et al. 2003). Selective serotonin reuptake inhibitors such as fluoxetine may modify depression by enhancing the serotonergic release of BDNF, which in turn may induce formation and stabilization of synaptic connectivity. Given the favorable therapeutic effect of SSRIs in autism, the same mechanisms may be involved. Chugani (2002) comments that the available studies provide a rationale for trials of serotonergic drugs in very young autistic children in an attempt to alter synaptic plasticity during postnatal development. Such trials are underway.

Available data does not explain the increase in serotonin synthesis in the dentate nucleus that is evident in Chugani's 11C-alphamethyltryptophan PET images (Chugani et al. 1997). The simplest interpretation would suggest that, because there may be a reciprocal relationship between at least some serotonin receptors and GABA$_A$ receptors, and that since the number of Purkinje cells (which are GABAergic) is decreased, the increase in serotonin synthesis may be compensatory. This is not established, however.

CEREBELLAR FUNCTION IN AUTISM

Role of Cerebellum in Cognition and Affect

Schmahmann and Sherman (1998) studied 20 adult patients with disease confined to the cerebellum, evaluating the nature and severity of the changes in neurological and mental function. They found behavioral changes to be clinically prominent in patients with lesions involving the posterior lobe of the cerebellum and the vermis. The changes were characterized by the following: impairment of executive functions such as planning, set-shifting, verbal fluency, abstract reasoning, and working memory; difficulties with spatial cognition including visual-spatial organization and memory; personality change with blunting of affect or disinhibited and inappropriate behavior; and language deficits including agrammatism and dysprosodia. The investigators named this newly defined clinical entity the "cerebellar cognitive affective syndrome." They suggested the constellation of deficits is indicative of disruption of the cerebellar modulation of neural circuits that link prefrontal, posterior parietal, superior temporal, and limbic cortices with the cerebellum.

Scott et al. (2001) examined the role of the cerebellum in the developing cognitive profiles of children with cerebellar tumors. MRI and longitudinal intellectual profiles were obtained on 7 children (2 females, 5 males; mean age at diagnosis was 3 years; mean age at first assessment was 7 years). The tumors were astrocytomas in 3 of the children, medulloblastomas in 2, a low-grade glioma in 1, and an ependymoma in 1. In right-handed children, the authors observed an association between greater damage to right cerebellar structures and a plateauing in verbal and/or literacy skills. In contrast, greater damage to left cerebellar structures was associated with delayed or impaired nonverbal/spatial skills. Long-term cognitive development of the children studied tentatively supported a role for the cerebellum in learning/development. The authors suggested that lateralized cerebellar damage may selectively impair the development of cognitive functions subserved by the contralateral cerebral hemisphere.

Anatomical data suggests crossed reciprocal connections between the cerebellum and higher order cortical association areas. In a study by Mottaghy et al. (1999), 1 left- and 1 right-handed female volunteer underwent functional magnetic resonance imaging in a conventional block design. Regions of activation were detected after performance of a silent verbal fluency task inside the scanner. In the right-handed volunteer, the investigators found an activation of the left frontoparietal cortex and the right cerebellar hemisphere, while in the left-handed volunteer the activation was seen in the right frontoparietotemporal cortex and the left cerebellar hemisphere. These initial results demonstrate that cerebellar activation is contralateral to the activation of the frontal cortex even under conditions of different language dominance. They provide evidence for the hypothesis of a lateralized organization of the cerebellum crossed to the cerebral hemispheres in supporting higher cognitive function. These findings are entirely congruent with the findings of Chugani et al. (1997) indicating impairment of dentatothalamocortical pathways, primarily from the right dentate to left cerebral hemisphere, in young autistic boys.

Role of Cerebellum in Attention

Courchesne and his group initiated studies designed to clarify the role of cerebellar abnormality in disturbances of attention in autism, particularly disturbances in the dynamic control of attention and the ability to shift attention (Allen & Courchesne 2003). Certainly, severe disturbances of attention characterize such children: it is extraordinarily difficult to engage their attention; attention to or persistence in a task may be fleeting; and once attention is fixated on an object of interest it is exceedingly difficult to shift it to any other object. To investigate links between the cerebellum and attention function, Courchesne and his associates undertook formal behavioral and neurophysiological studies of shifting attention (between auditory and visual modalities, between color and form, and between two visual spatial locations). Study groups were composed of autistic patients with parietal MRI abnormalities, autistic patients without parietal MRI abnormalities, patients with acquired neocerebellar abnormalities, or normal controls. The study tasks required subjects to rapidly shift attention back and forth between visual and auditory stimuli (or, in analogous tests, between color and form information or between different visual-spatial locations) when signaled by the appearance of the rare target stimuli. Following signals to shift attention, autistic and neocerebellar patients were slow to disengage attention and to reengage attention.

In another study of autistic subjects (Townsend et al. 2001), attention-related, late positive event–related potentials in the frontal lobe were delayed or missing during conditions in which attention was to peripheral visual fields, and the related parietal late positive response was smaller than normal. The authors argued indirectly that these potentials, thought to be cortically generated, reflect cerebellar influences.

In a behavioral and MRI study, Pierce and Courchesne (2001) found that children with autism spent significantly less time and less range in active exploration than did normal controls. Measures of decreased exploration were significantly correlated with the magnitude of cerebellar hypoplasia of vermal lobules VI-VII in the autistic children, but no relationship to vermal size was seen in the normal children. Limited environmental exploration is an obvious behavioral feature in autism; this documentation of a relationship to cerebellar vermis atrophy is of interest and may accord with indications of cerebellar involvement in attentional functions, for example.

In more recent studies, the Courchesne group has used fMRI to evaluate cerebellar function in autism. They found that autistic individuals, in performing a motor task, showed greater than normal cerebellar motor activation; however, in performing an attention task, autistic individuals showed significantly less cerebellar activation (Allen & Courchesne 2003). In another fMRI study, the group found that the pattern of activations was similar in both normal and autistic groups, but activations were less pronounced in the autistic group. Also demonstrated were greater activation in perirolandic and supplementary motor areas in the control group and greater activation in posterior and prefrontal cortices in the autism group. Notable were the less distinct regional activation/deactivation patterns in autism, compatible with the general hypothesis of disturbances of functional differentiation in the cerebrum in autism (Muller et al. 2001). No distinct cerebellar role was demonstrated in this study.

While it may be unwise to engage in too much speculation, the data just cited might be interpreted in part as showing compensatory overactivity in some areas of the autistic brain; it may be "trying harder": during motor tasks, the cerebellum and prefrontal areas both exhibited greater than normal activation. Both these areas have pathological abnormalities in autism. The ineffective attempt to employ or engage them might be a cause for the increased activation seen by fMRI.

Cerebellar Function in Language and Social Behavior in Autism

The investigations reviewed above, along with many others including the neuroanatomy of the cerebellum and its interconnections, evidence from functional neuroimaging and neurophysiological research, and advancements in clinical neurology and neuropsychology have established the view that the cerebellum participates in a much wider range of functions than conventionally accepted. It has become clear that the cerebellum importantly modulates cognitive functioning. Marien et al. (2001) review the recently acknowledged role of the cerebellum in cognition and address in more detail experimental and clinical data disclosing the modulatory role of the cerebellum in various nonmotor language processes such as lexical retrieval, syntax, and language dynamics. The authors advance the concept of a "lateralized linguistic cerebellum," suggesting that functional depression of supratentorial language areas due to reduced input via cerebellocortical pathways might represent the relevant pathomechanism for linguistic deficits associated with cerebellar pathology. Also, since memory is so closely linked to language function, it is noteworthy that another fMRI study found activation in cerebellar areas during encoding of a word-association task as opposed to retrieval (Mottaghy et al. 1999).

The Chugani group followed up its studies of dentatothalamocortical pathway disturbances in autistic boys by looking at possible effects of such disturbances on brain activations for language in autistic adults (Muller et al. 1998). Using [15(O)]-water PET, 4 autistic and 5 normal men were studied while listening to, repeating, and generating sentences. In the autistic group, activation in the right dentate nucleus and in the left frontal area 46 was lower during verbal auditory and expressive language and higher during motor speech functions than it was control group. The thalamus showed group differences concordant with area 46 for expressive language. The results suggest atypical functional specialization of the dentatothalamocortical pathways and are compatible with a model of cerebellar-cortical serotonergic disturbance in the developing autistic brain. Once again, the Chugani studies illustrate the importance of lateralization of function and of biochemical markers in studies of autistic brains.

Using functional MRI, Critchley et al. (2000) investigated high-functioning autistic people processing emotional facial expressions. Subjects with autistic disorder differed significantly from controls in the activity of cerebellar, mesolimbic, and temporal lobe cortical regions of the brain when processing facial expressions. In autistic persons, a cortical "face area" was not activated during explicit appraisal of expressions, nor was the left amygdala region and left cerebellum of these subjects activated during implicit processing of emotional facial expressions. Cerebellar activity appears to be an intrinsic part of the temporal and amygdalar system involved in processing facial emotion.

Cerebellar Function in Motility and Dyspraxia in Autism

This section is included to call attention to the motility problems seen in autism. There is, to my knowledge, a paucity of studies of motility disturbances in autism. Consequently, what follows are primarily my own clinical observations and impressions. I apologize to those who may have greater experience and understanding of this area. The current chapter is concerned with cerebellar involvement in autism, and it seems important to discuss motoric disturbances in connection with cerebellar dysfunction. However, to my knowledge, from my reading of the literature, there is no clear understanding of the role of cerebellar dysfunction in relation to the motor disturbances of autism.

Motility disturbances in autism, aside from the prominent twiddling, flapping, and tensing stereotypies that draw attention, are commonly overlooked. But both gross and fine motor disturbances of function are very common—although not universal—in autism and beg for further study. It is noteworthy that the discussion of such motoric abnormalities has largely been conducted in psychiatric, occupational therapy, and physical therapy arenas, rather than by neurologists (with notable exceptions). The pertinent disabilities are commonly referred to as dyspraxias, especially perhaps by speech pathologists, since abnormalities of speech often parallel those of general motility. Dyspraxic motor dysfunction appears to correlate with the general hypotonia exhibited by many autistic individuals. These disabilities are commonly discussed under the entities *clumsy child*, *developmental coordination disorder*, or related terms, and may accompany autistic spectrum disorders or occur without autism, though often with other areas of developmental problems.

From clinical observations, many autistic children have great difficulty hopping on one foot, walking on heels and toes, walking tandem, and holding arms outstretched on command or in response to demonstration. Likewise, they have great difficulty holding a pen, writing or drawing, or doing other skilled manual activities such as tying shoes, buttoning, and so on. (By contrast, others show great agility, balance, and motor control in general.) A rarer disorder, but seemingly related, is that of aberrant ocular smooth pursuit, which in occasional instances shows dramatic aberration. The motor clumsiness is recognized as part of Asperger's syndrome, but is not separable from autism as such.

Our question is whether any of this phenomenology derives from primary cerebellar dysfunction. The usual signs of cerebellar dysfunction are largely or completely missing. Ataxia, tremor, nystagmus, dysdiadochokinesia, and dysmetria are not seen. Speech, when present, is not scanning. A respected textbook of neurology (Victor & Ropper 2001) describes the cerebellum as "responsible for the regulation of muscular tone, the coordination of movements, especially skilled voluntary ones, and the control of posture and gait." Certainly autism is commonly, if not always, accompanied by diffuse muscular hypotonia, poor coordination of skilled voluntary movements, and awkwardness of posture and gait; the latter is particularly evident when stressed by asking the individual to hop, walk tandem, walk on heels or toes, and so on, as described above. Much of the deficit that is so evident almost certainly involves cerebellar dysfunction; but the point remains that this picture is quite different from that of pure cerebellar disease and must represent the result of defects of cerebellar-cerebral cortical integration. It is still quite obscure to neurologists and merits further study.

CEREBELLAR MUTISM AFTER POSTERIOR FOSSA SURGERY: A MODEL FOR AUTISM?

Cerebellar mutism after posterior fossa surgery may provide a valuable model of autism. Pollack et al. (1995) reviewed a surgical experience of 142 patients undergoing resection of infratentorial tumors, of whom 12 (8.5%) manifested cerebellar mutism. Each of the 12 had a lesion that involved the vermis (7 medulloblastomas, 3 astrocytomas, 2 ependymomas), and all had vermian incisions. All had normal speech preoperatively. In 10 of the 12, mutism developed in a delayed fashion (24 to 96 hours postoperatively). The speech disturbance was associated with poor oral intake in 9 children, urinary retention in 5, long-tract signs in 6, and bizarre personality changes, emotional lability, and/or decreased initiation of voluntary movements in all 12.

Neuropsychiatric testing confirmed impairments not only in speech but also in initiation of other motor activities. Ten children regained normal speech, bladder control, and neurological functioning, other than ataxia and mild dysarthria, within 1 to 16 weeks. Characteristically, affect and oral intake returned to their preoperative baseline before the speech difficulties began to resolve.

Three children underwent xenon computed tomographic blood flow studies, 1 underwent SPECT, and 1 underwent 18-FDG PET. All findings were normal. A detailed radiological review of 24 cases of vermian tumors without mutism identified only one factor that was significantly associated with the mutism syndrome, bilateral edema within the brachium pontis ($P < 0.01$). The authors suggest that the mutism syndrome results from transient impairment of the afferent and/or efferent pathways of the dentate nuclei involved in initiating complex volitional movements. All had marked neurobehavioral abnormalities. Eleven children exhibited an almost stereotypical response, remaining curled up in bed and whining inconsolably, without actually uttering intelligible speech. Nine had significant impairment in oromotor coordination and seemed unwilling to eat. Speech was profoundly abnormal during recovery. Three began speaking in a whispered voice and 4 others spoke in a high-pitched "whiny" voice. In all 12 children, speech exhibited a dysarthric quality before full recovery. Detailed neuropsychiatric testing during recovery demonstrated that initiation and completion of age-appropriate motor activities was also impaired. Several also had impairment in recent memory, attention span, and problem-solving ability.

ILLUSTRATIVE CASES

A 6-year-old girl had limited spontaneous initiation of both speech and movement. During recovery, speech was whispered and monosyllabic.

A 16-year-old boy awoke from anesthesia with clear speech, but by the third postoperative day, he developed mutism and a bizarre, depressed affect. He lay curled up in bed with his eyes closed, whining intermittently, refusing to follow commands, exhibiting poor oral intake, and experiencing urinary retention. Poor oral intake and bizarre personality changes each improved by the third postoperative week. Serial neuropsychiatric testing during his recovery phase initially found poor initiation and completion of age-appropriate motor and problem-solving activities, despite improvement in his mood.

In their discussion, the authors concluded that the critical anatomic area for postoperative mutism is not in the vermis. If so, the complication should be more common and more persistent after resection of midline cerebellar tumors. The vast majority of patients undergoing resection of an inferior vermian tumor experience no mutism. Rather, the critical site must reside more laterally in the cerebellum. Symptoms developed 1 to 3 days postoperatively, indicating that the structures responsible do not generally suffer direct injury or infarction intraoperatively. No evidence of discrete areas of infarction, hypoperfusion, or decreased metabolic activity was found within the cerebellar hemispheres, diencephalon, or cerebral cortex. Patients with mutism had a significantly increased incidence of bilateral edema within the cerebellar peduncles, implying that a critical pathway responsible for initiating speech and other complex voluntary movements travels within this structure.

The authors suggested the overall symptom complex may reflect the sequelae of injury to the afferent and/or efferent pathways to the dentate nuclei, which are involved in initiating volitional movements. This pathway includes projections from the premotor and supplementary motor cortices via the brachium pontis and projections back to these areas via the dentatothalamocortical system.

A single case of a 7-year-old boy who developed mutism after surgery for cerebellar medulloblastoma was studied using SPECT (single photon emission computed tomography) (Sagiuchi et al. 2001). During mutism, SPECT scanning revealed decreased cerebral blood flow in the bilateral thalami, bilateral medial frontal lobes, and left temporal lobe in addition to the cerebellar vermis and both cerebellar hemispheres, indicating bilateral crossed cerebellocerebral diaschisis. The authors postulated that circulatory disturbance in both cerebellar hemispheres secondary to tumor resection probably induced bilateral crossed cerebellocerebral diaschisis in both cerebral hemispheres, predominantly in the left, via the dentatothalamocortical pathway. With recovery of his mutism, blood flow increased in the right thalamus, bilateral medial frontal lobes, and left temporal lobe, with only slight decrease in blood flow persisting in the left thalamus. The findings suggested that mutism was associated with cerebral circulatory and metabolic hypofunction in the supplementary motor area mediated via the dentatothalamocortical pathway.

The parallel between the apparent disturbance of the dentatothalamic outflow tract occurring with cerebellar mutism, and the abnormality in that tract found by Chugani et al. (1997) using [11C] alpha-methyltryptophan PET, cannot escape notice. Likewise, the clinical syndromes of autism and cerebellar mutism have many cogent similarities, including language disturbance, dyspraxia, inattention, personality disturbances, emotional lability, and impairment of initiating voluntary activities. These findings suggested to us that serotonin synthesis might be decreased in cerebellar mutism as it appears to be in autism. Since SSRIs such as fluoxetine have shown a beneficial effect in some children with autism, we tried fluoxetine treatment of 2 patients with cerebellar mutism (Nabbout & DeLong 2002). The first, a 3-year-old boy, had typical mutism of 3 days duration. At that point, fluoxetine was started; he recovered fully, to the point of riding his tricycle around the ward, within 24 hours of beginning treatment. The second patient was an 8-year-old boy who had cerebellar mutism for 3 weeks without improvement. At that time, he was given fluoxetine, after which he recovered within 36 hours, speaking in sentences. These cases are anecdotal, of course, and since such cases occur only sporadically in any one institution, we still await opportunity to further test this result. We hope others may attempt such treatment so that it can be determined with certainty whether SSRIs ameliorate mutism.

Vandeinse and Hornyak (1997) studied 4 children, 3 of whom presented with a period of mutism following posterior fossa surgery and 1 who did not exhibit mutism. All 4, however, demonstrated a similar profile of significant high-level linguistic and cognitive deficit on formal speech-language and neuropsychological measures. The investigators compared the results to recent literature documenting the role of the cerebellum in language and cognition.

Riva and Giorgi (2000) studied intellectual, language, and executive functions of 26 children who had undergone surgery for removal of cerebellar hemisphere or vermal tumors. The children with right cerebellar tumors presented with disturbances of auditory sequential memory and language processing, whereas those with left cerebellar tumors showed deficits on tests of spatial and visual sequential memory. The vermal lesions led to 2 profiles: (1) postsurgical mutism, which evolved into speech disorders or language disturbances similar to agrammatism; and (2) behavioral disturbances ranging from irritability to behaviors reminiscent of autism.

CRITIQUE OF A CEREBELLAR HYPOTHESIS OF AUTISM

There is no longer any doubt that cerebellar damage causes cognitive impairments, particularly when the cerebellar deficit is present early in life. Thus, it is interesting to compare the cognitive deficits seen with congenital nonprogressive cerebellar ataxia with the picture of cognitive deficits seen in autism. The hypothesis is that the pattern of deficits would be similar if the cognitive deficits of autism derive primarily from cerebellar pathology. Steinlin et al. (1999) studied 11 patients (ages 8 to 28 years) with nonprogressive congenital ataxia using Wechsler's intelligence testing and additional tests of attention, memory, language, visual perception, and frontal functions. Seven of the 11 patients had an IQ of 60 to 92, with marked nonverbal deficits and subnormal-to-normal verbal performance (group A). Four patients had an IQ of 30 to 49 without pronounced profile asymmetry (group B). Four of the 7 group A patient had decreased alertness and sustained attention, but all had normal selective attention. In this group, tests of frontal functions and memory yielded higher verbal scores than nonverbal scores. Furthermore, group A patients did not exhibit deficits on the Aachener Naming Test (similar to the Boston Naming Test), but the majority did have marked difficulty with visuoconstructive tasks and visual perception. Group B was significantly abnormal in almost all subtests, having a less prominent but similar profile.

Thus, these patients have significant cognitive deficits with an asymmetric profile and better verbal than nonverbal performance. Notably, this profile is very different from that of autism, in which language is typically much more severely impaired than visuoconstructive tasks and visual perception, and selective attention is notably poor. (We should also note that the patients of Schmahmann and Sherman [1998], as well as the children with cerebellar tumors described by Scott et al. [2001] [see above], although showing symptoms consistent with autism, were not considered to show autism as such.)

Insofar as these findings may be compared with those of autism, they do not support a hypothesis that congenital (or gradually progressive early life) cerebellar damage per se can explain the findings characteristic of autism. However, the findings in cerebellar mutism, the alpha-methyltryptophan PET findings of Chugani et al., and the findings of Courchesne attributing attentional defects to cerebellar dysfunction might argue otherwise. The question certainly cannot be settled at our present state of knowledge. I would frame the question thus: Is the cerebellum the primary and causative site of the functional syndrome of autism, as it seemingly is of cerebellar mutism? Or is the cerebellar pathology of autism one part of a more widespread network of abnormalities that also includes primary abnormalities in medial temporal lobes (including the hippocampus and amygdala), sites within prefrontal lobes, and perhaps other regions as well? The latter, if less neat, would seem to be nearer to the mark.

REFERENCES

Allen G, Courchesne E (2003) Differential effects of developmental cerebellar abnormality on cognitive and motor functions in the cerebellum: an fMRI study of autism. *American Journal of Psychiatry* 160:262–273.

Chugani DC (2002) Role of altered brain serotonin mechanisms in autism. *Molecular Psychiatry* 7:S16–S17.

Chugani DC, Musik O, Rothermal R, Behen M, Chakraborty P, Mangner T, da Silva EA, Chugoni HT (1997) Altered serotonin synthesis in the dentatothalamocortical pathway in autistic boys. *Annals of Neurology* 42:666–669.

Critchley HD, Daly EM, Bullmore ET, Williams SC, Van Amelsvoort T, Robertson DM, Rowe A, Phillips M, McAlonan G, Howlin P, Murphy DG (2000) The functional neuroanatomy of social behaviour: changes in cerebral blood flow when people with autistic disorder process facial expressions. *Brain* 23:2203–2212.

DelBello MP, Strakowski SM, Zimmerman ME, Hawkins JM, Sax KW (1999) MRI analysis of the cerebellum in bipolar disorder: a pilot study. *Neuropsychopharmacology* 121: 63–68.

Fatemi SH (2002) The role of reelin in pathology of autism. *Molecular Psychiatry* 7:919–920.

Fatemi SH, Halt AR, Realmuto G, Earle J, Kist DA, Thuras P, Merz A (2002a) Purkinje cell size is reduced in cerebellum of patients with autism. *Cellular and Molecular Neurobiology* 22:171–175.

Fatemi SH, Halt AR, Stary JM, Kanodia R, Schulz SC, Realmuto GR (2002b) Glutamic acid decarboxylase 65 and 67 kDa proteins are reduced in autistic parietal and cerebellar cortices. *Biological Psychiatry* 52:805–810.

Fatemi SH, Stary JM, Halt AR, Realmuto GR (2001) Dysregulation of reelin and Bcl-2 proteins in autistic cerebellum. *Journal of Autism and Developmental Disorders* 31: 529–535.

Kates WR, Mostofsky SH, Zimmerman AW, Mazzocco MM, Landa R, Warsofsky IS, Kaufmann WE, Reiss AL (1998) Neuroanatomical and neurocognitive differences in a pair of monozygous twins discordant for strictly defined autism. *Annals of Neurology* 43:782–791.

Kaufmann WE, Cooper KL, Mostofsky SH, Capone GT, Kates WR, Newscoffer CJ, Bukelis I, Stemp MH, Lamm AE, Laubam DC (2003) Specificity of cerebella XXXX abnormalities in autism: aquontitavia 1DRS study. *Journal of Child Neurology* 18:463–470.

Kemper TL, Bauman ML (2002) Neuropathology of infantile autism. *Molecular Psychiatry* 7:S12–S13.

Lee M, Martin-Ruiz C, Graham A, Court J, Jaros E, Perry R, Iversen P, Bauman M, Perry E (2002) Nicotinic receptor abnormalities in the cerebellar cortex in autism. *Brain* 125:1483–1495.

Marien P, Engelborghs S, Fabbro F, De Deyn PP (2001) The lateralized linguistic cerebellum: a review and a new hypothesis. *Brain and Language* 79:580–600.

Mottaghy FM, Shah NJ, Krause BJ, Schmidt D, Halsband U, Jancke L, Muller-Gartner HW (1999) Neuronal correlates of encoding and retrieval in episodic memory during a paired-word association learning task: a functional magnetic resonance imaging study. *Experimental Brain Research* 128:332–342.

Muller RA, Chugani DC, Behen ME, Rothermel RD, Muzik O, Chakraborty PK, Chugani HT (1998) Impairment of dentatothalamocortical pathway in autistic men: language activation data from positron emission tomography. *Neuroscience Letters* 245:1–4.

Muller RA, Pierce K, Ambrose JB, Allen G, Courchesne E (2001) Atypical patterns of cerebral motor activation in autism: a function al magnetic resonance study. *Biological Psychiatry* 49:665–676.

Nabbout B, DeLong GR (2002) Fluoxetine treatment reversed cerebellar mutism in two children (Abstract). *Annals of Neurology*.

Persico AM, D'Agruma L, Maiorano N, Totaro A, Militerni R, Bravaccio C, Wassink TH, Schneider C, Malmed R, Trillo S, et al. (2001) Reelin gene alleles and haplotypes as a factor predisposing to autistic disorder. *Molecular Psychiatry* 6:150–159.

Pierce K, Courchesne E (2001) Evidence for a cerebellar role in reduced exploration and stereotyped behavior in autism. *Biological Psychiatry* 49:655–664.

Pollack IF, Polinko P, Albright AL, Towbin R, Fitz C (1995) Mutism and pseudobulbar symptoms after resection of posterior fossa tumors in children: incidence and pathophysiology. *Neurosurgery* 37(5):885–893.

Purcell AE, Jeon OH, Zimmerman AW, Blue ME, Pevsner J (2001) Postmortem brain abnormalities of the glutamate neurotransmitter system in autism. *Neurology* 57:1618–1628.

Riva D, Giorgi C. (2000) The cerebellum contributes to higher functions during development: evidence from a series of children surgically treated for posterior fossa tumours. *Brain* 123:1051–1061.

Saarelainen T, Hendolin P, Lucas G, Koponen E, Sairanen M, MacDonald E, Agerman K, Haapasalo A, Nawa H, Aloyz R, Ernfors P, Castren E (2003) Activation of the TrkB neurotrophin receptor is induced by antidepressant drugs and is required for antidepressant-induced behavioral effects. *Journal of Neuroscience* 23:349–357.

Sagiuchi T, Ishii K, Aoki Y, Kan S, Utsuki S, Tanaka R, Fujii K, Hayakawa K (2001) Bilateral crossed cerebello-cerebral diaschisis and mutism after surgery for cerebellar medulloblastoma. *Annals of Nuclear Medicine* 15:157–160.

Schmahmann JD, Sherman JC (1998) The cerebellar cognitive affective syndrome. *Brain* 121:561–579.

Scott RB, Stoodley CJ, Anslow P, Paul C, Stein JF, Sugden EM, Mitchell CD (2001) La-
    teralized cognitive deficits in children following cerebellar lesions. *Developmental
    Medicine and Child Neurology* 43(10):685–691.
Sparks BF, Friedman SD, Shaw DW, Aylward EH, Echelard D, Artru AA, Maravilla KR,
    Giedd JN, Munson J, Dawson G, Dager SR (2002) Brain structural abnormalities
    in young children with autism spectrum disorder. *Neurology* 59:184–192.
Steinlin M, Styger M, Boltshauser E. (1999) Cognitive impairments in patients with con-
    genital nonprogressive cerebellar ataxia. *Neurology* 53:966–973.
Townsend J, Westerfield M, Leaver E, Makeig S, Jung T, Pierce K, Courchesne E (2001)
    Event-related brain response abnormalities in autism: evidence for impaired
    cerebello-frontal spatial attention networks. *Cognitive Brain Research* 11:127–145.
Vandiense D, Hornyak JE (1997) Linguistic and cognitive deficits associated with cerebellar
    mutism. *Pediatric Rehabilitation* 1:41–44.
Victor M, Ropper AH (2001) *Adams and Victor's Principles of Neurology (7th ed.)* New
    York: McGraw-Hill.
Wassink TH, Schneider C, Melmed R, Trillo S, Montecchi F, Palermo M, Pascucci T,
    Puglisi-Allegra S, Reichelt KL, Conciatori M, Marino R, Quattrocchi CC, Baldi A,
    Zelante L, Gasparini P, Keller F (2001) Reelin gene alleles and haplotypes as a factor
    predisposing to autistic disorder. *Molecular Psychiatry* 6:150–159.
Zhang H, Liu X, Zhang C, Mundo E, Macciardi F, Grayson DR, Guidotti AR, Holden JJ
    (2002) Reelin gene alleles and susceptibility to autism spectrum disorders. *Molecular
    Psychiatry* 7:1012–1007.

Chapter 4

The Cranial Circumference in Autism

Michele Zappella

Leo Kanner (1943), in his original description of autism, noticed that Richard, the third of his 11 cases, had an enlarged head: 54.5 cm in circumference at 3 years of age and definitely macrocephalic. The occurrence of macrocephaly, usually described as cranial circumference above the 97°, was subsequently noticed in single cases of autism, but it became the object of systematic study only in the 1990s. Macroencephaly was studied initially in a series of cases of cerebral gigantism (Sotos syndrome) with autism (Zappella 1990), and subsequently in large series of subjects with idiopathic autism where it was found present in 14% (Lainhart et al. 1997; Deutsch & Joseph 2003) to 26.6% (Bailey et al. 1995) of subjects. A large but normal head was even more common (Coleman 1976; Bolton et al. 1994; Bailey et al. 1995; Davidovitch et al. 1996; Lainhart et al. 1997), suggesting a shifting of the entire distribution toward larger sizes. Cranial circumference is therefore one of the few physical findings that varies significantly from the norm in autism and its most current "endophenotypes."

In a study conducted on 137 individuals with idiopathic autism, Miles et al. (2000) found 23.4% of subjects had macrocephaly. This subgroup was not significantly different from the normocephalic subgroup in sex ratio, IQ, severity of autism, morphological abnormalities, seizures, or recurrence risk. The head circumference of parents, none of whom had autism, was skewed toward macrocephaly slightly more in the macrocephalic than in the normocephalic, suggesting that some genes that predispose to macrocephaly may also predispose to autism. Fidler et al. (2000) also found a prevalence of macrocephaly among the nonautistic relatives of autistic probands. In other words, macrocephaly may be a genetic attribute that is fundamental to a subgroup of nonsyndromic autism and, as a consequence, a possibly useful phenotypic marker for undiscovered autism gene(s).

It was soon evident that macrocephaly was more frequent at a younger age, occurring in 37% of those younger than 16 years versus 22% of those in a more extensive age group (Bolton et al. 1994). The same result was found in a study of twins by Bailey et al. (1995), which showed that 42% of those twins under the age of 16 had macrocephaly, while macroencephaly was found in only 26% of twins in a more extensive age group (Bailey et al. 1995). Aylward et al. (2002) used coronal MRI scans to compare 67 children and adults with autism to matched controls and found that the average brain volume of children 12 years of age and younger was larger than the average brain volume of controls, but the investigators did not find this effect in autistic subjects older than 12 years of age. These studies suggest some kind of early overgrowth syndrome that then begins to lag typical cranial circumference growth curves in later childhood.

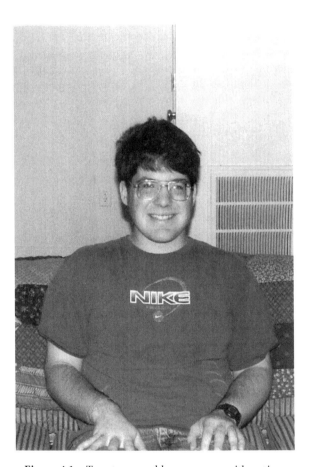

Figure 4.1   Twenty-year-old young man with autism.

Macrocephaly usually is not present at birth and develops during the early years of life; Stevenson et al. (1997) found later macrocephaly in 24% of 100 persons with autism whose head size had been normal at birth. It has been postulated that the development of macrocephaly in infants may be an early concomitant sign of autism. Accelerated head circumference growth trajectories occurring between the 2nd and 14th months of life were found in 59% of young autistic children but only 6% in normal babies (Courchesne et al. 2003; Lainhart 2003). It would be of interest to see if children whose cranial circumference moves from within normal limits at birth to macrocephaly within the first 3 years of life are more likely to have a pattern of autistic regression than those with more stable cranial growth curves; this question awaits research.

However, sometimes enlarged head circumference and macrocephaly can be found at birth. Bolton et al. (2001) did a case-controlled, catch-up study of a cohort of boys with infant macrocephaly and showed that the condition was a risk factor for autism spectrum disorders. In a study by Gillberg and DeSouza (2002), 11 out of 43 individuals (25%) with Asperger syndrome and 4 out of 42 (10%) of individuals with autism had macrocephaly at birth; it was noted that newborn cranial circumference and later IQ were not correlated.

An increase in head width but not length has been noted by Deutsch and Joseph (2003), who found that children with discrepantly high nonverbal abilities had a larger head circumference; they speculated that this might be consistent with an enlargement of parietotemporal cortex and related to the skills mediated by those brain regions. Localized studies of regional cerebral, individual lobe, and even gyri volumes have begun in an attempt to define the areas of enlargement (Piven et al. 1996; Carper et al. 2002; Bigler et al. 2003) but methodological differences, possible heterogeneity of populations, and age factors have not led to consistent results. Analyzing grey matter and white matter changes, such as the volume of white or grey matter in toddlers (Courchesne et al. 2001) or the presence of late myelinating white matter (Herbert et al. 2004), may prove more fruitful.

In addition to being linked to nonsyndromic autism, macrocephaly is found in other neurological conditions associated with autism. These disorders usually belong to overgrowth syndromes in which infants are large for gestational age, may or may not experience excessive postnatal growth, and exhibit increased weight, length or head circumference, and/or asymmetric enlargement, singly or in combination (Cohen 2003).

What are the possibilities regarding the size of the brain when macrocephaly is present? The variations are megaloencephaly, hydrocephalus and/or ventriculomegaly, and benign cranial tumours, each with completely different theoretical implications. Factors that might cause megaloencephaly in nonsyndronic autism are discussed in chapter 2. Ventriculomegaly and/or hydrocephalus and tumors are discussed below in the context of specific syndromes.

To further confuse the situation, some patients who meet autism criteria are microcephalic (Fombonne et al. 1999). In the Miles et al. (2000) study of cranial circumferences in a population of children with idiopathic autism, those who had microcephaly were more likely to have abnormal physical morphology, structural brain malformations, lower IQ, and seizures. This suggests that children with microcephaly and autism are more likely to be at risk for an MCA/MR syndrome, just as is also seen in some of the children with macrocephaly.

SOTOS SYNDROME

Sotos syndrome is an autosomal dominant overgrowth syndrome. The initial association of Sotos syndrome with autism was noticed in the 1970s in one patient (Zappella & Boscherini 1973) and subsequently confirmed in more subjects: in these cases, mental retardation was also present (Morrow et al. 1990; Zappella 1990). Behavioral abnormalities, including attention deficits, drooling, and in many children a persistent hypotonic posture and gait that may improve in subsequent years, are common in this syndrome. Separation anxiety, anxious behavior in new situations, and difficulties in social contact have been frequently observed: as a consequence, these subjects are usually alone and have problems in making friends (Sarimski 2003).

Sotos syndrome is characterized by megaloencephaly, peculiar facial features such as a broad forehead, antimongolian slant of the eyes, prominent chin, gigantism, large hands and feet, and advanced bone age. Clumsiness and poor coordination are common. Febrile seizures occur in numerous cases, and overall 50% have convulsions. IQ/DQ vary to a large extent (40-129), and the mean value has been estimated to be 78 (Cole & Hughes 1994). In childhood, these subjects often show a delay in language, commonly beginning after 2 and a half years of age, and in motor development; but in some instances, this initial delay is followed by a normal or near-normal intelligence in subsequent years.

Cerebral abnormalities usually involve midline structures and are common at RMI. They include dilatation of the cerebral ventricles, prominent trigones and occipital horns, and thinning of the posterior part of the corpus callosum. In some cases, prominent cortical sulci, cavum septum pellucidum, and cavum velum interpositum are also found. These data suggest an inadequate development of the cerebral white matter of the posterior part of the brain. Prominent sulci, macrocisterna magna, heterotopias, and macrocerebellum can also be observed. Abundant ventricular and extracerebral fluid suggest that these subjects have brains of normal size in a large heads (Schaefer et al. 1997).

The major cause of Sotos syndrome is haploinsufficiency of the *NSD1* gene at 5q35 (Imaizumi et al. 2002; Kurotaki et al. 2003). A preferential paternal origin of microdeletions has been observed (Miyake et al. 2003).

COLE-HUGHES MACROCEPHALY SYNDROME

Basing their study on cases that had been excluded from a previous study of Sotos syndrome, Cole and Hughes (1991) identified in 6 individuals a new syndrome characterized by postnatal progressive macrocephaly in a context of familial macrocephaly and inherited through an autosomal dominant pattern. The patients had a typical face characterized by a square outline with frontal bossing, a "dished out" mid-face, biparietal narrowing, and a long philtrum. Also present was marked obesity, variable developmental delay, and, occasionally, delayed bone age. Naqvi et al. (2000) described patients who had Cole-Hughes syndrome and autistic characteristics; these patients seemed to manifest a distinct behavioral phenotype associated with the Cole-Hughes syndrome.

FRAGILE X SYNDROME

Macrocephaly is a possible, nonspecific feature of fragile X syndrome, a common neurodevelopmental disorder with a prevalence of 1 in 4000 and the most common genetic cause of mental retardation. In typical adult males, the head circumference is increased. Other symptoms include a long, narrow face, prominent long ears, strabismus, a thick nasal bridge, a prominent jaw, and macroorchidism after puberty. This disorder is almost always due to an expansion of a CGG-repeat in the 5' untranslated region of the *FMR1* gene. In subjects with the full mutation, mental retardation of various degrees is common in males, while in females, physical, cognitive, and behavioral abnormalities are less severe (Stoll 2001).

The behavioral phenotype of fragile X syndrome is very much like a child with autism. It includes pronounced gaze aversion, perseveration, stereotypies, need for sameness, and language delay with echolalia. However, although social anxiety with unfamiliar adults and peers occurs, the majority do have emotional relationships with their parents and other familiar adults and develop concern for others, thus lacking the core symptom of autism. A small minority do develop full autism criteria, more than can be accounted for by chance (Feinstein & Reiss 1998).

ORSTAVIK 1997 SYNDROME

Orstavik et al. (1997) identified a syndrome that included autism in two sisters with macrocephaly, epilepsy, mental retardation, and dysmorphic features (high and broad forehead, deep set eyes, short philtrum, bushy eyebrows, and hairy upper lips). (It is called the Orstavik 1997 syndrome because although Orstavik and colleagues identified another syndrome in 1998, it was a deglutition dysfunction syndrome without autistic features.) Steiner et al. (2003) also identified the Orstavik 1997 syndrome in two sisters who presented in a similar phenotype except for the absence of epilepsy. These authors pointed out that variability in clinical expression may occur, since autistic features were very marked in the two sisters yet not presented in an otherwise affected brother.

NEUROFIBROMATOSIS TYPE 1

Macrocephaly in the absence of hydrocephalus is found in 30% to 50% of individuals with neurofibromatosis 1. The diagnosis is made from skin lesions of 6 or more café au lait spots, axillary freckling, cutaneous neurofibromatosis, and pathognomic Lisch nodules (seen with a slit lamp after 20 years of age). In addition to the nervous system, it is associated with complications affecting almost every system in the body, including the eyes, endocrine system, skeleton, and circulation. The *NF1* gene found on the long arm of chromosome 17 (17q11.2) encodes the protein neurofibromin.

Neurofibromatosis type 1 can be regarded as an overgrowth syndrome by virtue of several of its features: macrocephaly, the presence of tumors, and, on occasion, hemihyperplasia of a limb or digit. It was increased about 150 fold in a population of autistic patients (Cohen 2003). However, neurofibromatosis 1 is a relatively common syndrome, with an estimated incidence of between 1 in 2,500 and 1 in 3,000. That is why it is hard to be sure that, in any one case, the reports of neurofibromatosis 1 and autism reveal an etiological connection. The neurofibromatous tumors in the brain may or may not be involved in clinical symptoms. The literature describes a number of children who are initially diagnosed with autism but are later found to have neurofibromatosis (Gillberg & Forsell 1984; Williams & Hersh 1998).

HYPOMELANOSIS OF ITO

Hypomelanosis of Ito (HI) or *incontinentia pigmenti achromians* is a neurocutaneous syndrome characterized by macular hypopigmented whorls, streaks, and patches usually distributed on the trunk, where they should not cross the midline, or the limbs. HI affects both sexes with a possible preponderance in girls. It is the third most frequent neurocutaneous disease, following neurofibromatosis type 1 and tuberous sclerosis, and it is accompanied by abnormalities of the CNS in over half of the cases. Macrocephaly is a common occurrence in this syndrome and was present in 16% of the cases reported by Pascual-Castroviejo et al. (1998), who also described autism in 10% of their cases. The occurrence of autism in HI series is probably related to the number of cases of autism seen in a single service, and it was therefore higher in a study conducted on this topic in Siena's service of child neuropsychiatry (Zappella 1992). In this study of 25 children with HI, 5 children (20%) had macrocephaly; however, only 1 out of the 15 children had both an autistic disorder and HI.

PTEN HAMARTOMA-TUMOR SYNDROME

Mutations of the *PTEN* gene can result in developmental syndromes; the mutations are also associated with macrocephaly, hamartomas, and neoplasias. The Cowden syndrome and Bannayan-Riley-Ruvalcaba syndrome probably should be considered as one disease entity (Marsh et al. 1999), as they are both caused by germline mutations in the *PTEN* gene at a chromosome 10q22-23 locus. The literature describes children who have Cowden syndrome or Bannayan-Riley-Ruvalcaba syndrome and who meet the criteria of autism, but only after an autistic regression (Butler et al. 2005). Goffin et al. (2001) described a boy with Cowden syndrome, autism, and macrocephaly with a broad and high forehead and hypotonia that resolved with age; this phenotype is similar to a description of a boy with autism and Bannayan-Riley-Ruvalcaba syndrome (Zori et al. 1998).

OCCULT OR MILD HYDROCEPHALUS

Sometimes the apparent macrocephaly of a child with autism reflects a developmental problem with absorption or blocking of cerebral spinal fluid, resulting in a diminution of brain tissue around the ventricles, or ventriculomegaly. One of the first series of cases of autism evaluated from a biological point of view revealed a child with occult hydrocephalus (Schain and Yannet 1960). Since then there have been many such cases published, and the one consistent finding is an occult or mild widening of the ventricular system and/or hydrocephalus; fully developed or severe hydrocephalus has not been reported. In the case reported by Knobloch and Pasamanick (1975), the etiology of the hydrocephalus was the Dandy-Walker syndrome, which occurs secondarily to meningitis or a papilloma of the choroid plexus. But in most reported cases, the underlying factor leading to the hydrocephalus is unknown.

CONCLUSION

The presence in an infant of abnormal crossing of cranial growth parameters by head measurements (an actual measurement out of the normal range) raises the possibility of a developing central nervous system disorder. One of the possible disorders in both macrocephaly and microcephaly is a disease entity of the autistic syndrome.

A number of studies on nonsyndromic autism and Asperger syndrome have found a significant subgroup of young children with macrocephaly. However, it is an early age phenomenon, with the rate of cranial growth slowing in later childhood. In addition, several overgrowth syndromes can present with both macrocephaly and autism. Macrocephaly in children with autism can reflect either megaloencephaly, occult/mild hydrocephalus, or benign cranial tumours.

A brief medical examination of family members is indicated in all young children developing progressive macrocephaly and a mild or moderate delay in psychomotor development (Goffin et al. 2001). Parents that have normal intelligence and social skills may still have medical signs and symptoms that can help identify their child's specific diagnosis, such as one of the neuroepidermal disorders, a *PTEN* syndrome, and so on.

REFERENCES

Aylward EH, Minshew NJ, Field K, Sparks BF, Singh N (2002) Effects of age on brain volume and head circumference in autism. *Neurology* 59:175–183.

Bailey A, Le Couteur A, Gottesman I, Bolton P, Simonoff E, Yuzda E, Rutter M (1995) Autism as a strongly genetic disorder: evidence from a British twin study. *Psychological Medicine* 25:63–77.

Bigler ED, Tate DF, Neeley ES, Wolfson LJ, Miller MJ, Rice SA, Cleavinger H, Anderson C, Coon H, Ozonoff S, Johnson M, Dinh E, Lu J, McMahon W, Lsainhart JE (2003) Temporal lobe autism and mocrocephaly. *American Journal of Neuroradiology* 24: 2066–2076.

Bolton P, MacDonald H, Pickles A, Rios P, Goode S, Crowson M, Bailey A, Rutter M (1994) A case-control family history study of autism. *Journal of Child Psychology and Psychiatry* 35:877–900.

Bolton PF, Roobol M, Allsopp L, Pickles A (2001) Association between idiopathic infantile macrocephaly and autism spectrum disorders. *Lancet* 358:726–727.

Butler MG, Dasouki MJ, Zhou XP, Talebizadeh Z, Brown M, Takahashi TN, Miles JH, Wang CH, Stratton R, Pilarski R, Eng C (2005) Subset of individuals with autism spectrum disorders and extreme macrocephaly associated with germline PTEN tumour suppressor gene mutations. *Journal of Medical Genetics* 42:318–321.

Carper RA, Moses P, Tigue ZD, Courchesne E (2002) Cerebral lobes in autism: early hyperplasia and abnormal age effects. *Neuroimage* 16:1038–1051.

Cohen MM (2003) Mental deficiency, alterations in performance, and CNS abnormalities in overgrowth syndromes. *American Journal of Medical Genetics* 117C:49–56.

Cole TRP, Hughes HE (1991) Autosomal dominant macrocephaly: benign familial macrocephaly or a new syndrome? *American Journal of Medical Genetics* 41:115–124.

Cole TRP, Hughes HE (1994) Sotos syndrome: a study of the diagnostic criteria and natural history. *Journal of Medical Genetics* 31:20–32.

Coleman M (Ed) (1976) Patient Code Appendix. The Autistic Syndromes. Amsterdam: North-Holland Publishing Co.

Courchesne E, Carper R, Akshoomoff N (2003) Evidence of brain overgrowth in the first year of life in autism. *Journal of the American Medical Association* 290:337–344.

Courchesne E, Karns CM, Davis HR, Ziccardi R, Carper RA, Tigue ZD, Chisum HJ, Moses P, Pierce K, Lord C, Lincoln AJ, Pizzo S, Schreibman L, Haas RH, Akshoomoff NA, Courchesne RY (2001) Unusual brain growth patterns in early life in patients with autistic disorder. An MRI study. *Neurology* 57:245–254.

Davidovitch M, Patterson B, Gartside P (1996) Head circumference measurement in children with autism. *Journal of Child Neurology* 11:389–393.

Deutsch CK, Joseph RM (2003) Brief report: cognitive correlates of enlarged head circumference in children with autism. *Journal of Autism and Developmental disorders* 33: 209–215.

Feinstein C, Reiss AL (1998) Autism: the point of view from fragile X. *Journal of Autism and Developmental Disorders* 28:393–405.

Fidler DJ, Bailey JN, Smalley SL (2000) Macrocephaly in autism and other pervasive developmental disorders. *Developmental Medicine and Child Neurology* 42:737–740.

Fombonne E, Roge B, Claverie J, Courty S, Fremolle J (1999) Microcephaly and macrocephaly in autism. *Journal of Autism and Developmental Disorders* 29:113–119.

Gillberg C, De Souza L (2002) Head circumference in autism, Asperger syndrome and ADHD: a comparative study. *Developmental Medicine and Child Neurology* 44(5): 296–300.

Gillberg C, Forsell C (1984) Childhood psychosis and neurofibromatosis—more than a coincidence. *Journal of Autism and Developmental Disorders* 14.1–8.

Goffin A, Hoefsloot LH, Bosgoed E, Swillen A, Fryns JP (2001) PTEN mutation in a family with Cowden syndrome and autism. *American Journal of Medical Genetics* 105:521–524.

Herbert MR, Ziegler DA, Makris N, Filipek PA, Kemper TL, Normandi JJ, Sanders HA, Kennedy DN, Caviness VS Jr. (2004) Localization of white matter volume increase in autism and developmental language disorder. *Annals of Neurology* 55:530–540.

Imaizumi K, Kimura J, Matsuo M, Kurosawa K, Masumo M, Niikawa N, Kuraki Y (2002) Sotos syndrome associated with de novo balanced reciprocal translocation (t(5;8) 8q 35; q24). *American Journal of Medical Genetics* 107:58–60.

Kanner L (1943) Autistic disturbances of affective contact. *The Nervous Child* 2:217–250.

Knobloch H, Pasamanick B (1975) Some etiologic and prognostic factors in early infantile autism and psychosis. *Journal of Pediatrics* 55:182–191.

Kurotaki N, Harada N, Shimokawa O, Miyake N, Kawame H, Uetake K, Makita Y, Kondoh T, Ogata T, Hasegawa T, Nagai T, Ozaki T, Touyama M, Shenhav R, Ohashi H, Medne L, Shiihara T, Ohtsu S, Kato Z, Okamoto N, Nishimoto J, Lev D, Miyoshi Y, Ishikiriyama S, Sonoda T, Sakazume S, Fukushima Y, Kurosawa K, Cheng JF, Yoshura K, Ohta T, Kishino T, Niikawa N, Matsumoto N (2003) Fifty microdeletions among 112 cases of Sotos syndrome: low copy repeats possibly mediated the common deletion. *Human Mutation* 22:378–387.

Lainhart JE (2003) Increased head growth during infancy in autism. *Journal of the American Medical Association* 290:393–394.

Lainhart JE, Piven J, Wzorek M, Landa R, Santangelo SL, Coon H, Folstein SE (1997) Macrocephaly in children and adults with autism. *Journal of the American Academy of Child and Adolescent Psychiatry* 36:282–290.

Marsh DJ, Kum JB, Lunetta KL, Bennett MJ, Gorlin RJ, Ahmed SF, Bodurtha J, Crowe C, Curtis MA, Dasouki M, Dunn T, Feit H, Geraghty MT, Graham JM Jr., Hodgson SV, Hunter A, Korf BR, Manchester D, Miesfeldt S, Murday VA, Nathanson KL, Parasi M, Pober B, Romano C, Tolmie JL, Trembath R, Winter RM, Zackai EH, Zori RT, Weng LP, Dahia PLM, Eng C (1999) PTEN mutation spectrum and genotype-phenotype correlations in Bannayan-Riley-Rucalcaba syndrome suggest a single disease entity with Cowden syndrome. *Human Molecular Genetics* 8:1461–1472.

Miles JH, Hadden LL, Takahashi TN, Hillman RE (2000) Head circumference is an independent clinical finding associated with autism. *American Journal of Medical Genetics* 95:339–350.

Miyake N, Kurotaki N, Sugawara H, Shimokawa O, Harada N, Kndoh T, Tsukahara M,

Ishikiriyama S, Sonoda T, Miyoshi Y, Sakazume S, Fukushima Y, Ohashi H, Nagai T, Kawame H, Kurosawa K, Touyama M, Shiihara T, Okamoto N, Nishimoto J, Yoshiura K, Ohta T, Kishino T, Niikawa N, Matsumoto N (2003) Preferential paternal origin of microdeletions caused by prezygotic chromosome or chromatid rearrangements in Soto's syndrome. *American Journal of Human Genetics* 72:1331–1337.

Morrow JD, Whitman BY, Accardo PJ (1990) Autistic disorder in Sotos syndrome. *European Journal of Pediatrics* 149:567–569.

Naqvi S, Cole T, Graham JM (2000) Cole-Hughes macrocephaly syndrome and associated autistic manifestations. *American Journal of Medical Genetics* 94:149–152.

Orstavik KH, Stromme P, Ek J, Tirvik A, Skjeldal OH (1997) Macrocephaly, epilepsy, dysmorphic features and mental retardation in two sisters: a new autosomal recessive syndrome? *Journal of Medical Genetics* 34:849–851.

Pascul-Castroviejo I, Roche C, Martinez-Bermejo A, Arcas J, Lopez-Martin V, Tendero A, Esquiroz JLH, Pascual-Pascual SI (1998) Hypomelanosis of Ito. A study of 76 infantile cases. *Brain and Development* 20:36–43.

Piven J, Arndt S, Bailey J, Andreasen N (1996) Regional brain enlargement in autism: a magnetic resonance imaging study. *Journal of the American Academy of Child and Adolescent Psychiatry* 35:530–536.

Sarimski K (2003) Behavioural and emotional characteristics in children with Sotos syndrome and learning disabilities. *Developmental Medicine and Child Neurology* 45:172–178.

Schaefer GB, Bodensteiner JB, Buehler BA (1997) The neuroimaging findings in Sotos syndrome. *American Journal of Medical Genetics* 68:462–465.

Schain R, Yannet H (1960) Infantile autism: an analysis of 50 cases and a consideration of certain relevant neuropsychological concepts. *Journal of Pediatrics* 57:560–567.

Steiner CE, Mantovani Guerreiro M, Marques-de-Faria P (2003) On macrocephaly, epilepsy, autism, specific facial features and mental retardation. *American Journal of Medical Genetics* 120A: 564–565.

Stevenson RE, Schroer RJ, Skinner C, Fender D, Simensen RJ (1997) Autism and macrocephaly. *Lancet* 349:1744–1745.

Stoll C (2001) Problems in the diagnosis of fragile X syndrome in young children are still present. *American Journal of Medical Genetics* 100:110–115.

Williams PG, Hersh JH (1998) Brief report: the association of neurofibromatosis 1 and autism. *Journal of Autism and Developmental Disorders* 28:567–571.

Woodhouse W, Bailey A, Rutter M, Bolton P, Baird G, LeCouteur A (1996) Head circumference in autism and other pervasive developmental disorders. *Journal of Child Psychology and Psychiatry* 37:665–671.

Zappella M (1990) Autistic features in children affected by cerebral gigantism. *Brain Dysfunction* 3:241–244.

Zappella M (1992) Hypomelanosis of Ito is frequently associated with autism. *European Child and Adolescent Psychiatry* 1:170–177.

Zappella M, Boscherini B (1973) Considerations apropos of 7 cases of cerebral gigantism (sotos syndrome). Pediatric 28:419–428. (French)

Zori RT, March DJ, Graham GE, Marliss EB, Eng C (1998) Germline PTEN mutation in a family with Cowden syndrome and Bannayan-Riley-Ruvalcaba syndrome. *American Journal of Medical Genetics* 80:399–402.

Chapter 5
Other Neurological Signs and Symptoms in Autism

Mary Coleman

Whether a child has syndromic autism or nonsyndromic autism is not the only important distinction to be made in the process of reaching a diagnosis. It also is important to determine if the child does or does not have neurological signs and symptoms. In the 60 years since autism was first described, it has become very clear that it is a behaviorally valid syndrome. Initially, the children were diagnosed based on behavioral and developmental symptoms, and at first it was not apparent that they had any significant number of neurological signs or symptoms. However, as these children were examined more closely and as the syndrome was extended to more and more disease entities with no criteria of exclusion, the role of neurological signs and symptoms has become ever more prominent. Most striking of all has been the documentation of the frequency of seizure disorders.

EPILEPSY

It is now clear that children with autism are at heightened risk for epilepsy. This risk of developing seizures was already apparent in the very first group of children described by Kanner (1971); 2 of the initial 11 children became epileptic. The prevalence of epilepsy among children with autism now is estimated to be about 30% (Minshew 1991; Tuchman & Rapin 2002); EEG abnormalities occur in even more children, up to 43% of children with autism in some series (Hashimoto 2001). Seizure disorders can occur in any IQ range among children with autism but are more common among individuals with lower IQ (Volkmar & Nelson 1990). Children with Asperger syndrome are in the higher IQ range and less likely to have epilepsy than children with autism, although some cases have been reported. The children with autism who test in the severely retarded range are at even higher risk for epilepsy than other children who have severe mental retardation but do not have autistic features (Gillberg et al. 1986). Other factors known to predispose a child with autism to seizures are motor deficits, such as cerebral palsy, and severe auditory agnosia (Tuchman et al. 1991). One study in autism linked the probability of a seizure disorder to the severity of behavioral symptoms (Olsson et al. 1988).

Seizure disorders may begin at any age in children with autism, but there are ages of greatest risk. Besides infantile spasms of the extended neonatal period, the two other age groups with peaks of seizure-onset are early childhood (under 5 years of age) and adolescence (above 10 years of age). The highest rates of epilepsy are found in surveys that include adolescents and adults (Giovanardi-Rossi et al. 2000).

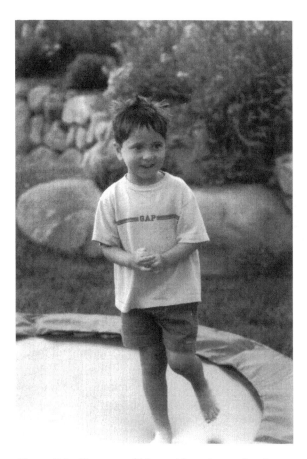

Figure 5.1   Five-year-old boy with autism and epilepsy.

Epilepsy is defined as two or more unprovoked seizures of any type. All major seizure types have been described in the medical literature in children with autism or PPD-NOS (Tuchman et al. 1991). These types include infantile spasms, atonic seizures, the myoclonic epilepsies, atypical absence, complex partial seizures, and generalized tonic-clonic seizures. Seizure manifestations in a child with autism may have unusual presentations; complex partial seizures in particular can be disguised in many ways, such as in the form of fears, difficulty talking, absences, etc. For example, spitting can be a manifestation of temporal lobe epilepsy (Renier 2004). There are even cases of intractable epilepsy, where the severity of the seizures is said to preclude a diagnosis of autism, leading instead to a diagnosis of PDD-NOS (Mann et al. 2004); this type of diagnosis is an example of how the failure to have exclusion requirements for the diagnosis of autistic disorders results in the poorly defined PDD-NOS label.

West syndrome refers to infantile spasms accompanied by a hypsarrhythmic EEG. Patients with infantile spasms have a 2-16% chance of later developing autism; the average percentage is thought to be approximately 10%. However, the percentage jumps above 50% if these infants exhibit bitemporal hypometabolism in a PET scan (Chugani et al. 1996). A population-based study of pre-pubertal children with autism or autistic-like conditions found complex partial seizures were present in 71% of those with an onset of seizures in early childhood (Olsson et al. 1988). Grand mal/tonic-clonic seizures are the most frequent form of seizures in the general population, and they are relatively more frequent in older children and adolescents with autism. Some children with autism have more than one seizure type.

Landau-Kleffner syndrome is an acquired epileptic aphasia affecting children usually between 2 to 5 years of age who have already developed speech. In the classical type, the aphasia is acquired and other higher cortical functions usually do not deteriorate. "Epilepsy with continuous spike-waves during slow wave sleep" may be a variation of the syndrome; intellectual deterioration occurs, and often symptoms reminiscent of autism appear. Because the prognosis of Landau-Kleffner can be limited, early aggressive treatment, such as adequate doses of valproic acid/divalproex or corticosteroids, is indicated.

A subgroup comprising possibly a third of autistic toddlers regress in language, sociability, play, and often cognition (Rapin 1995). Does a seizure problem ever cause this autistic regression? Statistically, the answer is an overwhelming "no". Yet the question of autistic regression related to abnormal EEG or clinical seizures has been raised in a very few cases (Deonna et al. 1993; Nass et al. 1998). A prolonged sleep EEG that includes a study of sleep stages III and IV has been recommended for children without seizures who have regressed or who have fluctuating deficits, and for mute and poorly intelligible children who might have verbal auditory agnosia (Tuchman & Rapin 1997). When a child regresses in language, classic Landau-Kleffner syndrome can be distinguished from autism by the absence of all or most of the autistic behavioral profile.

Epilepsy-Autism Combinations

The specific etiology of seizures due to an underlying epileptic disorder has not yet been demonstrated in the majority of patients with seizures; in that sense, epilepsy is a vast syndrome like autism. Both of these huge syndromes await major clarifications. Many of the reports of behavioral symptoms associated with a known epilepsy syndrome are still in the anecdotal range and await validated measures of behavior.

The higher prevalence of epilepsy in autism is probably best explained by the reality that many different diseases underlie the presentation of autistic symptoms. Autism is a collection of different, often unknown, disease entities that share a distinctive pattern of behavior; many of these disease entities are seizure-free, others are not. In spite of a large and growing differential diagnosis of possible rare combinations of autism and epilepsy (table 5-1), most children with both syndromes still do not receive an etiological diagnosis. Thus, speculation about the mechanism that causes epilepsy in most patients with autism is premature. The role of GABA receptors, the alterations in synaptic transmission or ion channels, abnormal calcium/magnesium levels or the presence of heterotopic neurons need to be studied disease by disease. One interesting general association, however, was noted by Tuchman and Rapin (2002), who pointed out that the association of severe receptive-language disorders with epilepsy and with autism may not be fortuitous, because all three implicate temporal-lobe dysfunction.

The known diseases that can include a combination of autism and seizures in their phenotype are usually classified in two general groups: some of them are classified as idiopathic epilepsy (Besag 2004), while others are part of an established syndrome with stigmata that includes epilepsy within its phenotype (table 5-1). Some of the genes that have been implicated in idiopathic epilepsies encode voltage gated ion channels (channelopathies). In contrast, syndromes with epilepsy as a main feature can be caused by genes that are involved in functions as diverse as cortical development, mitochondrial function, and cell metabolism (Steinlein 2004).

An example of a channelopathy where autistic symptoms can be seen is the Dravet syndrome, also known as severe myoclonic epilepsy in infancy. It is a rare disease, and for a child with the disease to develop autism is even rarer; Harkin et al. (2002) described one such child with a mutation in the $GABA_A$ receptor gamma2 subunit gene. The more frequent mutation found in this patient group is found in the neuronal voltage-gated sodium channel alpha subunit type 1 (*SCN1A*) gene (Claes et al. 2003, Ceulemans et al. 2004). A lariat branchpoint mutation of the *SCN2A* gene has been described in one multiplex autism family (Weiss et al. 2003).

The tuberous sclerosis complex is an example of a syndrome in which epilepsy is a main feature and autistic symptoms are found. This is a neurocutaneous syndrome, many of which have autism and seizures (Pascual-Castroviejo et al.

Table 5-1   Disease entities reported in the literature
to be present in one or more children who have both
epilepsy and autistic symptoms

A. Epilepsy syndromes

    Epilepsy with continuous spike wave in slow-wave sleep
    Dravet syndrome—severe myoclonic epilepsy of infancy
    HEADD syndrome
    Landau-Kleffner acquired epileptic aphasia
    Lennox-Gastaut syndrome
    Orstavik 1997 syndrome
    Pyridoxine-dependent seizures
    West syndrome

B. Other syndromes

    Adenylosuccinate lyase deficiency
    Angelman syndrome
    ARX partial duplication syndrome
    Chromosome 15q11-q13 duplication syndrome
    Chromosome 1q43 deletion
    Creatine transporter defect
    Classic Kanner autism
    Cortical dysplasias
    Cytochrome C oxidase deficiency
    D-glyceric aciduria
    Dysembryoplastic neuroepithelial tumors (DNETs)
    Fragile X syndrome
    Hippocampal sclerosis (bilateral)
    Hypocalcinuria subgroup
    Hypomelanosis of Ito
    PKU autism
    Rasmussen encephalitis
    Rett syndrome
    Sanfilippo syndrome, type A
    Sotos syndrome
    Succinic semialdehyde dehydrogenase deficiency
    Temporal sclerosis (medial)
    Tuberous sclerosis
    X-linked creatine transporter defect

1998), a member of the group of phakomatoses. It is an autosomal dominant disorder characterized by benign tumors (hamartomas) called tubers, although the most disabling aspect of this central nervous system disease may be the white matter lesions (see chapter 2). Malformations occur in one or more body systems, including the skin. This prevalence of this disease entity occurs in 0.01% of the general population, but it is found in 1% to 4% of children with autism, with a higher percentage among those having a seizure disorder (Smalley 1998).

Tuberous sclerosis complex is a genetically heterogenous disorder due in most cases to the *TSC1* and *TSC2* genes. Families segregating to *TSC1* and *TSC2* look clinically similar, and autism can be a behavioral feature of mutations in both. Unfortunately, some of the affected children are simply called "autistic" during the earlier years of their life (Reich et al. 1997); after 5 years of age, a characteristic acne-like lesion on their faces (adenoma sebaceum) may suggest the underlying diagnosis. The first sign of tuberous sclerosis complex may be the presentation of infantile spasms. In a follow-up study of 214 children with infantile spasms, Riikonen and Amnell (1981) found that 25% of the children who had a combination of infantile spasms, autism, and no changes in muscle tone also had the tuberous sclerosis complex. As they advance through childhood, other seizure types present; by the time they reach adulthood, 84% of the children with the tuberous sclerosis complex have experienced one or more types of seizures.

Treatment

The goal of pharmacotherapy to treat seizures themselves in children with autism is to achieve seizure control with optimal cognitive and physical function using the simplest possible antiepileptic drug (AED) regimen. Like with the treatment of other groups of patients with epilepsy, monotherapy with one AED to control seizures is preferred.

In the case of infantile spasms, ACTH is often the preferred treatment. However, a new drug, vigabatrin, appears to be particularly effective in the treatment of infantile spasms in children with tuberous sclerosis, although it is not an FDA-approved medication at this time owing to potentially irreversible retinal toxicity and vision loss (Mackay et al. 2004).

For older children with complex partial seizures or tonic-clonic grand mal seizures, a number of options exist. Both older therapies, such as valproic acid/divalproex, carbamazepine, and corticosteroids, as well as newer AEDs, such as lamotrigine, topiramate, gabapentin, oxcarbazepine, and tiagabine, can be tried. Individual patient responsiveness will determine which AED is used consistently.

A minority of children with autism should be monitored for the presence of hypocalcinuria (Coleman 1994); chronic administration of anticonvulsants can further adversely affect calcium levels. The anticalcium mechanism involved in some anticonvulsant drugs is believed to be the induction of hepatic enzymes that increase the catabolism of vitamin D and its biologically active products.

AEDs generally act on diverse molecular targets largely through effects on voltage-gated sodium and calcium channels, or by promoting inhibition mediated by $GABA_A$ receptors. The subtle biophysical modifications in channel behavior that are induced by AEDs are often functionally opposite to defects in channel properties caused by mutations associated with epilepsy (Rogawski & Loscher 2004).

Some children with autism are placed on a psychopharmaceutical therapy (see chapter 10). If a child also has epilepsy, it is important that drugs that change seizure threshold not be selected for that child.

Finally, it should be kept in mind that although a child has both an autistic syndrome and an epilepsy syndrome, the two syndromes are not necessarily directly related; because both syndromes are relatively common, in some patients it may just be a miserable coincidence.

STEREOTYPIES AND OTHER ABNORMAL MOVEMENTS

Abnormal movements, called hyperkinesias in neurology, are for the most part involuntary contractions of voluntary muscles. Some of the movements defined by classical neurology—such as tics, chorea, and athetosis—can be observed in individuals with autism. But most of the abnormal movements seen in patients with autism/Asperger fall under the category of stereotypies, also known as adventitious movements. Stereotypies are abnormal repetitive, unvarying behaviors that appear to have no goal or function. Although such abnormal repetitive behaviors are not pathognomic of autism, their occurrence and severity are more frequent in autism than in mental retardation (Bodfish et al. 2000).

Many stereotypies are seen in autism (Walker & Coleman 1976; Gardenier et al. 2004). They are hand flapping, patting, tapping, rubbing, clasping, wringing, hand and thumb sucking, and finger flicking. Hands covering the ears and the twirling/spinning of objects are common. Smelling, licking, spitting, and mouthing of objects and other people are seen. Children with autism often posture, rock or twirl their bodies, or jump for no apparent reason. Head rocking can progress to head banging. Facial grimacing, eye squinting, and even phonic tics can be observed. The most distressing of the stereotypies are self-injurious behaviors, such as biting the back of the hand, wrist, or arm and the poking or hitting of the eyes.

Regarding treatment, occasionally, an abnormal EEG, if found, leads to a trial of anticonvulsants. A number of standard antipsychotic medicines can be tried (chapter 10). An extensive literature also describes behavior conditioning that attempts to ablate or ameliorate these stereotypies.

But the pathophysiology of stereotypies and their relationship to other movement disorders is poorly understood. The neurological substratum underneath such adventitious movements is not established in humans. A distinct possibility is the presence of abnormalities of basal ganglia-thalamocortical projections directed primarily (although not exclusively) to the frontal lobe and involving the premotor and prefrontal cortices. Theoretically, stereotypies could arise anywhere within such circuits. It has been proposed that such circuits might be dysfunctional at the basal ganglia level in autism because the basal ganglia are dysfunctional with so many other neurologically defined movement disorders. Classic basal ganglia signs can be observed in at least 10% of children with autism (Walker & Coleman 1976). Both serotonin and dopamine pathways likely are involved.

In animals, dopamine appears to be the overriding culprit: microinjection of dopaminergic agents into rodent striatum has induced or ablated stereotypic movements (Graybiel et al. 2000). Not enough work has even begun to be completed in handicapped children, but a MRI/PET study relates stereotypical behaviors in children with the tuberous sclerosis complex to functional imbalance in subcortical circuits (Asano et al. 2001).

The role of the frontal cortex in stereotypies and perserverative behavior is another possibility. Stereotypies and obsessive-compulsive behaviors are considered to be mutually exclusive categories of behavior, with likely different neural substrates. However, in at least some patients with autistic symptoms, executive frontal control causing a dysfunctional motor circuit can not yet be ruled out, if only because there is so much evidence by imaging studies of frontal lobe involvement (see chapter 2). In one study, measures of stereotyped behavior were significantly positively correlated with frontal lobe volume and significantly negatively correlated with area measures of cerebellar vermis lobules VI-VII (Pierce & Courchesne 2001).

Additional insight might be gained by looking at neurologically defined movement disorders such as the tics sometimes seen in children with autism or Asperger syndrome (Ringman & Jankovic 2000; chapter 8). In Tourette's syndrome, activity appears to be positively coupled between the motor and lateral orbitofrontal circuits in contrast to a negative correlation in controls; the connectivity of the ventral striatum, part of the basal ganglia, is the most severely affected (Jeffries et al. 2002).

Under the *DMS-IV* classification, behaviors as diverse as stereotypies, cognitive inflexibility, and a need for sameness are grouped together (Militerni et al. 2002). As the dysfunctional neural circuits become more clearly defined in each subgroup of individuals with autism/Asperger, motor and cognitive networks are likely to be separated from each other.

CHANGES IN MUSCLE TONE

Muscle tone is defined as the tension of muscles when they are relaxed, or as their resistance to passive movement when voluntary control is absent. The entire range of increased, normal, and decreased muscle tone has been reported in children with autism and Asperger syndrome, undoubtedly depending upon the pathophysiology of the underlying illnesses. Muscle tone can be difficult to appraise clinically and minor impairments are especially hard to identify except by a skilled examiner. In many patients with autism, changes in muscle tone are subtle or borderline, making it difficult to be sure. Questionable abnormalities of gait are a clinical sign that raise questions about changes in muscle tone (Hallett et al. 1993; Smith 2000).

Many possible factors can impair muscle tone. Normal tone is dependent upon a complex system: the integrity of the muscle, the myoneural junction, the peripheral nerves, the alpha and gamma motor neurons, the interneurons in the spinal cord, as well as all the central connections above these levels. Many, perhaps even the majority, of children with autism have normal muscle tone, but adequate studies are not available. However, in a number of different groups of patients with autistic symptoms, abnormal muscle tone has been reported.

Hypertonicity usually is caused by impulses from supraspinal regions. A great range of hypertonicity has been reported in autism. At one extreme is mild hypertonus as exemplified by toe-walking, an early sign noted in some children with autism. Usually these children have subtle increases in tone and do not have evidence of pyramidal responses, such as ankle clonus or the Babinski sign. At the other extreme are children with the spasticity of cerebral palsy who also are found to have classical symptoms of autism. Spasticity is a state of sustained increase in tension of a muscle when it is passively lengthened. Spastic cerebral palsy, a nonprogressive disorder of posture or movement due to lesions in the developing brain, occurs in about 2 per 1000 live births. The reported percentage of children with cerebral palsy and autistic symptoms is 1% to 10% (Fombonne et al. 1997; Nordin & Gillberg 1996). Since autism and cerebral palsy are among the most common of the developmental disorders, it is not known if the presence of both syndromes in any individual child is coincidental or not. A variable and asymmetrical spasticity has been reported in children with Angelman syndrome (Beckung et al. 2004), one of the forms of syndromic autism.

In between these two extremes, different degrees of hypertonus can be found. The rigidity seen from involvement of the basal ganglia or other parts of the extrapyramidal system is a form of hypertonus. Extrapyramidal rigidity shows resistance to passive movement but often to a lesser degree than is found in spasticity. There has been little examination of this question in autism except by Vilensky et al. (1981), who did a kinesiologic analysis of gaits of children with autism and reported that they had some resemblance to the gait of rigid adults with Parkinson.

Catatonic rigidity also is a form of hypertonus and has been reported in a number of patients with autism. From a neurological point of view, catatonic rigidity is a waxy or lead-pipe type of resistance to passive movement; the term catalepsy is used when it may be possible to mold an extremity into any position in which it remains for some time. The term "catatonia" has been used more generally for accompanying catatonic stupor or excitement; sometimes the term has been used to include extreme slowness, passivity, and lack of spontaneous action. Catatonia was first described in patients with Asperger syndrome in 1981 (Wing) and in autism in 1991 (Realmuto & August). It appears from 10 to 19 years of age and affects about 6% of patients with an autistic syndrome. Catatonia has since been described as part of the fuller motor, behavioral, and affective complex of catatonia in some adolescents and adults with autism by Wing and Shah (2000). Dhossche (2004) has raised the question of whether autism could be an early childhood expression of adolescent/adult catatonia in some patients since the mutism, echopraxia/echolalia, and stereotypies of the catatonia complex are the same symptoms that can be seen in autism. Hare and Malone (2004) have suggested that autistic catatonia may include a complex of very slow voluntary motor movements, as well as stopping or freezing in the course of movement and requiring prompting, which may or may not help.

Hypotonicity has been reported in small groups of children with autism. Hypotonus usually arises from impairment of the lower levels of the system: the muscles themselves, the peripheral nerves, or the spinal connections and pathways. However, it also can occur from central connections such as poor feedback from higher sensory systems or inadequate impulse from the cerebellum. Little or no resistance to passive extension or flexion is found in a tonus examination of a child with hypotonia.

Neonatal hypotonia is unusual in case histories of children with later autistic symptoms, but there are some exceptions. The most severe cases of chromosome 15q11-q13 duplication syndrome can have profound hypotonia (Mann et al. 2004). Most children with Rett Complex have a brief period of normal development before their symptoms present (see chapter 7); however, infant hypotonia has been described (Heilstedt et al. 2002).

Poor muscle tone can be due to many factors. In children with autism, cerebellar dysfunction is a reasonable possibility and can be checked by neurological examination (Haas et al. 1996). When hypotonia is due to impairment of the muscle, there is a possibility of a mitochondrial disease (Clark-Taylor & Clark-Taylor 2004; Pons 2004). Actually, when a child with autistic symptoms has hypotonia, there is a significant chance that this child's underlying diagnosis can be determined today. Besides the hypotonia commonly seen in the easier to diagnose MC/MR syndromes, children with autism may be affected by a chromosomal or genetic disease, a metabolic dysfunction, or a mitochondrial disease (see table 5-2).

MUTISM

One of the most haunting questions in autism is why some of the children with autism are mute even though they can demonstrate a surprising level of knowledge through independent typing and other means. Children with a history of regression sometimes speak a few words before the autistic regression, and then become mute. Also unanswered is why some apparently mute children with autism finally begin to speak, but at extremely late ages (Windsor et al. 1994). Estimates of mutism in autism vary widely, undoubtedly depending upon how the patient population was selected. The estimates range from as low as 18% (Coleman 1976) to as high as 61% (Fish et al. 1966). Occasionally a child has deaf-mutism. Some of the speaking children with autism have very limited vocabularies, perhaps only a few single words. The percentage of children with mutism has been declining in recent years as more and more high functioning children are classified as having an autistic spectrum disorder.

Table 5-2   Differential diagnosis of
nonsyndromic autism and hypotonia

Chromosomal syndromes:

Chromosome 1q43 deletion
Chromosome 15q11-q13 duplications

Metabolic syndromes:

Adenylosuccinate lyase deficiency
D-glyceric aciduria
Succinic semialdehyde dehygrogenase deficiency

Nuclear genetic syndromes:

Rett Complex

Mitochondrial dysfunction syndromes:

mtDNA syndromes
HEADD syndrome

Kanner (1943) described the language characteristics of the first 11 children whom he diagnosed as autistic, including 3 who were mute. He described a mutism that was rarely interrupted by the production of a full sentence and usually occurred in situations that the child perceived to be highly stressful. There are known variations of mutism in which the child speaks only to certain people (elective mutism) or only in certain conditions (selective mutism).

More recently, it has been assumed that mutism in autism was a symptom of a major global developmental delay problem because children who have both autism and mutism tend to be lower functioning (Miranda-Linne & Melin 1997; Carter et al. 1998) not only in terms of language, but also in the behavioral repertoire, such as self-stimulation (Chock & Glahn 1983). It is not known if most mute patients with autism (who do not have a known MR/MCA syndrome) might have a similar underlying pathophysiology from one disease entity or whether mutism in autism is a final common clinical expression of a number of different underlying diseases. A theory arose that mute patients were more likely to have a prenatal infectious etiology, but this has not been supported by a study of the seasonality hypothesis in either the mute or the verbal groups (Landau et al. 1999). In some cases, mutism in children with autism has been associated with other neurological findings, such as catatonia (Realmuto & August 1991). Individual evaluation of language networks might be another approach in mute children, since it has been discovered that some children with autism have unique neural circuitry based on aberrant and individual-specific neural sites (Pierce et al. 2001).

Gesture can be as affected as language in autism; all the communicative skills are diminished. Of particular interest to evaluating the problems in autism are the studies showing that language and gesture may be mediated by common neural systems (Bates & Dick 2002). Language and gesture milestones advance together in typical children growing up. It has been shown that there is a close correlation between the first word production and what is called "gestural naming," usually in the 12 to 18 month age group. In studies of young autistic children, word production does not begin until recognitory gestures have appeared (Happé & Frith 1996). Further evidence for language-gesture links in early development comes from a study of handedness, which shows a right-hand bias in typical children before they begin to speak; the right-handed bias is greatest for gestures with communicative or symbolic content (Bates et al. 1986). A whole topic in itself is the extensive literature on the problem of brain lateralization, or failure of lateralization, in autism.

In infants, linguistic knowledge is not thought to be innate and is not localized in a clear and compact place in the brain, but the infant brain is not a *tabula rasa* either: it is already highly differentiated at birth, and certain regions are biased from the beginning toward modes of information processing that are particularly useful for language. However, if there is a developmental problem, the infant brain is thought to be highly plastic, which permits alternative "brain plans" for language to emerge if the standard situation does not hold (Bates 1999). Since social interaction with another human being affects speech learning, children with autism are at risk especially if they prefer nonspeech signals to "motherese."

Some mute individuals with autism clearly have an oral dyspraxia; they have hypomobile, atrophic tongues, suggestive of cranial nerve involvement. But the neural networks that control speech are difficult to evaluate in mute patients with autism. Perhaps one reason there is so little consistent work is that the circuits underlying vocal control are extremely complex. They consist of essentially three components: laryngeal activity, supralaryngeal (articulatory) activity, and respiratory movements (Jurgens 2002). Voluntary control of vocalization, in contrast to involuntary vocal reactions such as shrieks of pain, requires the intactness of the forebrain. The motor neurons controlling vocalization are located in nuclei of the pons, medulla, and ventral horn of the spinal cord and need facilitation and coordination by many additional nuclei ranging from the supplementary motor area of the frontal lobe all the way down to the cerebellum.

In adults and older children, mutism results from the interruption of neural pathways of previously acquired language, and evidence often points toward frontal interruption of those networks in adults. It is known that left-sided anterior cerebral artery infarction can result in mutism. Bilateral anterior cerebral artery infarction affect the dorsal part of the medial prefrontal region as a whole (including the anterior cingulate), which forms a bottleneck region where systems concerned with movement, emotion, attention, and working memory interact. A bilateral injury there can cause akinetic mutism (Kumral et al. 2002). It has been suggested that akinetic mutism is a specific condition characterized by injury of the frontal neuronal systems that promote executive function (Tengvar et al. 2004). Surgical injury to the medial frontal lobe for resection of a low-grade glioma often results in transient postoperative speech disorders, including complete mutism. In a study by Krainik et al. (2003), speech deficit was directly related to the resection of the supplementary motor area of the dominant hemisphere for language, as demonstrated by fMRI.

Children who already have developed speech and then suffer from severe traumatic head injury can experience posttraumatic mutism, perhaps involving mesencephalic structures. The 7 children described in the paper by Dayer et al. (1998) recovered verbal production in between 5 to 94 days. Another example of mutism occurring in children who previously had language is cerebellar mutism, which usually follows surgical or infectious injury of the cerebellum. Mutism can be evoked by surgical injury to the dentatothalamofrontal tract itself (Wang et al. 2002); this circuit has been implicated in autism (Chugani et al. 1997). Although initial mutism and the subsequent dysarthria are the most feared sequelae of cerebellar astrocytoma surgery, Asperger syndrome has recently been added to the list of sequelae (Aarsen et al. 2004).

In children, the mutism associated with surgical cerebellar lesions or infectious injury to the cerebellum is usually reversible owing to the phenomenon of diaschisis. Diaschisis is an example of how complex it can be to locate an exact lesion site when studying mutism; it refers to the effects of a lesion in one part of the brain on other regions that are both remote and not directly involved in the primary lesion. In diaschisis, normal input traveling from one cortical region to another is interrupted; it produces a disruption of cerebral oxygen metabolism, glucose metabolism, and blood flow in the secondarily affected cortical area (Meyer et al. 1993). As the primary lesion heals, a partial or complete return of function occurs in that remote, temporarily deactivated region. A chronic syndrome associated with cerebellar malfunction is the cerebellar cognitive affective syndrome (CCAS). In children, it sometimes includes symptoms associated with autism, including language disorder (see chapter 3). Originally described in adults, the syndrome consists of linguistic difficulties, personality changes, impaired spatial cognition, and disturbances of executive function.

One of the most unexpected outcomes of the study of language in child development is that of children born with hemihydranencephaly. This is a rare condition characterized by complete or almost complete destruction of half the cerebral cortex, leaving only a membranous sac containing cerebrospinal fluid but preserving the meninges, basal ganglia, pons, medulla, and cerebellum on the affected side. Such patients with half of their cerebral cortex missing constitute an experiment of nature with implications for speech development. It is of great interest that language development has been recorded in patients with both left and right hemihydranencephaly. The destruction of one or the other of the cerebral hemispheres that occurs soon after the completion of neurogenesis in the second trimester demonstrates that each cortex contains sufficient circuitry for the potential of language development (Greco et al. 2001). The relatively good outcome in hemihydranencephaly is thought to be due in part to neuronal plasticity (Porro et al. 1998). These children are classified as mentally retarded; surprisingly, it is often only a mild retardation.

The experience with hemihydranencephaly raises the possibility that the dysfunction of developing language networks might be bilateral in children with autism who remain mute. In autism, these bilaterally affected circuits include gesture, as well as language networks, and failures in timely cerebral lateralization occur. Some of the areas of malfunction in autism that might be bilateral could be those that affect neurotransmission, such as genetically programmed synaptogenesis, the levels of ions or neurotransmitters, the presence of ventriculomegaly, or inadequate myelination. But so little is known; this is a major area for research.

REFERENCES

Aarsen FK, Van Dongen HR, Paquier PF (2004) Long-term sequelae in children after cerebellar astrocytoma surgery. *Neurology* 62:1311–1316.

Asano E, Chugani DC, Muzik O, Behen M, Janisse J, Rothermel R, Manger TJ, Chakraborty PK, Chugani HT (2001) Autism in tuberous sclerosis complex is related to both cortical and subcortical function. *Neurology* 57:1269–1277.

Bates E (1999) Language and the infant brain. *Journal of Communication Disorders* 32:195–205.

Bates E, Dick F (2002) Language, gesture and the developing brain. *Developmental Psychobiology* 40:293–310.

Bates E, O'Connell B, Vaid J, Sledge P, Oakes L (1986) Language and hand preference in early development. *Developmental Neuropsychology* 2:1–5.

Beckung E, Steffenburg S, Kyllerman M (2004) Motor impairments, neurological signs, and developmental level in individuals with Angelman syndrome. *Developmental Medicine and Child Neurology* 46:239–243.

Besag FM (2004) Behavioral aspects of pediatric epilepsy syndromes. *Epilepsy Behavior* Suppl 1:S3–13.

Bodfish JW, Symons FJ, Parker DE, Lewis MH (2000) Varieties of repetitive behavior in autism; comparison to mental retardation. *Journal of Autism and Developmental Disorders* 30:237–243.

Carter AS, Volkmar FR, Sparrow SS, Wang JJ, Lord C, Dawson G, Fombonne E, Loveland K, Mesibov G, Schopler E (1998) The Vineland Adaptive Behavior Scales: supplementary norms for individuals with autism. *Journal of Autism and Developmental Disorders* 28:287–302.

Ceulemans BP, Claes LR, Lagae LG (2004) Clinical correlations of mutations in the *SCN1A* gene: from febrile seizures to severe myoclonic epilepsy in infancy. *Pediatric Neurology* 30:236–243.

Chock PN, Glahn TJ (1983) Learning and self-stimulation in mute and echolalic autistic children. *Journal of Autism and Developmental Disorders* 13:365–81.

Chugani DC, Muzik O, Rothermel R, Behen M, Chakraborty P, Mangner T, da Silva EA, Chugani HT (1997) Altered serotonin synthesis in the dentatothalamocortical pathway in autistic boys. *Annals of Neurology* 42:666–9.

Chugani HT, Da Silva E, Chugani DC (1996) Prognostic implications of bitemporal hypometabolism on positron emission tomography. *Annals of Neurology* 39:643–649.

Claes L, Ceulemans B, Audenaert D, Smets K, Lofgren A, Del-Favero J, Ala-Mello S, Basel-Vanagaite L, Plecko B, Raskin S, Thiry P, Wolf NI, Van Broeckhoven C, De Jonghe P (2003) De novo *SCN1A* mutations are a major cause of severe myoclonic epilepsy of infancy. *Human Mutations* 21:615–621.

Clark-Taylor T, Clark-Taylor BE (2004) Is autism a disorder of fatty acid metabolism? Possible dysfunction of mitochondrial ß-oxidation by long chain acyl-CoA dehydrogenase. *Medical Hypotheses* 62:970–975.

Coleman M (Ed.) (1976) Patient Code Appendix. *The Autistic Syndromes.* Amsterdam: North-Holland Publishing Co.

Coleman M (1994) Clinical presentations of patients with autism and hypocalcinuria. *Developmental Brain Dysfunction* 7:63–70.

Dayer A, Roulet E, Maeder P, Deonna T (1998) Post-traumatic mutism in children: clinical characteristics, pattern of recovery and clinicopathological correlations. *European Journal of Pediatric Neurology* 2:109–116.

Deonna T, Ziegler AL, Moura-Serra J, Innocenti G (1993) Autistic regression in relation to limbic pathology and epilepsy: report of two cases. *Developmental Medicine and Child Neurology* 35:166–176.

Dhossche DM (2004) Autism as early expression of catatonia. *Medical Science Monitor* 10: RA31–39.

Fish B, Shapiro T, Campbell M (1966) Long-term prognosis and the response of schizophrenic children to drug therapy. *American Journal of Psychiatry* 123:32–39.

Fombonne E, du Mazaubrun C, Cans C, Grandjean H (1997) Autism and associated medical disorders in a French epidemiological survey. *Journal of the American Academy of Child and Adolescent Psychiatry* 36:1561–1569.

Gardenier NC, MacDonald R, Green G (2004) Comparison of direct observational methods for measuring stereotypic behavior in children with autism spectrum disorders. *Research in Developmental Disabilities* 25:99–118.

Gillberg C, Persson E, Grufman M, Themnér U (1986) Psychiatric disorders in mildly and severely mentally retarded urban children and adolescents: epidemiological aspects. *British Journal of Psychiatry* 149:68–74.

Giovanardi-Rossi P, Posar A, Parmeggiani A (2000) Epilepsy in adolescents and young adults with autistic disorder. *Brain Development* 22:102–106.

Graybiel AM, Canales JJ, Capper-Loup C (2000) Levodopa-induced dyskinesias and dopamine-dependent stereotypies: a new hypothesis. *Trends in Neuroscience* 23:S71–77.

Greco F, Finocchiaro M, Pavone P, Trifiletti RR, Parano E (2001) Hemihydranencephaly: case report and literature review. *Journal of Child Neurology.* 16:218–21.

Haas RH, Townsend J, Courchesne E, Lincoln AJ, Schreibman L, Yeung-Courchesne R

(1996) Neurologic abnormalities in infantile autism. *Journal of Child Neurology* 11: 84–92.

Hallett M, Lebiedowska MK, Thomas SL, Stanhope SJ, Denckla MB, Rumsey J (1993) Locomotion of autistic adults. *Archives of Neurology* 50:1304–1308.

Happé F, Frith U (1996) The neuropsychology of autism. *Brain* 119:1377–1400.

Hare DJ, Malone C (2004) Catatonia and autistic spectrum disorders. *Autism* 8:183–195.

Harkin LA, Bowser DN, Dibbens LM, Singh R, Phillips F, Wallace RH, Richards MC, Williams DA, Mulley JC, Berkovic SF, Scheffer IE, Petro S (2002) Truncation of the GABA(A)-receptor gamma2 subunit in a family with generalized epilepsy with febrile seizures plus. *American Journal of Human Genetics* 70:530–536.

Hashimoto T, Sasaki M, Sugai K, Hanaoka S, Fukumizu M, Kato T (2001) Paroxysmal discharges on EEG in young autistic patients are frequent in the frontal regions. *Journal of Medical Investigation* 48:175–180.

Heilstedt HA, Shahbazian MD, Lee B (2002) Infantile hypotonia as a presentation of Rett syndrome. *American Journal of Medical Genetics* 111:238–242.

Jeffries KJ, Schooler C, Schoenbach C, Herscovitch P, Chase TN, Braun AR (2002) The functional neuroanatomy of Tourette's syndrome: an FDG PET study III: functional coupling of regional cerebral metabolic rates. *Neuropsychopharmacology* 2002 Jul; 27(1):92–104.

Jurgens U (2002) Neural pathways underlying vocal control. *Neuroscience Biobehavioral Review* 26:235–258.

Kanner L (1943) Autistic disturbances of affective contact. *Nervous Child* 2:217–250.

Kanner L (1971) Follow-up study of eleven children originally reported in 1943. *Journal of Autism and Childhood Schizophrenia* 1:119–145.

Krainik A, Lehericy S, Duffau H, Capelle L, Chainay H, Cornu P, Cohen L, Boch AL, Mangin JF, Le Bihan D, Marsault C (2003) Postoperative speech disorder after medial frontal surgery: role of the supplementary motor area. *Neurology* 60:587–594.

Kumral E, Bayulkem G, Evyapan D, Yunten N (2002) Spectrum of anterior cerebral artery territory infarction: clinical and MRI findings. *European Journal of Neurology* 9:615–624.

Landau EC, Cicchetti DV, Klin A, Volkmar FR (1999) Season of birth in autism: a fiction revisited. *Journal of Autism and Developmental Disabilities* 29:385–393.

Mackay MT, Weiss SK, Adams-Webber T, Ashwal S, Stephens D, Ballaban-Gill K, Baram TZ, Duchowny M, Hirtz D, Pellock JM, Shields WD, Shinnar S, Wylie E, Snead OC 3rd; American Academy of Neurology; Child Neurology Society (2004) Practice parameter; medical treatment of infantile spasms: report of the American Academy of Neurology and the Child Neurology Society. *Neurology* 62:168–181.

Mann SM, Wang NJ, Liu DH, Wang L, Schultz RA, Dorrani N, Sigman M, Schanen NC (2004) Supernumerary tricentric derivative chromosome 15 in two boys with intractable epilepsy: another mechanism for partial hexasomy. *Human Genetics* 115:104–111.

Meyer JS, Obara K, Muramatsu K (1993) Diaschisis. *Neurological Research* 15:362–366.

Militerni R, Bravaccio C, Falco C, Fico C, Palmermo MT (2002) Repetitive behaviors in autistic disorder. *European Child and Adolescent Psychiatry* 11:210–218.

Minshew NJ (1991) Indices of neuronal function in autism: clinical and biological implications. *Pediatrics* 87:774–780.

Miranda-Linne FM, Melin L (1997) A comparison of speaking and mute individuals with autism and autistic-like conditions on the Autism Behavior Checklist. *Journal of Autism and Developmental Disorders* 27:245–64.

Nass R, Gross A, Devinsky O (1998) Autism and autistic epileptiform regression with occipital spikes. *Developmental Medicine and Child Neurology* 40:453–458.

Nordin V, Gillberg C (1996) Autism spectrum disorders in children with mental and physical disability or both. I. Clinical and epidemiological aspects. *Developmental Medicine and Child Neurology* 38:297–313.

Olsson I, Steffenburg S, Gillberg C (1988) Epilepsy in autism and autistic-like conditions: a population-based study. *Archives of Neurology* 45:666–668.

Pascual-Castroviejo I, Lopez-Rodriguez L, de la Cruz Medina M, Salamanca-Maesso C, Roche Herrero C (1988) Hypomelanosis of Ito. Neurological complications in 34 cases. *Canadian Journal of Neurological Science* 15:124–129.

Pierce K, Courchesne E (2001) Evidence for a cerebellar role in reduced exploration and stereotyped behavior in autism. *Biological Psychiatry* 49:655–664.

Pierce K, Muller RA, Ambrose J, Allen G, Courchesne E (2001) Face processing outside the fusiform "face area" in autism: evidence from functional MRI. *Brain* 124:2059–2073.

Pons R, Andreu AL, Checcarelli N, Vila MR, Englestad K, Sue CM, Shungu D, Haggerty R, DeVivo DC, DiMauro S (2004) Mitochondrial DNA abnormalities and autistic spectrum disorders. *Journal of Pediatrics* 144:81–85.

Porro G, Wittebol-Post D, de Graaf M, van Nieuwenhuizen O, Schenk-Rootlieb AJ, Treffers WF (1998) Development of visual function in hemihydranencephaly. *Developmental Medicine and Child Neurology* 40:563–567.

Rapin I (1995) Autistic regression and disintegrative disorder: how important is the role of epilepsy? *Seminars in Pediatric Neurology* 2:278–285.

Realmuto GM, August GJ (1991) Catatonia in autistic disorder: a sign of comorbidity or variable expression? *Journal of Autism and Developmental Disorder* 21:517–528.

Reich M, Lenoir P, Malvy J, Perrot A, Sauvage D (1997) Bourneville's tuberous sclerosis and autism. (French) *Archives de Pediatre* 4:170–175.

Renier WO (2004) Compulsive spitting as a manifestation of temporal lobe epilepsy. *European Journal of Paediatric Neurology* 8:61–62.

Riikonen R, Amnell G (1981) Psychiatric disorders in children with earlier infantile spasms. *Developmental Medicine and Child Neurology* 23:747–760.

Ringman JM, Jankovic J (2000) Occurrence of tics in Asperger's syndrome and autistic disorder. *Journal of Child Neurology* 15:394–400.

Rogawski MA, Loscher W (2004) The neurobiology of antiepileptic drugs. *Nature Reviews Neuroscience* 5:553–564.

Smalley SL (1998) Autism and tuberous sclerosis. *Journal of Autism and Developmental Disorders* 28:407–414.

Smith IM (2000) Motor functioning in Asperger's syndrome. In Klin A, Volkmar FR, Sparrow SS (Eds) *Asperger's Syndrome.* New York: The Guildford Press.

Steinlein OK (2004) Genetic mechanisms that underlie epilepsy. *Nature Reviews Neuroscience* 5:400–408.

Tengvar C, Johansson B, Sorensen J (2004) Frontal lobe and cingulate cortical metabolic dysfunction in acquired akinetic mutism: a PET study of the interval form of carbon monoxide poisoning. *Brain Injury* 18:615–625.

Tuchman RF, Rapin I (1997) Regression in pervasive developmental disorders: seizures and epileptiform electroencephalogram correlates. *Pediatrics* 99:560–565.

Tuchman R, Rapin I (2002) Epilepsy in autism. *The Lancet Neurology* 1:352–358

Tuchman RF, Rapin I, Shinnar S (1991) Autistic and dysphasic children. 2. Epilepsy. *Pediatrics* 88:1291–1225.

Vilensky JA, Damasio AR, Maurer RG (1981) Gait disturbance in patients with autistic behavior; a preliminary study. *Archives of Neurology* 38:646–649.

Volkmar FR, Nelson DS (1990) Seizure disorders in autism. *Journal of the American Academy of Child and Adolescent Psychiatry* 29:127–129.

Walker HA, Coleman M (1976) Chapter 12. Characteristics of adventitious movement in autistic children. In Coleman M (Ed) *The Autistic Syndromes*. Amsterdam: North-Holland Publishing Co.

Wang MC, Winston KR, Breeze RE (2002) Cerebellar mutism associated with midbrain cavernous malformation. Case report and review of the literature. *Journal of Neurosurgery* 96:607–610.

Weiss LA, Escayg A, Kearney JA, Trudeau M, MacDonald BT, Mori M, Reichert J, Buxbaum JD, Meisler MH (2003) Sodium channels SCN1A, SCN2A, SCN3A in familiar autism. *Molecular Psychiatry* 8:186–194.

Windsor J, Doyle SS, Siegel GM (1994) Language acquisition after mutism: a longitudinal case study of autism. *Journal of Speech and Hearing Research* 37:96–105.

Wing L (1981) Asperger's syndrome: a clinical account. *Psychological Medicine* 11:115–129.

Wing L, Shah A (2000) Catatonia in autistic spectrum disorders. *The British Journal of Psychiatry* 176:357–362.

Chapter 6

The Epidemiology of Autism

Christopher Gillberg

For a long time, childhood autism was considered to be an extremely rare dis-order, with its prevalence rate usually reported at a fraction of a 10th of 1% (Lotter 1966; Brask 1970; Sponheim & Skjeldal 1998). It is only in the past few years that autism has been reported to be, if not common, certainly not a very rare disorder (Gillberg & Wing 1999). The most recent estimates of the prevalence of autism have ranged from 0.5% to 1.1%, that is, 20-100 times higher than those suggested in text books even in the mid 1990s (Lord & Rutter 1994). However, for a quarter of a century, and independently, Wing and Gillberg have argued that autism is much more common than originally believed (Wing & Gould 1979; Gillberg 1983; Gillberg 1991; Gillberg et al. 1991; Wing 1996).

The present chapter aims to review the major epidemiological studies per-formed in the field of autism (including so-called ASDs). However, only studies published in the English language and meeting certain criteria for inclusion will be referred to.

CRITERIA FOR INCLUSION OF EPIDEMIOLOGICAL STUDIES IN PRESENT REVIEW

This review includes only studies that have been published in the English language up until the end of 2003. (Some reference will also be made to yet unpublished studies performed by the author in the past few years.)

All studies meet the following additional criteria:

1. Screening among a wider population should have been performed, and more than one register or one type of school must have been in-cluded in the screening stage of the study.

2. Clinical evaluation of individual cases should have been performed; studies accepting cases *only* on the basis of registered diagnoses are not included.
3. Studies excluding cases with a known or presumed etiology are not included.
4. Diagnostic criteria and meticulously described assessment methods must be included.

STUDIES PUBLISHED IN THE 1960s

The first autism epidemiology studies were published in the 1960s (table 6-1). Lorna and John Wing supervised a study by Victor Lotter from Middlesex, England, that appeared in 1966 and for many years was the standard by which all other autism studies were measured. Lotter found a very low rate of "nuclear autism" (2.0 in 10,000 school-age children) and a similar rate of "non-nuclear autism" (Lotter 1966).

Even before Lotter's study, Michael Rutter had published a study from Aberdeen, Scotland on the prevalence of psychotic disorders in children of school age (Rutter 1967). One needs to keep in mind that, at the time, psychotic disorders in childhood were conceptualized as including autism and similar conditions, and that autism was considered the most common and typical form of "childhood psychosis." Lotter (1966) found that approximately 4 in 10,000 children had childhood psychosis/autism.

STUDIES PUBLISHED IN THE 1970s

Three important papers on the epidemiology of autism were published in the 1970s (table 6-1). The first U.S. study appeared in 1970 and reported the lowest rate in the history of autism (0.7 in 10,000 children) (Treffert 1970). In the same year, a Danish pioneer in the field, Birthe Brask, published her account of a

Table 6-1 Prevalence studies for autism and other ASD: age specific rates per 10,000 children (age ranges vary) 1966–1980

	Authors	Year publ	Area Studied	Rate of autism/other ASD	Criteria used for autism/other ASD
1	Lotter	1966	Middlesex, England	4.5/-	Kanner/-
2	Brask	1970	Aarhus, Denmark	4.3/-	Kanner/-
3	Treffert	1970	Wisconsin, USA	0.7/2.4	Kanner/DSM-II
4	Wing & Gould	1979	Camberwell, England	4.6/15.7	Kanner/Triad

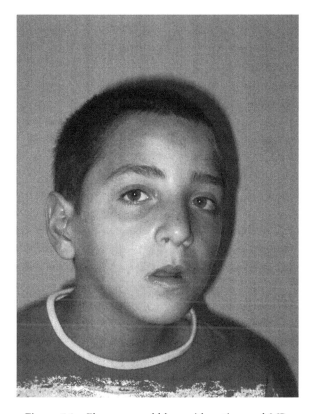

Figure 6.1   Eleven-year-old boy with autism and MR.

Jutland autism prevalence study, reporting that 4.3 in 10,000 children suffered from autism (Brask 1970).

The ground-breaking epidemiological studies of Lorna Wing and her collaborators started to appear in the late 1970s. Wing, for the first time in the history of autism, had taken the view that autism might not be a discrete disease entity that presented only in "classic" forms. She studied "social impairment" across the board of all those with any kind of registered disability/handicap in the southeast London borough of Camberwell and found almost 5.0 in 10,000 with autism (slightly under half of whom had core autism) and another 16 in 10,000 who had the triad of social, communicative, and imagination/behavioural impairment considered crucial for a diagnosis of autism but who did not meet the clinical prototype of "classic" autism. Thus, Wing suggested that more than 20 in 10,000 (0.2%) children had either autism or something similar (possibly an "ASD") (Wing & Gould 1979).

STUDIES PUBLISHED IN THE 1980s

In the early 1980s, Gillberg (1983) published the first modern account of multiple comorbidities in a population sample of individuals with child psychiatric disorders. He noted that children with a combination of deficits in attention, motor control, and perception (individuals who would nowadays be diagnosed as suffering from attention deficit/hyperactivity disorder [ADHD] and developmental coordination disorder [DCD]) very often had the triad of symptoms referred to by Lorna Wing, and, in the parlance of the time, he called these problems "psychotic behaviour." In recent years, cases with these types of problems would almost definitely be referred to as suffering from "ASDs." The total population prevalence of psychotic behaviour/ASDs in 7-year-old children was 0.69%, according to the results of that study. The individuals thus classified have since been reevaluated on several occasions and found to meet currently accepted diagnostic criteria for Asperger syndrome, atypical autism, and autistic disorder. On the basis of this study, the first-ever epidemiological estimate of Asperger syndrome in the general population was made (a minimum of 0.26% of 7-year-olds) (Gillberg & Gillberg 1989).

Gillberg's group also published two general population studies focused specifically on infantile autism/autistic disorder, which both found relatively low rates of autism (0.02% and 0.07%, respectively) (Gilllberg 1984; Steffenburg & Gillberg 1986) (table 6-2).

Several other international publications reporting on the rate of autism—mostly based on the Rutter (1978), *DSM-III* (American Psychiatric Association 1980), and *DSM-III-R* (American Psychiatric Association 1987) criteria for the condition—appeared in the 1980s, with most studies documenting rates that were marginally to considerably higher than those reported in the 1960s and 1970s (0.03 through 0.16%).

STUDIES PUBLISHED IN THE 1990s

In the early 1990s, Gillberg and his group published a paper based on a population study performed in 1988, in which the question was raised: "Is autism more common now than 10 years ago?" (Gillberg et al. 1991). This study was met with skepticism, and other autism experts in the field queried whether the Gothenburg group might have started to overdiagnose autism. Nevertheless, most of the studies published during the rest of this decade found prevalence rates for autism and its spectrum disorders that were much higher than reported in the earliest studies (table 6-3). In a review study toward the end of the decade, Gillberg and Wing (1999) concluded that autism was "not a rare disorder," and that the prevalence rate from 1966 onward had gone up by a yearly steady increase of approximately 3-4%.

Table 6-2 Prevalence studies for autism and other ASD: age specific rates per 10,000 children (age ranges vary) 1981–1990

	Authors	Year publ	Area studied	Rate of autism/other ASD	Criteria used for autism/other ASD
1	Hoshino et al.	1982	Fukushima, Japan	5.0/-	Kanner
2	Bohman et al.	1983	Västerbotten, Sweden	3.0/2.6	Rutter/Rutter
3	Ishii & Takahashi	1982	Toyota, Japan	16.0/-	Rutter/-
4	McCarthy et al.	1984	E Health Bd, Ireland	4.3/-	Kanner/-
5	Gillberg	1984	Göteborg, Sweden	2.0/1.9	*DSM-III/DSM-III*
6	Gillberg et al.	1987	Göteborg, Sweden	3.3/14.3	*DSM-III*/Triad
7	Steffenburg & Gillberg	1986	Göteborg, Sweden	4.7–2.8	*DSM-III/DSM-III*
8	Steinhausen et al.	1986	W Berlin, Germany	1.9/-	Rutter/-
9	Matsuishi et al.	1987	Kurume City, Japan	15.5/-	*DSM-III*/-
10	Burd et al.	1987	Dakota, USA	1.2/2.1	*DSM-III/DSM-III*
11	Tanoue et al.	1988	Ibaraki, Japan	13.8/-	*DSM-III*
12	Bryson et al.	1988	Nova Scotia, Canada	10.1/-	*DSM-III-R*/-
13	Ritvo et al.	1989	Utah, USA	4.0/-	*DSM-III*/-
14	Sugiyama & Abe	1989	Nagoya, Japan	13.0/-	*DSM-III*/-
15	Cialdella & Mamelle	1989	Rhone, France	5.1/5.2	*DSM-III/DSM-III*

STUDIES PUBLISHED FROM 2000

Almost all autism epidemiology studies published in the past 5 years have yielded prevalence rates of more than 0.1% for "autistic disorder" and of 0.3-0.7% for other disorders in the autism spectrum (including Asperger syndrome and atypical autism) (table 6-4). However, it is only the rate of "autistic disorder" and that of the wider range of "ASDs" (including autistic disorder) that can be regarded as relatively well established.

Rates for Asperger syndrome, and particularly for atypical autism (or PDD-NOS) and childhood disintegrative disorder, are much more uncertain (table 6-5). In the case of Asperger syndrome, only a handful of studies have been published using specific criteria, but these criteria have varied from one study to another. Nevertheless, all four Scandinavian studies that have used Gillberg and Gillberg's (1989) operationalized criteria for the disorder (based on Asperger's original descriptions of his patients) have yielded fairly consistent findings of 0.2-

Table 6-3   Prevalence studies for autism and other ASD: age specific rates per 10,000 children (age ranges vary) 1991–2000

	Authors	Year publ	Area studied	Rate of autism/ other ASD	Criteria used for autism/other ASD
1	Gillberg et al.	1991	Göteborg, Sweden	8.4/3.2	*DSM-IIIR/DSM-IIIR*
2	Fombonne & du Mazaubrun	1992	4 regions, France	4.9/-	*ICD-10/-*
3	Honda et al.	1996	Yokohama, Japan	21.1/-	*ICD-10/-*
4	Fombonne et al.	1997	3 departments, France	5.4/10.9	*ICD-10/ ICD-10*
5	Arvidsson et al.	1997	Molnlycke, Sweden	31.0/15.0	*ICD-10/ ICD-10*
6	Webb et al.	1997	S Glamorgan, Wales	7.2/-	*DSM-III-R/-*
7	Sponheim & Skjeldal	1998	Akershus, Norway	3.8/1.4	ICD-10/ ICD-10
8	Kadesjö et al.	1999	Karlstad, Sweden	60.0/60.0	*ICD-10*/Gillberg[1]
9	Magnusson & Saemundsen	2001	Iceland	8.6/4.6	*ICD-10/ ICD-10*
10	Baird et al.	2000	SE Thames, England	30.8/27.1	*ICD-10/ ICD-10*
11	Powell et al.	2000	W Midlands, England	16.2/17.5	*DSM-IIIR, ICD-10*
12	Kielinen et al.	2000	N Finland	12.2/1.7	*DSM-IV/DSM-IV*

0.5% of the general population of school age children having this variant of an ASD. For atypical autism/PDD-NOS the situation is more difficult still, given that the so-called operationalized criteria for this category according to the *ICD-10/ DSM-IV* are extremely vague and really nowhere near true operationalization. The general population rate for childhood disintegrative disorder has recently been estimated to be 0.17 in 10,000 children or 50-100 times less than that for autistic disorder.

SUMMARY OF PREVALENCE STUDY FINDINGS

The most recent estimates of the prevalence of ASDs in the general population (including autistic disorder, Asperger syndrome, and atypical autism/PDD-NOS) converge around a rate of 0.6% to 1.1% of school age children. This is 20-100 times higher than the rate suggested by the early studies performed approximately 40 years ago. Autistic disorder probably contributes 20–40% of the total prevalence of reported ASD. Most of what we currently regard as state-of-the-art

Table 6-4 Prevalence studies for autism and other ASD: age specific rates per 10,000 children (age ranges vary) 2001–2003

	Authors	Year publ	Area studied	Rate of autism/ other ASD	Criteria used for autism/other ASD
1	Bertrand et al.	2001	Brick Township, USA	40.0/27.0	*DSM-IV/DSM-IV*
2	Chakrabarti & Fombonne	2001	Staffs, England	16.8/45.8	*DSM-IV/DSM-IV*
3	Croen et al.	2002	California, USA	11.0/-	*DSM-IIIR, DSM-IV*
4	Yeargin-Allsopp et al.	2003	Atlanta, USA	34.0 all	*DSM-IV*

knowledge about autism is based on what we know about autistic disorder. This knowledge cannot automatically be generalized and applied to ASD. For instance, the old "truth" that 70-90% of all individuals with autism also suffer from mental retardation does not apply to Asperger syndrome or PDD-NOS. Rather, the rate of mental retardation across all ASDs is probably in the range of 15%-20% if all variants of disorders in the spectrum are taken into account.

Girls are much underrepresented in all the autism prevalence studies reviewed here. However, there is a tendency in recent studies to indicate the male excess of cases to be slightly less pronounced. It is possible that in the near future—with autism know-how becoming more and more widespread in the educational and medical communities—many more girls with ASD will be recognized and diagnosed.

POSSIBLE REASONS FOR THE APPARENT INCREASE IN PREVALENCE RATE OF AUTISM

A number of possible explanations exist for the apparent increase in the rate of autism (spectrum disorders) in the community. The explanatory models are not exclusive; each of the following factors is likely to have contributed to the change in reported autism prevalence rates over the past 40 years.

Conceptual Change

Autism has been reconceptualized several times over the past 40 years. Once believed to be a discrete disorder, perhaps even a well-delineated disease entity (Kanner 1943; Rutter 1978), autistic disorder/childhood autism is now recognized as only one of several behavioral presentations of a condition that belong in a spectrum that also includes Asperger syndrome, atypical autism, and childhood disintegrative disorder. Some authors (Gillberg & Coleman 2000) have even proposed that autism might be better framed as a final common behavioral pathway

Table 6-5   Prevalence studies for autism and other ASD (including Asperger syndrome): age specific rates per 10,000 children (age ranges vary) 1989–2003

	Authors	Year publ	Area studied	Rate of autism/ other ASD (including Asperger syndrome)	Criteria used for autism/other ASD/Asperger syndrome
1	Gillberg*	1983	Göteborg, Sweden	69.0	Wing's ASD triad
2	Gillberg & Gillberg*	1989	Göteborg, Sweden	26.0 (+43.0)	Gillberg[1]
3	Ehlers & Gillberg**	1993	Göteborg, Sweden	36.0 (+36.0)	Gillberg[1]
4	Fombonne et al.	2003	Great Britain	26.1	DSM-IV
5	Scott et al.	2002	Cambridge, England	57.0	DSM-IV
6	Baker	2002	Australian Cap Territ	5.0	DSM-IV
7	Webb et al.	2003	Cardiff, Wales	20.0	ICD-10

"Other ASD" includes subgroups of the autism spectrum other than "autism". These differ among the studies listed

* This study looked only at Asperger syndrome and other ASDs (in brackets) in a total population study focusing on children with deficits in attention, motor control, and perception

** The rate in brackets is for children with marked social impairment but not the full picture of Asperger syndrome; autistic disorder not included.

[1] Gillberg's criteria for Asperger syndrome (Ehlers & Gillberg 1993)

of a whole host of different disorders and variations in brain development ("autistic syndromes") rather than as a "spectrum," with its implication of cases being readily referable to specific sections on a continuum ranging from mild to severe.

The fact that researchers and clinicians now view autism as a broader group of conditions that will inevitably affect a larger group of individuals is probably the major reason for the perceived increase in the rate of autism in the general population.

This aspect is well illustrated by the Gillberg study (1983) in which the investigator reported that 0.7% of the general population of 7-year-olds suffered from "psychotic behaviour" in the 1970s. With the conceptual change, the individuals diagnosed as having "psychotic behavior" would be diagnosed today as having an ASD (including autistic disorder). At the time of the publication of these data, Gillberg also reported that 0.02% of the general population of school age children from the same geographical region as suffered from "infantile autism" (Gillberg 1984). The two studies were published before the conceptual change occurred; infantile autism was seen as a discrete entity that was (probably) not on a spectrum with "psychotic behavior."

Change in Diagnostic Criteria over Time

It is clear that autism diagnostic criteria have changed considerably over the past decades, and, in particular, over the past 25 years. The diagnostic criteria of the *DSM-III* were very vague compared to the detailed criteria of the *DSM-III-R*. Nevertheless, the *DSM-III* was more stringent in that it demanded the problems be very severe for a diagnosis to be made. The *DSM-III-R* and *DSM-IV* criteria are both strictly operationalized and circumscript in terms of the algorithms used for diagnosis under the various pervasive developmental disorder categories. Experience has shown the *DSM-IV* (and the almost identical *ICD-10*) criteria to be more inclusive than the *DSM-III*. Lorna Wing rediagnosed her cases in the original Camberwell study using *ICD-10* criteria rather than the Kanner-Lotter gestalt that she had used in the original publication from the 1970s (Wing & Gould 1979; Gillberg & Wing 1999). This produced a 3-fold increase in the rate of diagnosed autism.

On the basis of this and other findings and clinical experience, it is clear that the change in diagnostic criteria over time has contributed substantially to the higher rate of autism reported in more recent studies (table 6-6).

Better Autism Awareness in the Community

Although no formal studies of this aspect have been conducted, it is generally agreed that knowledge about the existence of the syndrome of autism among lay people and nonspecialist doctors and psychologists has increased dramatically in recent years. This would lead to many more parents attending clinics with their children enquiring specifically about the possibility that their child might be suffering from an ASD, as well as doctors and other specialists being more alert to

Table 6-6 Age-specific rates per 10,000 by diagnostic criteria used: means and ranges (includes only studies giving rates for autism separately from other ASD)

Criteria	No of studies of autism	Mean rate for autism	Range of rates	No of studies of other ASD	Range of rates
Kanner	6	3.9	0.7–5.0	-	-
DSM-II	-	-	-	1	2.4
Rutter	3	7.0	1.9–16.0	1	2.6
DSM-III	9	7.0	1.2–15.5	5	1.9–5.2
DSM-III-R	3	8.6	7.2–10.1	1	3.2
DSM-IV/ICD-10	14	21.0	3.8–60.0	10	1.4–58.0
Triad *	-	-		2	14.3–15.7
Gillberg **	-	-		1	60.0

* Triad of impairments (Wing & Gould 1979). The rates are for children with IQ <70.
** Gillberg's criteria for Asperger syndrome—first version (Ehlers and Gillberg, 1993). The rate is for children of all levels of IQ.

the possibility that the child might actually suffer from one of the conditions in the spectrum.

The Development of Autism Diagnostic Services

Virtually no diagnostic centers with specific autism competency could be found in the western world (or elsewhere) 40 years ago. Nowadays, autism diagnostic services are available in many countries. Also, legislation and federal/national guidelines for diagnosing and intervening in autism are available in many western countries, including the United States and Canada, the UK, and some of the Scandinavian countries. The availability of diagnostic services has contributed greatly to the increase in autism prevalence, at least to that portion contributed by cases filed on a register (Gillberg et al. 2004).

Increase in Environmental Risk Factors Possibly Contributing to Autism Pathogenesis

Some environmental risk factors, such as maternal use of valproic acid or abuse-level quantities of alcohol in pregnancy and extreme prematurity, have all been associated with an increased risk of autism in children (Gillberg & Coleman 2000). Given that these risk factors have become more prevalent in recent years, it would be expected that they would contribute toward a somewhat (in some populations considerably) higher rate of autism in the general population.

Decrease in Environmental Risk Factors Possibly Contributing to Autism Pathogenesis

A number of environmental biological risk factors associated with the development of autism in children have been drastically reduced or eliminated in many populations over the past 40 years. These include thalidomide embryopathy and congenital rubella infection. The disappearance of such risk factors in the general population would have decreased the number of new autism cases to some extent.

Possible Links of Autism with Immigrant Status of One or Both Parents

It has been reported for many years that autism is statistically associated with migrant status of one or both parents in some populations (Gillberg et al. 1987). This was first noted by Lotter (1978) in his study of the prevalence of autism in Africa. He—and indeed others—noted that the link was particularly strong if parents had migrated over long distances. Many possible explanations have been forwarded to account for this statistical link, but it now seems that one of the most likely reasons is intimately linked with genetic rather than environmental factors. Men or women with ASDs (carrying a much increased risk of having offspring affected by ASDs) might not be able to find a partner to have a child with in his or her own culture, where others are likely to perceive of him or her as strange or even disabled. With increased globalization, such men and women are more likely to travel to distant regions of the globe, where the likelihood of finding a partner may be much greater, because a potential partner may ascribe his or her social oddities and communication problems to him or her coming from a different culture rather than to any kind of major oddity or disability. Other possible factors that could account for a link between autism and parent migrant status are (1) the fetus being subjected to viral infections to which mothers arriving in a new country would not be immune (i.e., rubella embryopathy), (2) dietary incompatibilities, (3) whole extended families with genetic autism emigrating from their native country, (4) language confusion during the first years of development in children genetically predisposed to problems in the social-communication domain, and (5) combinations of any or all of these.

Possible Links with Specific Genetic-Social Changes

Simon Baron-Cohen has suggested that recent reports of increased rates of autism in the general population may actually mirror real increases associated with a particular genetic-social mechanism. In the past, people with ASDs could have been prevented from becoming parents by way of their social oddities, communication problems, and, often, academic failure. With the advent of computers, many people in the autism spectrum found an outlet for their particular kind of intelligence/cognitive style. Many, who in the past could not make a living on their own, found jobs and a new social standing among age peers. This would have strongly increased their likelihood of finding a partner and becoming a parent, which, in turn, because of genetic factors, would often result in the offspring having ASDs (Baron-Cohen 2004). Evidence suggests that many adults with ASDs are computer engineers or self-made experts in the field of computers (Baron-Cohen et al. 2001; Cederlund & Gillberg 2004).

THE RATE OF AUTISM AS IT RELATES TO NEUROLOGICAL PROBLEMS

Several recent studies have suggested that, even with the much higher prevalence reported in recent autism studies, many cases in the spectrum may still actually be missed. This would be most likely to affect those people with ASDs who have another neurological or diagnosed medical condition such as epilepsy, cerebral palsy, tuberous sclerosis, etc. In their study of autism in patients with epilepsy and mental retardation, Steffenburg et al. (1996) showed that even in a geographical region where both autism and epilepsy had been screened for meticulously over a period of decades, autism in patients with epilepsy very often remains undiagnosed. The same applies to cerebral palsy ataxia (Ahsgren & Gillberg 2005) and tuberous sclerosis (Ahlsén et al. 1994). In such cases, where a neurological condition had already been diagnosed, the physician in charge of the care of the individual patient often felt that a "proper" diagnosis (epilepsy, cerebral palsy, tuberous sclerosis) had already been made that there was no need to look specifically for further problems, or that the obvious (and usually extremely handicapping) autistic problems would somehow be subsumed under the neurological diagnosis and were just another sign of brain dysfunction in the affected individual. Thus, rather than finding a higher rate of autism associated with medical disorders in specialized autism clinics, one would expect to find a particularly low rate of such disorders in child psychiatry or tertiary referral autism diagnostic centers (Gillberg & Coleman 1996).

Epilepsy

Several studies have now demonstrated that the rate of ASDs in individuals with epilepsy is much higher than in the general population. This is particularly the case if mental retardation coexists with the epileptic disorder (Steffenburg et al. 1996, 2003). However, the rate of ASDs including Asperger syndrome is probably much higher than in the general population even when there is no associated mental retardation, as evidenced by the very common occurrence of Asperger syndrome in individuals of normal or near normal intelligence undergoing evaluation for epilepsy surgery (Taylor et al. 2000).

Conversely, the rate of epilepsy in autism and other ASDs is extremely high. In "classic" autistic disorder, the rate is approximately 20% by early childhood (Volkmar & Nelson 1990; Olsson et al. 1988), 25–35% by late adolescence (Rutter 1970; Gillberg 1984) and almost 40% by approximately 30 years of age (Danielsson et al., unpublished data, 2004). In Asperger syndrome, the rate of epilepsy is much lower, but even in classic cases of this condition in which the patients' IQs are in the normal or above-average range, the rate is several times higher than in the general population, ranging from approximately 3% to 10% (Cederlund & Gillberg 2004).

The types of epilepsy most commonly encountered in autism are infantile spasms and complex partial epilepsies of various kinds (Steffenburg et al. 2003; Danielsson et al., unpublished data, 2004).

Cerebral Palsy

Very few studies that have looked specifically at the rate of ASDs in cerebral palsy have been published. One recent study of cerebral palsy ataxia found an extremely high rate of autistic disorder and atypical autism in children with this variant of cerebral palsy and found that approximately 1 in 4 of children with ataxia meeting criteria for typical or atypical autism (Ahsgren & Gillberg 2005). It is interesting to note that although the study was primarily designed to determine the contribution of cerebellar dysfunction to the development of symptoms of autism, only a weak such link was found.

Very few studies have included any detail on the occurrence of cerebral palsy in autism. One study of Asperger syndrome in 23 individuals (including as controls 23 high-functioning subjects with autism) found 1 individual with cerebral palsy (hemiplegia) and coloboma of 1 of the eyes (Gillberg et al. 1991).

Tuberous Sclerosis and Other Medical Disorders Sometimes Associated with Autism and Other ASDs

The rate of autism and atypical autism in tuberous sclerosis is extremely high, ranging from approximately 1 in 4 to approximately 1 in 2 individuals showing symptoms of the neurological disorder before 5 years of age (Hunt & Dennis 1987; Ahlsén et al. 1994). Conversely, approximately 1 in 20 individuals with classic autism exhibit the syndrome of tuberous sclerosis. (But often such individuals must be examined in detail in order for the diagnosis to be revealed.)

The reasons for the link between autism and tuberous sclerosis are likely to be complex; both genetic and specific brain dysfunction localization factors probably play a major role. First, there are at least 2 genetic variants of tuberous sclerosis, one on chromosome 9 and another on chromosome 16. An autism genetic susceptibility area has been identified in the same region on chromosome 16. This autism-gene region of interest overlaps with a region that has also been established as an important area for genes relevant for ADHD. The fact that when children with tuberous sclerosis have major behaviour problems, they usually involve both ASD and ADHD is of special interest in this context. Second, it has been shown repeatedly that when tubers are located in the frontotemporal regions of the brain and when they are numerous, the risk that the child with tuberous sclerosis will suffer from ASD is very much increased.

The link between herpes encephalitis and autism is probably mediated through frontotemporal brain damage (Gillberg & Coleman 2000). Brainstem damage is implied by the linking of thalidomide embryopathy, Möbius, and CHARGE syndromes with ASD. In the case of thalidomide embryopathy, the timing of the insult to the developing nervous system (around day 21 postconception) can be inferred from the nature of the limb and eye anomalies typical of those with thalidomide intrauterine exposure who develop autism (Strömland et al. 1994).

CONCLUSION

Autistic disorder is not extremely rare, occurring in approximately 0.2% of the general population of children. Spectrum disorders, including Asperger syndrome, are probably considerably more common that "classic" autism. The link between ASD and male gender remains strong in recent prevalence studies, but it is likely that females are currently underdiagnosed. The link between autism and various other types of brain disorders and brain damaging factors is strong, although the pattern is different and more complex once the whole spectrum of clinical presentations of autism is taken into account. The pathogenesis of ASD will not be fully understood unless the much higher prevalence of these conditions is recognized and factored into all models of etiology.

REFERENCES

Ahlsén G, Gillberg IC, Lindblom R, Gillberg C (1994) Tuberous sclerosis in Western Sweden. A population study of cases with early childhood onset. *Archives of Neurology* 51:76–81.

Ahsgren I, Gillberg C (2005) Ataxia, autism, and the cerebellum. A clinical study of 32 cases of congenital ataxia. *Developmental Medicine and Child Neurology*, in press.

American Psychiatric Association (1980) *Diagnostic and Statistical Manual of Mental Disorders* (3rd ed.). Washington, DC: APA.

American Psychiatric Association (1987) *Diagnostic and Statistical Manual of Mental Disorders.* (3rd ed., revised). Washington, DC: APA.

Arvidsoon T, Danielsson B, Forsberg P, Gillbert C, Johansson M, Källgren G (1997) Autism in 3-6-year-old children in a suburb of Göteborg, Sweden. *Autism*, 1(2), 163–173.

Baird G, Charman T, Baron-Cohen S, Cox A, Swettenham J, Wheelwright S, Drew A (2000) A screening instrument for autism at 18 months of age: a 6-year follow-up study. *Journal of the American Academy of Child Adolescent Psychiatry* 39:694–702.

Baker HC (2002) A comparison study of autism spectrum disorder referrals 1997 and 1989. *Journal of Autism and Developmental Disorders* 32:121–125.

Baron-Cohen S (2004) Autism: research into causes and intervention. *Pediatric Rehabilitation* 7:73–78.

Baron-Cohen S, Wheelwright S, Skinner R, Martin J, Clubley E (2001) The autism-spectrum quotient (AQ): evidence from Asperger syndrome/high-functioning autism, males and females, scientists and mathematicians. *Journal of Autism and Developmental Disorders* 31:5–17.

Bertrand J, Mars A, Boyle C, Bove F, Yeargin-Allsopp M, Decoufle P (2001) Prevalence of autism in a United States population: the Brick Township, New Jersey, investigation. *Pediatrics* 108:1155–61.

Bohman M, Bohman IL, Björk Sjoholm E (1983) Childhood psychosis in a northern Swedish county: some preliminary findings from an epidemiological survey. In MH Schmidt, & H Remschmith (Eds), *Epidemiological Approaches in Child Psychiatry* (pp. 164–173). Stuttgart: Georg Thieme.

Brask BH (1970) A prevalence investigation of childhood psychosis. Paper presented at the 16th Scandinavian Congress of Psychiatry.

Bryson SE, Clark BS, Smith IM (1988) First report of a Canadian epidemiological study of autistic syndromes. *Journal of Child Psychology and Psychiatry* 29:433–445.

Burd L, Fisher W, Kerbeshian J (1987) A prevalence study of pervasive developmental disorders in North Dakota. *Journal of the American Academy of Child Adolescent Psychiatry* 26:700–703.

Cederlund M, Gillberg C (2004) One hundred boys with Asperger Syndrome. A clinical study of background and associated factors. *Developmental Medicine and Child Neurology*, 46:652–660.

Chakrabarti S, Fombonne E (2001) Pervasive developmental disorders in preschool children. *JAMA* 285:3093–3099.

Cialdella P, Mamelle N (1989) An epidemiological study of infantile autism in a French department (Rhone): a research note. *Journal of Child Psychology and Psychiatry* 30: 165–175.

Croen LA, Grether JK, Hoogstrate J, Selvin S (2002) The changing prevalence of autism in California. *Journal of Autism and Developmental Disorders* 32:207–215.

Danielsson S, Billstedt E, Gillberg IC, Gillberg C, Olsson I (2004) Epilepsy in young adults with autism spectrum disorders and learning disability: A long-term follow-up population-based study, unpublished.

Ehlers S, Gillberg C (1993) The epidemiology of Asperger syndrome. A total population study. *Journal of Child Psychology and Psychiatry* 34:1327–1350.

Fombonne E, du Mazaubrun C (1992) Prevalence of infantile autism in four French regions. *Society of Psychiatry and Psychiatry and Epidemiology* 27:203–210.

Fombonne E, du Mazaubrun C, Cans C, Grandjean H (1997) Autism and associated medical disorders in a French epidemiological survey. *Journal of the American Academy of Child and Adolescent Psychiatry* 36:1561–1569.

Fombonne E, Simmons H, Ford T, Meltzer H, Goodman R (2003) Prevalence of pervasive developmental disorders in the British nationwide survey of child mental health. *International Review of Psychiatry* 15:158–165.

Gillberg C (1983) Perceptual, motor and attentional deficits in Swedish primary school children. Some child psychiatric aspects. *Journal of Child Psychology and Psychiatry* 24:377–403.

Gillberg C (1984) Infantile autism and other childhood psychoses in a Swedish urban region. Epidemiological aspects. *Journal of Child Psychology and Psychiatry* 25:35–43.

Gillberg C, Coleman M (1996) Autism and medical disorders. A review of the literature. *Developmental Medicine and Child Neurology* 38:191–202.

Gillberg C, Steffenburg S, Börjesson B, Andersson L. (1987) Infantile autism in children of immigrant parents. A population-based study from Göteborg, Sweden. *British Journal of Psychiatry* 150:856–858.

Gillberg C, Steffenburg S, Schaumann H (1991) Is autism more common now than 10 years ago? *British Journal of Psychiatry* 158:403–409.

Gillberg C, The Emanuel Miller Memorial Lecture (1991) Autism and autistic-like conditions: subclasses among disorders of empathy. *Journal of Child Psychology and Psychiatry* 33:813–842.

Gillberg C, Wing L (1999) Autism: Not an extremely rare disorder. *Acta Psychiatrica Scandinavica* 99:399–406.

Gillberg C, Coleman M (2000) *The Biology of the Autistic Syndromes.* London: Cambridge University Press.

Gillberg C, Cederlund M, Zeiljon L (2004) The Autism Epidemic. The registered prevalence of autism in a Swedish urban area. *Journal of Autism and Developmental Disorders,* in press.

Gillberg IC, Gillberg C (1989) Asperger syndrome-some epidemiological considerations: a research note. *Journal of Child Psychology and Psychiatry* 30(4):631–638.

Honda H, Shimizu Y, Misumi K, Niimi M, Ohashi Y (1996) Cumulative incidence and prevalence of childhood autism in children in Japan. *British Journal of Psychiatry* 169(2), 228–235.

Hoshino Y, Kumashiro H, Yashima Y, Tachibana R, Watanabe M (1982) The epidemiological study of autism in Fukushima-ken. *Folia Psychiatry Neurology Japan* 36:115–124.

Hunt A, Dennis J. (1987) Psychiatric disorder among children with tuberous sclerosis. *Developmental Medicine and Child Neurology* 29:190–198.

Ishii T, Takahashi O (1982) Epidemiology of autistic children in Toyota City, Japan. Prevalence, World Child Psychiatry Conference, Dublin.

Kadesjö B, Gillberg C, Hagberg B (1999) Brief report: autism and Asperger syndrome in seven-year-old children: a total population study. *Journal of Autism and Developmental Disorders* 29:327–31.

Kanner L (1943) Autistic disturbances of affective contact. *Nervous Child*, 2, 217–250.

Kielinen M, Linna SL, Moilanen I (2000) Autism in Northern Finland. *European Child and Adolescent Psychiatry* 9:162–7.

Lord C, Rutter M (1994) Autism and pervasive developmental disorders. In Rutter M, Taylor E, Hersov L (Eds) *Child and Adolescent Psychiatry. Modern Approaches (3rd ed)* (pp. 569–93). Oxford: Blackwell.

Lotter V (1966) Epidemiology of autistic conditions in young children. *Social Psychiatry* 1: 124–137.

Lotter V (1978) Childhood autism in Africa. *Journal of Child Psychology and Psychiatry* 19: 231–244.

Magnusson P, Saemundsen E (2001) Prevalence of autism in Iceland. *Journal of Autism and Developmental Disorders* 31:153–63.

Matsuishi T, Shiotsuki Y, Yoshimura K, Shoji H, Imuta F, Yamashita F (1987) High prevalence of infantile autism in Kurume City, Japan. *Journal of Child Neurology* 2:268–271.

McCarthy P, Fitzgerald M, Smith MA (1984) Prevalence of childhood autism in Ireland. *Irish Medical Journal* 77:129–130.

Olsson I, Steffenburg S, Gillberg C (1988) Epilepsy in autism and autistic-like conditions: a population-based study. *Archives of Neurology* 45:666–668.

Powell JE, Edwards A, Edwards M, Pandit BS, Sungum-Paliwal SR, Whitehouse W (2000) Changes in the incidence of childhood autism and other autistic spectrum disorders in preschool children from two areas of the West Midlands, UK. *Developmental Medicine and Child Neurology* 42:624–628.

Ritvo ER, Jorde LB, Mason-Brothers A, Freeman BJ, Pingree C, Jones MB, McMahon WM, Petersen PB, Jenson WR, Mo A (1989) The UCLA-University of Utah epidemiologic survey of autism: recurrence risk estimates and genetic counseling. *American Journal of Psychiatry* 146:1032–1036.

Rutter M (1967) Psychotic disorders in early childhood. In Coppen A, Walk A (Eds) *Recent developments in schizophrenia. British Journal of Psychiatry. Special Publication* (pp. 133–58). Ashford, Kent: Headley Bros.

Rutter M (1970) Autistic children: infancy to adulthood. *Seminars in Psychiatry* 2:435–450.

Rutter M (1978) Diagnosis and definition. In Rutter M, Schopler E (Eds) *Autism. A Reappraisal of Concepts and Treatment* (pp. 1–25). New York: Plenum Press.

Scott FJ, Baron-Cohen S, Bolton P, Brayne C (2002) Brief report: prevalence of autism spectrum conditions in children aged 5–11 years in Cambridgeshire, UK. *Autism* 6: 231–237.

Sponheim E, Skjeldal O (1998) Autism and related disorders: epidemiological findings in a Norwegian study using ICD-10 diagnostic criteria. *Journal of Autism and Developmental Disorders* 28:217–227.

Steffenburg S, Gillberg C (1986) Autism and autistic-like conditions in Swedish rural and urban areas: a population study. *British Journal of Psychiatry* 149:81–87.

Steffenburg S, Gillberg C, Steffenburg U (1996) Psychiatric disorders in children and adolescents with mental retardation and active epilepsy. *Archives of Neurology* 53:904–912.

Steffenburg S, Steffenburg U, Gillberg C (2003) Autism spectrum disorders in children with active epilepsy and learning disability: comorbidity, pre- and perinatal background and seizure characteristics. *Developmental Medicine and Child Neurology* 45: 724–730.

Steinhausen HC, Gobel D, Breinlinger M, Wohlleben B (1986) A community survey of infantile autism. *Journal of the American Academy of Child Psychiatry* 25:186–189.

Strömland K, Nordin V, Miller M, Åkerström B, Gillberg C (1994) Autism in thalidomide embryopathy: A population study. *Developmental Medicine and Child Neurology* 36: 351–356.

Sugiyama T, Abe T (1989) The prevalence of autism in Nagoya, Japan: a total population study. *Journal of Autism and Developmental Disorders* 19:87–96.

Tanoue Y, Oda S, Asano F, Kawashima K (1988) Epidemiology of infantile autism in southern Ibaraki, Japan: differences in prevalence in birth cohorts. *Journal of Autism Developmental Disorders* 18:155–166.

Taylor RB, Wennberg RA, Lozano AM, Sharpe JA (2000) Central nystagmus induced by deep-brain stimulation for epilepsy. *Epilepsia* 41:1637–1641.

Treffert DA (1970) Epidemiology of infantile autism. *Archives of General Psychiatry* 22:431–438.

Volkmar FR, Nelson DS (1990) Seizure disorders in autism. *Journal of the American Academy of Child and Adolescent Psychiatry* 29:127–129.

Webb EV, Lobo S, Hervas A, Scourfield J, Fraser WI (1997) The changing prevalence of autistic disorder in a Welsh health district. *Developmental Medicine and Child Neurology* 39:150–152.

Webb E, Morey J, Thompsen W, Butler C, Barber M, Fraser WI (2003) Prevalence of autistic spectrum disorder in children attending mainstream schools in a Welsh education authority. *Developmental Medicine and Child Neurology* 45:377–384.

Wing L. (1996) *The Autism Spectrum.* London: Constable

Wing L, Gould J (1979) Severe impairments of social interaction and associated abnormalities in children: epidemiology and classification. *Journal of Autism and Developmental Disorders* 9:11–29

Yeargin-Allsopp M, Rice C, Karapurkar T, Doernberg N, Boyle C, Murphy C (2003) Prevalence of autism in a US metropolitan area. *JAMA* 289:49–55.

Chapter 7

Disease Entities with a Temporary Autistic Phase: The Autistic Features of Rett Syndrome

Yoshiko Nomura

Autism can be defined as a syndrome, with specific symptom complexes involving mainly psychobehavioral and mental deviations that have heterogeneous etiologies (Gillberg & Coleman 2000a; Rapin 2002). Thus, autistic spectrum disorders can be differentiated based on their biological etiologies. Although the most commonly observed category is *autistic disorder* (sometimes referred to as early infantile autism, childhood autism, or Kanner's autism) (*DSM-IV* 1994), autistic symptoms are observed in other disorders, which include Rett syndrome (RTT), fragile X syndrome, Angelman's syndrome, tuberous sclerosis, other genetic and certain acquired conditions (Rett 1977; Hagberg et al. 1983; Nomura et al. 1984; Zappella 1985; Olsson 1987; Tranebjaerg & Kure 1991; Tuchman et al. 1991; Nordin & Gillberg 1996a,b; Mazzocco et al. 1998; Gillberg & Coleman 2000b,c; Veiga & Toralles 2002; Mount et al. 2003a,b).

The essential features of autistic disorder are characterized by markedly abnormal or impaired development in social interaction and communication, and a markedly restricted repertoire of activity and interests, that emerge during infancy or early childhood (*DSM-IV*). The autistic features seen in the disorders mentioned above sometimes do not meet the full diagnostic criteria for autism but manifest them only transiently in the course of the disorder, as seen in RTT, or they may only meet part of the criteria, as observed in most patients with fragile X syndrome. In this chapter, the autistic symptoms observed in RTT are delineated, and the pathophysiology of such symptoms is discussed in reference to Kanner's autism.

The autistic behaviors of RTT are consistent in most patients but manifested transiently during the early stage of its clinical course. Furthermore, some features seen in RTT seem to differ from Kanner's autism in their character and the clinical course. This suggests that, despite the phenotypical similarities, the underlying pathophysiological mechanisms or the neuronal networks responsible for the each characteristic symptom are different between RTT and Kanner's autism.

RETT SYNDROME (RTT)

In 1966, Andreas Rett first described RTT (Rett 1966a,b; 1969), which caused great interest because of the syndrome's unique clinical features and pathophysiology. The characteristic symptoms and signs of RTT occur in an age-dependent manner and consist of autistic tendency, hypotonia of antigravity muscles, delayed or abnormal locomotion in infancy followed by stereotyped hand movements with loss of the purposeful hand use, dystonic increase of the muscle tone, scoliosis, mental retardation, abnormal respiratory pattern, and epilepsy

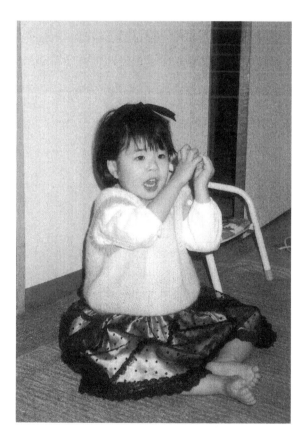

Figure 7.1   Wringing of the hands seen in Rett syndrome is a stereotypy. This 3-year-old girl has an R168X mutation of the MECP2 gene.

from early to later childhood (Rett 1977; Hagberg 1980; Hagberg et al. 1983; Nomura et al. 1984). Each of these symptoms changes along the course of the syndrome; for example, the pattern of hand stereotypy goes from simple to complex and then to simple and slow again as the patients grew older (Nomura et al. 1984; Nomura & Segawa 1990a). Based on these clinical characteristics, some diagnostic criteria have been proposed (Hagberg et al. 1985; The Rett Syndrome Diagnostic Criteria Work Group 1988; *DSM-IV*; *ICD-10*).

As for the onset of the symptoms of RTT, in the diagnostic criteria shown in 1985 by Hagberg et al., it was stressed that the child is normal for the first 6 to 18 months, and in those of *DSM-IV*, the child is normal for the first 5 months. However, we have noted that the autistic symptoms and hypotonia of the postural muscles are present even from early infancy, and that RTT is a neurodevelopmental disorder with its onset very early in infancy (Nomura et al. 1984; Nomura & Segawa 1990b; Nomura & Segawa 2001).

We also have suggested that the autistic symptoms and hypotonia of the postural muscles might be pathognomonic symptoms of RTT, indicating the involvement of the monoaminergic neurons of the brainstem and the midbrain (Nomura et al. 1984, 1985; Nomura & Segawa 2001). The monoaminergic neurons of the brainstem and the midbrain, with the axons projecting to the various levels of the higher neuronal system that are hierarchically arranged, play important roles in functional maturation of the higher neuronal system by modulating the synaptogenesis in an age-dependent manner (Morrison et al. 1984; Segawa 2001c) and are also considered candidate neurons for the pathogenesis of autism (Segawa 1982, 1998). It is postulated that the age-dependent occurrence of the particular symptoms observed in both RTT and Kanner's autism is based on early dysfunction of these neurons. The discovery of the causative gene for RTT, methyl-CpG-binding protein 2 (*MECP2*) (Amir et al. 1999), presents a further basis for exploring the pathophysiology of this disorder (Wan et al. 1999).

AUTISTIC FEATURES OF RTT

In his initial report, Andreas Rett called the disorder "cerebral atrophy associated with hyperammonaemia," and mentioned "hypomimia or amimia (lack of facial expression) and alalia (lack of speech)" as main symptoms, in addition to "hyperammonaemia, stereotyped movement patterns in arms and hands, enhanced reflex activity, spastic increase in tone, gait apraxia, tendency to cerebral convulsive attacks, high grade of mental retardation, gynaecotropy (only females), and progression of the disease" (Rett 1977). He also described the modulation of the autistic symptoms with age as follows.

> Smiling initially developed in a fairly normal manner, although it was impossible to relate this to environmental events. After third year, however, there was only sporadic smiling, usually very short lived and apparently unmotivated. Even during

the initial stage of disease when these children were able to respond to affective stimuli with appropriate mimicry, this capacity was gradually lost as the disease progressed. Thus facial expression is diminished and in the later stages lost entirely. In some older children, a mask-like face is present. (Rett 1977, 309, 311)

Although Rett did not use the term "autism" in his earlier essay, the features "hypomimia or amimia, and alalia," which describe the lack of the responsiveness to environments, and the lack of development of speech indicate the autistic feature as part of the main symptoms in RTT.

In 1978, independently from Andreas Rett, Ishikawa et al. described 3 interesting cases as "A new syndrome (?) of progressive psychomotor deterioration with peculiar stereotyped movement and autistic tendency: a report of three cases" in a short abstract form (Ishikawa et al. 1978). These cases are thought to be RTT cases.

Hagberg et al. (1983) reported 35 cases with the title of "A progressive syndrome of autism, dementia, ataxia, and loss of purposeful hand use in girls: Rett's syndrome." It was mentioned that the stagnation of developmental acquisitions occurred after normal development during the first 7 to 18 months, and a rapid deterioration of behavior and mental status followed, resulting in marked dementia to profound imbecility associated with severe autistic behavior within less than 18 months. The syndrome was further described as follows.

> The patients showed no sustained interest in persons or objects, although they were able to see and to visually follow them. Their responses to environmental stimuli were stereotypic, and interpersonal contact was either absent or very limited. All patients manifested great anxiety and apparent fear when confronted with an unfamiliar situation, or even without evident stimulation. (Hagberg et al. 1983, 473)

It was also pointed out that "spontaneous motor activity was stereotypic and monotonous," and that "in many patients, teeth grinding, facial grimacing, and other stereotypic motions were observed" (475). It was further mentioned that "There was no parallel between the severity of the motor disability and the degree of dementia and autism. Autistic traits in fact became less prominent in most of the patients followed to at least the age of 15 years than they had been during the initial phase of the disorder."

Olsson and Rett (1990) pointed out that the diagnosis of autism in RTT was thought to arise from the features of total aloofness, almost complete gaze and hearing avoidance, and a lack of means to communicate.

Thus, the autistic feature is considered to be one of the cardinal symptoms of RTT that appeared from very beginning of the description of this disorder.

As for the timing of the onset of autistic behaviors in RTT, it had been stressed that onset is rather acute and occurs in midinfancy to early childhood after seemingly normal development (Rett 1977; Hagberg et al. 1983). However, autistic behavior appears insidiously from early in infancy, with a delay in the development of sleep-wake (S-W) rhythm and an abnormality of postural muscle tone being the earliest signs of RTT (Nomura et al. 1984; Nomura & Segawa 1990b).

We conducted careful evaluation of the early behavioral characteristics of RTT by using the battery of the behavioral checklists that have been used widely in Japan to check the autistic behaviors in infancy and early childhood (table 7-1). Our results revealed the following (Nomura & Segawa 1990b): All the autistic behavioral abnormalities, with the exception of two behaviors, seen before 1 year of age were observed in more than half of the cases. "Lack of following" was present in the highest frequency, in over 80% of RTT children. The characteristic symptoms of "pervasive lack of social association," such as "aloneness or indifference," "expressionless face," and "lack of anticipatory motor adjustment" were present in approximately two thirds of the cases. The two less frequently observed behaviors were "hyposensitivity to sound" and "lack of stranger anxiety," which were seen in only a third of the cases. The autistic behaviors seen in after 1 year

Table 7-1   Checklists of Autistic Behavior

Abnormal behavior before 1 year old

    Lack of social smiling
    Hypersensitivity to sound
    Hyposensitivity to sound
    Lack of babbling
    Lack of stranger anxiety
    Aloneness or indifference
    Lack of following
    No response to calling
    Expressionless face
    No response to peek-a-boo
    Lack of anticipatory motor adjustment
    Lack of eye-to-eye contact

Abnormal behavior after 1 year old

    Never uses finger pointing
    Speech delay
    Loss of verbal expression
    Difficulty copying movements made by other people
    Autostimulation behavior
    Extreme withdrawal
    Dislikes any intervention while playing
    No symbolic play
    Insistence on sameness
    Hyperactivity
    Sudden laughing and crying without any apparent reason
    Irregular and disturbed nocturnal sleep

of age also were observed in various frequencies in the cases with RTT; "speech delay" and "no symbolic play" were observed in 100% of the cases, "never uses finger pointing" and "difficulty in copying movements made by other people" in 90%, "loss of verbal expression," "autostimulation," and "sudden laughing and crying without any apparent reason" in approximately two thirds of the cases, "extreme withdrawal" and "insistence on sameness" in 50%, and "hyperactivity" and "irregular and disturbed nocturnal sleep" in less than 50%. Thus, our study showed that the autistic features are the initial symptoms to be present from early infancy in RTT, which may be very subtle and often unnoticed (Nomura et al. 1984; Nomura & Segawa 1990 a,b). The earliest autistic features consist of "being very quiet, sleeping longer, and responding less to environmental stimulation," and because of these features, the infant appears to be "a good baby" instead of having any suspected underlying disorder.

Gillberg studied the early signs of RTT by using a questionnaire originally developed to evaluate early symptoms in infantile autism. Considerable overlap between early symptoms in RTT and infantile autism was seen, although clear differentiating features already were present in the first few years of life (Gillberg 1987).

It has been mentioned that in spite of the severe social withdrawal, active bodily turning away does not seem to be present in RTT (Olsson & Rett 1985).

The autistic features appearing in early childhood, particularly in the regressive stage of RTT, are marked. They are almost pervasive and complete before 2 years of age (Zappella 1985; Gillberg 1986).

Hagberg and Witt-Engerström classified the clinical course of RTT into stagings 1 to 4, and pointed out that the autistic features appear in stage 1, at ½–1½ years of age, as "changes in communication, eye contact, unspecified personality deviation and diminishing play interest," in stage 2, at 1–4 years of age, as "severe dementia" overcoming the autistic features, and in stage 3, during the preschool-early school years, as "not a major problem." Thus, the autistic symptoms appear during stage 1 and are followed by severe dementia and become less noticeable in stage 2; emotional contact improving in stage 3 (Hagberg & Witt-Engerström 1986).

Hence, the appearance of autistic features in early stage of RTT and its modulation with age have been pointed out by various authors, who also noted that, in RTT, the autistic traits are later accompanied by a high degree of developmental retardation (Rett 1977; Hagberg et al. 1983; Nomura et al. 1984; Olsson & Rett 1985; Gillberg 1986; Witt-Engerström & Gillberg 1987; Witt-Engerström 1992).

CHARACTERISTICS OF AUTISTIC FEATURES OF RTT IN CONTRAST TO KANNER'S AUTISM

According to the *DSM-IV*, pervasive developmental disorders (PPD) are characterized by pervasive impairment in several areas of development, which include reciprocal social interaction skills, communication skills, and the presence of stereotyped behavior, interests, and activities.

These three characteristics are seen in RTT. However, associated behavioral symptoms, such as hyperactivity, aggressiveness, or self-injurious behaviors are seen in only a few patients with RTT. Peculiar responses to sensory stimuli, such as high threshold to pain stimulation, are seen with some girls with RTT. Based on the clinical characteristics, it has been suggested that RTT represents a qualitative subtype of autism (Olsson & Rett 1985, 1987, 1990; Gillberg 1986, 1987, 1989).

In early childhood, particularly above the age of 1 year, children with RTT are often diagnosed as autistic owing to stereotyped movements, poor interaction with their social environments, and smiling or laughing without apparent reasons; sometimes it is not possible to differentiate RTT from other autistic syndromes. Very often the initial diagnosis of infantile autism/childhood psychosis before 2 years of age turns out to be RTT (Witt-Engerström & Gillberg 1987). In particular, the deterioration of a number of RTT patients was erroneously diagnosed as autism (Buccino & Weddell 1989).

However, there are differences between the behavior manifested by RTT and infantile autism patients; in RTT, a profound regression of motor, as well as verbal skills, occurs with the passage of years, whereas infantile autism does not result in motor impairment (Olsson & Rett 1987). The differential diagnosis must be based on the evaluation of both motor and behavioral skills.

Percy et al. (1988, 1990) have reported qualitative and quantitative differences in the autistic features of RTT and infantile autism. RTT appears to fulfill the Rendle-Short criteria for the diagnosis of autism, but the pattern of the behavior is qualitatively different from that exhibited by children with autism; that is, RTT patients exhibit ataxia, breath-holding, hyperventilation, bruxism, simplicity of stereotypies, and hand apposition, while children with autism demonstrate complex stereotypies and verbal but not motor regression. The more typical features of autism, namely, poor eye-to-eye contact, lack of sustained interest, speech disturbance, and repetitive truncal rocking motions were poor discriminators between the two groups. Percy et al. (1988) also stressed the necessity of analysis of the motor-behavioral features to reach to the correct diagnosis.

Mazzocco et al. (1998) attempted to delineate clinical similarities and differences between RTT and Kanner's autism based on the criteria of DSM-III-R. They noted that RTT patients fulfilled the criteria of the onset before the end of second year of life—disturbance of social interaction with poor environmental contact, no language and senseless sounds—but that they did not show discomfort in response to changes in daily schedules or environment, which are dramatic in Kanner's autism. They, too, mentioned a difference in motor symptoms, that is, the stereotypy with loss of purposeful hand use is particular for RTT. The authors also thought that in spite of their inability to interact with the environment, RTT patients try to communicate.

Full-blown symptoms appear at 2–3 years of age in Kanner's autism, but in RTT, other neurological symptoms and profound dementia become obvious after 2 years of age. When compared to Kanner's autism and organic brain damage that occurs in infancy, RTT is characterized by definite signs of dementia with almost overall developmental retardation that is more profound than in any other autistic syndrome, and RTT patients do not show several attributes regularly found in autistic children (Olsson & Rett 1985).

As to the outcome of the autistic features of RTT, it is said that either they improve or are masked by the following profound dementia. The possibility of later improvement of autistic features in RTT has been discussed as the point of differentiation from Kanner's autism, but Gillberg et al. (1990a) pointed out that they were not inclined to agree with that, because the autistic behavior also improves in Kanner's autism. Gillberg (1989) described 4 girls and 1 boy with PDD who met the *DSM-III-R* criteria for autistic disorder and also all showed the essential symptoms of RTT and stated that the symptomatic similarities might come from common pathophysiological abnormalities at the brainstem level.

Gillberg et al. (1990b) also reported an interesting family with 1 individual with RTT and 2 with autism. The affected family members were females and second cousins, and, in those three, RTT, autism with mild ataxia and autism with profound mental retardation occurred separately. The authors suggested that considerable overlap between the two disorders occurs, that a possible pathophysiological association between autism and RTT exits, and that these diseases may be closely related genetic disorders or may constitute relatively homogeneous phenotypes with several possible etiologies.

Thus, the autistic feature and its age-dependent modification seem to be distinctive between RTT and autism and may reflect the differences in the involved aminergic neurons, a subject that is discussed later in this chapter in the section entitled "Pathophysiological considerations of the autistic feature in RTT." Differences also appear in neurological findings, sleep parameters, and also in neuropathological findings.

NEUROLOGICAL FINDINGS IN THE EARLY STAGE OF RTT

The neurological characteristics of RTT in early infancy reveal hypotonia of the postural or antigravity muscles and abnormality in locomotion as in autism. However, in RTT these characteristics are more severe and present as a delay in rolling over in more than half of patients and abnormalities in crawling in almost all patients. The abnormality of the crawling consisted of either never having crawled, delayed in attaining crawling, or an abnormal pattern with total flexure posture (Nomura et al. 1984, 1987; Nomura & Segawa 1990a; Segawa 2001a). There is a discrepancy in locomotion in RTT, that is, though they can not crawl, RTT patients can walk. The gait, however, is abnormal, with wide-based posture, rocking of the trunk from side to side, and no coordinated movement of the upper extremities. This gait disturbance is an abnormality in locomotion but not gait apraxia. The rocking of the trunk is not a sign of ataxia, because without this children can not advance the gait forward. RTT patients, as well as patients with autism, can walk better on their toes (Segawa 2001a). This implicates that the abnormal locomotion of RTT is due to abnormal hypofunctioning of the brainstem aminergic neurons, which control the locomotion center in spinal cord level by sending descending projections (Miller & van der Burg 1973). These neurons are affected in both disease entities, but more severely in RTT.

The different age-dependent appearance of characteristic neurological symptoms and signs in RTT compared to autism suggests a difference in the involvement of aminergic neurons in these disorders.

EVALUATION OF SLEEP PARAMETERS AND SLEEP-WAKE (S-W) RHYTHM IN RTT

The S-W rhythm in RTT is abnormal, as is also seen in autism. However, in contrast to autism, children with RTT have a delay in decrement of the daytime sleep from late infancy to childhood, and they attain circadian S-W rhythm in infancy, although it is delayed.

Polysomnography (PSG) has revealed normal development of the parameters of REM sleep stage (sREM) that mature before the 36th week of gestation, but abnormal or failed development of the sleep parameters that occur during the critical period of development, from 4 months to 6 months. These abnormalities are the leakage of atonia of sREM into nonREM (NREM) sleep and the cooccurrence of twitch movements (TMs) of the mentalis muscle and rapid eye movements (Kohyama et al. 2001; Segawa et al. 1987). The former implicates abnormalities of the serotonergic (5HT) neurons modulating the antigravity muscles, and the latter of the noradrenergic (NA) neurons (Segawa et al. 1987).

In RTT, the numbers of TMs of the mentalis muscle, which are modulated by nigrostriatal dopaminergic (DA) system, decrease before 6 years of age and increase above 6 years of age (Nomura & Segawa 1986). These features and age variations are similar to those observed in autism. However, in RTT, these modulations of DA activities appear to be more marked and are correlated to the clinical symptoms, that is, increase in muscle tone and development of the characteristic stereotyped movement following loss of purposeful hand use (Segawa 2001a).

DIFFERENCES BETWEEN THE MORPHOLOGY OF THE BRAINS OF RTT AND AUTISTIC PATIENTS

The so-called acquired microcephalus in RTT represents the stagnation of the cranial circumference starting in late infancy. This pattern of the head growth reflects some devastating changes that take place in the brain development of

RTT at this period. This is in contrast to the cranial size of autistic patients, which is said to be large, particularly in children younger than 12 years of age (Bailey et al. 1993; Piven et al. 1996, 1997; Courchesne et al. 2003).

Neuropathological findings of RTT are also informative. The brain weight is not greater than that of normal 1-year-old children. There are no findings suggesting malformation or neuronal degeneration. Decreased amounts of the melanin pigments in substantia nigra seem to be the consistent findings (Jellinger & Seitelberger 1986; Jellinger et al. 1988; Armstrong 1992). Neither consistent cell loss or atrophy, nor apparent abnormality in myelin, are found. Reduced size of the individual neurons has been demonstrated, with increased cell-packing density throughout the cortical and subcortical regions and particularly in the medial temporal lobe and hippocampus, most prominently in CA4 and CA3 (Kemper & Bauman 1998). Furthermore, the findings seem to correlate with the clinical severities. It also has been shown that, in the cerebellum, Purkinje cells are reduced in the number, but the cerebellar vermis and deep cerebellar nuclei are normal. The changes in the inferior olivery nucleus were not consistent among the cases; no retrograde cell loss was identified but folds were simplified. The lack of glial hyperplasia and absence of retrograde cell loss in olivery nucleus, which are characteristic of postnatal insult, suggest lesions are acquired early in the development (Bauman et al. 1995; Bauman 1996).

Armstrong (Armstrong 1992, 2001; Armstrong et al. 1995, 1998) showed reduced arborization of basal dendrites of the pyramidal neurons of the layer 3 and 5 in the frontal, motor, and inferior temporal regions of the cerebral cortex, and of layer 4 of the subiculum. The arborization of apical dendrites of layer 5 of the motor cortex was also reduced, while those of the hippocampal and the occipital regions rather were spared. These reductions of dendritic branching suggested reduced synaptic input. This was confirmed by Belichenko and Dahlstrom (1995) using confocal laser scanning microscopy. Belichenco et al. (1996, 1997) showed decreased synapses in the speech area 4, 45, 22, 40 by the decrease of synaptophysin staining.

Abnormalities of other specific proteins and neurotransmitters have been studied to elucidate the pathogenic mechanism of RTT. The substantia nigra of RTT showed a decrease in tyrosine hydroxylase (TH) activities without glial cell infiltration (Itoh & Takashima 2002), which is similar to the abnormalities observed in the neuron after cytotoxic lesion of the pedunculopontine nuclei (PPN) (Kojima et al. 1997). Besides these, abnormalities of the NMDA receptors in the basal ganglia and the cortex that show alteration with age have been identified (Johnston et al. 2001).

These neuropathological findings in RTT reflect a maturational curtailment rather than a degenerative process (Bauman et al. 1995). Furthermore, they reveal that the brain of RTT is not one of simple developmental arrest, but rather one that undergoes selective and specific changes in particular regions during critical periods of maturation (Armstrong 2001).

In regard to the neuropathological findings of Kanner's autism, relatively few studies have been performed and the results have been inconsistent. In contrast to RTT, Kemper and Bauman (1998) showed that, in autism, selective and severe abnormalities in the forebrain were confined to the limbic system, hippocampal field CA1-4, subiculum, entorhinal cortex, mammillary body, several nuclei of the amygdala, and septal nucleus; these abnormalities included reduced size of the individual neuron with increased packing density. In the CA1 and CA4 area of hippocampus and the entorhinal cortex, neurons were small with decreased dendritic branches (Raymond et al. 1996).

In autism, the cerebellum is characterized by fewer Purkinje cells than are present in the cerebellum of control subjects. The deep cerebellar nuclei, which have no neuronal connection to the affected Purkinje cells, appeared hypertrophic in childhood and then became atrophic by adulthood. Kemper and Bauman (1998) commented that the neuropathological changes of autism originate in the prenatal period, with the process continuing into adult life.

Bauman (1996) reviewed the neuropathology of autism and RTT, and reported a distinct RTT pathology compared to autism. However, the reduced size of the neurons and increased cell-packing, particularly in the medial temporal lobe, cerebellar, and olive, were present both in RTT and Kanner's autism, and the marked reduction in Purkinje cell number seen in the posterior inferior region of the cerebellar hemisphere was observed in RTT, as well as in autism. Bauman et al. (1995) suggested that the presence in RTT of neuronal abnormalities that are similar to those that occur in autism might explain the early appearance of autism-like features in RTT.

PATHOPHYSIOLOGICAL CONSIDERATIONS OF AUTISTIC FEATURES IN RTT

The autistic features of RTT are present from early in infancy and are character-ized by poor response to environmental stimulation. In early childhood, these behavioral characteristics become associated with lack of communication and stereotyped movements. Here, stereotyped movement means rocking the body back and forth, not the hand movement characterized in RTT (Nomura et al. 1984; Nomura & Segawa 1990a; Segawa 2001a). However, with age, severe mental retardation and motor symptoms, the pathognomonic pattern of the stereotypy and underlying dystonic posture, come to the foreground, and autistic behaviors become unremarkable in RTT (Nomura et al. 1984; Nomura & Segawa 1990a; Segawa 2001a).

Neurological findings suggest similarities and differences between the respon-sible neurons and their neuronal systems in RTT and autism. In both RTT and autism, characteristic neurological abnormalities and symptoms appear in infancy and early childhood. These neurological findings suggest lesions in the brainstem and midbrain. However, the difficulties in closing eyes or mouth on command (orofacial apraxia), and in pronation/supination movement of the arm (limbkinetic apraxia), seen in autism imply the abnormalities in development of functional specialization of the cortex are not observed in RTT. The speech disturbance in autism that is echolalia and pronominal reversals, and the delay in determination of hand dominancy that suggests a delay in the hemispheric lateralization, are characteristic features of autism; these are not observed in RTT patients. This suggests the profound involvement of the cortex in RTT.

The circadian S-W rhythm develops by 4 months of age, and atonia of the mental muscle also begins to appear only in REM sleep (sREM) at approximately this month of age. From 4 months of age, arrangement of day sleeping starts and it appears once each in the morning and the afternoon at approximately the 7th month and once in the afternoon at approximately one and half years of age. The time spent sleeping during the day gradually decreases with age. This is controlled by the brainstem aminergic neurons, particularly the serotonergic (5HT) neurons specific for each sleep parameter (Segawa 1980, 2003).

Thus, the abnormality in the development of the circadian S-W rhythm and the presence of the atonic NREM in autism suggests hypofunction of 5HT neurons, which mature by 4 months of age, and abnormalities of the day sleeping organization and atonic NREM in RTT indicate a disturbance of neurons that mature at approximately 4 months of age and later. Experiments on rodents reveal that disturbance of the development of the circadian S-W rhythm, as well as early lesion in the 5HT neurons cause failure in social relationship, adaptation of the novel environment, and cognitive function after maturation.

In autism, improvement of the abnormal S-W cycle helps induce determination of hand dominancy and, if it occurs in early childhood, improves language development. This suggests that human development of the circadian S-W in early infancy has importance for development of the functional lateralization of the cortex.

Another experiment using rodents showed that early lesion of noradrenergic (NA) neurons causes failure in head growth (Brenner et al. 1983). It is interesting that the NA neurons have no axonal projection to the occipital lobe. This may simulate the stagnation of the head growth in RTT, in which disturbance of the dendritic formation is mild or spared in the occipital cortex (Armstrong 2001). Enhanced rote memory is due to the lesion of the dorsal bundle of the locus coeruleus to the forebrain, that is, loss of the dorsal bundle extinction effect (Tanaka et al. 1987). This might be related to the insistence on sameness and be part of the difficulty in adjusting to novel environments. These features are observed in autism but not in RTT. This suggests a difference of the involved NA neurons in these disorders.

The neuronal system controlling atonia in sREM is also the system inhibiting posture (Mori et al. 1992) and is enhanced by carbachol and inhibited by 5HT or NA. Neurons of the 5HT and NA types enhance the postural control and help make locomotion possible. Atonic NREM implies hypofunctioning of the brainstem aminergic neurons, particularly 5HT neurons, which prevent the leakage of the atonia of sREM into NREM sleep, and abnormalities of the neurons or neuronal systems involving in the posture and locomotion.

The importance of locomotion in the pathophysiology of RTT appears in the neuropathological findings of the substantia nigra, which are thought to be caused by dysfunction of the PPN. The hypofunction of the DA neuron is shown by the results of PSG studies (Nomura et al. 1984; Nomura & Segawa 1986).

The number of TMs of the mentalis muscle, which reflect the activities of nigrostriatal DA neurons, decrease in early childhood, while they increase in later ages. This suggests a decrease in the DA activities followed by exaggeration of the transmission, which could be explained by the occurrence of the DA receptor upward regulation (Nomura & Segawa 1986, 2001; Segawa & Nomura 1990, 1992). This may cause dysfunction of the basal ganglia and developing dystonic hypertonus via its descending output, as well as loss of purposeful hand use by the dysfunctioning supplementary motor area (SMA) and the premotor cortex via the ascending pathway through the thalamus. The appearance of the DA receptor supersensitivity may cause the development of stereotyped hand movement and regression of higher cortical function through dysfunctional feedback from the frontal cortex.

PSG of autism implies a similar modulation of the DA neurons exist in autism. However, this abnormality may involve mainly the limbic DA neurons. Thus, as for the PPN, those neurons projecting to the DA neurons of the ventral tegmental area may be affected predominantly with development of receptor supersensitivity. This abnormality causes hyperkinesia and stereotypy and also aggressiveness or panic state, with hypofunctioning of the 5HT and the NA neurons. This is shown in experiments on rats with 5HT and NA neuron lesions and is associated with enhanced DA transmission that resulted in the grooming of mice (friendliness) in a comfortable situation but the killing of mice (muricide) in an isolated situation, in spite of the fact that mice are not a source of food for rats (Valzelli & Garattini 1972). Similar conditions lead rats to the unexpected aggressive behavior toward their peers (S. Ueda, personal communication, 2003).

Experimental results also suggest differences of the involved aminergic neurons between RTT and autism (Segawa 1979, 2001a, 2001b).

THE CAUSATIVE GENE FOR RTT, METHYL-CPG-BINDING PROTEIN 2 (*MECP2*), AND AUTISTIC FEATURES OF RTT

Since *MECP2* was identified as the causative gene for RTT in 1999, extensive studies regarding not only the role of *MECP2* as the etiology of RTT (Hoffbuhr et al. 2001), but also the role of *MECP2* in the normal development of the brain have been in progress (Samaco et al. 2004). *MECP2* binds to single CpG base pairs via a methyl binding domain, recruits histone deacetylase via a transcription repression domain, and silences methylated chromatin. The defects in *MECP2* might affect specific target genes and lead to excessive transcription of certain genes at specific areas and specific time. *MECP2* is expressed ubiquitously but most highly in the brain and particularly in nuclei of neuronal cells. Developmentally, it shows dramatic changes in its expression.

Mutations in *MECP2* are found in approximately 80% of classic RTT cases (Bienvenu et al. 2000). Mutations in *MECP2* are also found in various clinical conditions. Those include mild learning disability, mild mental retardation, autism in females, and mental retardation X-linked to severe neonatal encephalopathy in males (Lam et al. 2000; Orrico et al. 2000; Hammer et al. 2002, 2003; Zoghbi 2003). Among *MECP2* negative cases with phenotypical similarities to RTT, mutations of CDKL5 (cyclin-dependent kinase-like 5) have been reported recently (Tao et al. 2004; Weaving et al. 2004).

In addition to the mutational pattern and the location of the mutation, X chromosome inactivation patterns also contribute to the heterogeneity of the clinical manifestations of RTT (Amir et al. 2000). A study was done on the preserved-speech variant group of RTT, a mild RTT variant that is also the allelic to RTT (De Bona et al. 2000) and in which autistic behavior is common. Zappella et al. (2003) reported 2 preserved speech patients (R133C and R453X) who initially developed the first three stages of the staging by Hagberg and Witt-Eugerstrom (1986) and were severely retarded with autistic behavior, but later improved to an IQ of 45 and lost autistic features. Thus, Zappella et al. (2003) suggested that *MECP2* mutations can be found in the RTT girls with an IQ of 45 and a clinical history of preserved speech, but *MECP2* mutations are not found in those whose autism remains stable many years.

Autism cases without Rett features were examined for a mutation in *MECP2*, the results were negative (Vourc'h et al. 2001; Zappella et al. 2003). This tended to confirm that autism and RTT are distinct disease entities, as predicted from the clinical analysis. Brain samples from persons with autism, pervasive developmental disorder, and Prader-Willi and Angelman syndromes were studied and showed significant differences in *MECP2* expression from age-matched controls caused by different transcriptional and posttranscriptional mechanisms; this raised the question of defective developmental expression in autism spectrum disorders in addition to RTT (Samaco et al. 2004). Recent studies of *MECP2* mutations in autism, schizophrenia, and other psychiatric diseases showed a higher frequency of missense and 3'-UTR variants in autism. These results suggest a possible association between *MECP2* mutations and autism (Shibayama et al. 2004).

The reason why autistic features were stressed in RTT is because the pathophysiology of both RTT and Kanner's autism share part of the complex pathophysiological mechanisms during the maturation of the nervous system. However, the role of *MECP2* and its putative target genes in relation to autism behaviors have not yet been identified. On the other hand, molecular or cytogenetic research in autism have provided other molecular bases of autism, such as candidate chromosomal abnormalities (e.g., extra copies of 15q11-q13) (Thomas et al. 2003) and autism loci, including the *UBE3A* and *ATP10C* genes (Kashiwagi et al. 2003).

CONCLUSION

RTT and Kanner's autism share phenotypic characteristics in the early stage of the development. The earliest autistic features that are usually very subtle and overlooked are "quietness and sleeping longer in daytime" from early infancy. These are present in both disorders; however, they have not been emphasized in most of the literature. In late infancy to early childhood, full-blown autistic features develop in both disorders, although there are some qualitative and quantitative differences.

Neurophysiological evaluation of RTT suggests that its pathophysiology lies in the hypofunction of the 5HT neuron followed by DA receptor upward regulation and later involves abnormal higher neuronal systems. The age-dependent appearance of the pathognomonic symptoms in RTT and Kanner's autism implies the significant roles of monoaminergic systems, which send axon to and modulate the synaptogenesis of the higher neuronal systems arranged hierarchically. Neuropathological studies have shown no degenerative changes in RTT brain but have revealed developmental curtailment occurring during the early period of brain maturation. The causative gene of RTT, *MECP2*, was found, but its exact mechanism remains to be clarified. The role of *MECP2* in the pathophysiology of autism also presents an interesting issue to explore, because *MECP2* shows specific spatial and temporal appearance in the brain throughout the course of its maturation.

Children with RTT may show only selected features of classic autism. Also, they may have only a transient course of the autistic symptoms, a modification or extinction of autistic characteristics with aging. The same phenomenon of modification of autistic symptoms with age can be seen in a number of other disease entities as well. When this is the usual clinical course, it is an important part of the background information in evaluating therapy claims.

Acknowledgment

The author appreciates Dr. Masaya Segawa, Director of Segawa Neurological Clinic for Children, for his critical review and discussion on this chapter.

REFERENCES

American Psychiatric Association (1994) *Diagnostic and Statistical Manuel of Mental Disorders* (4th ed.). Washington, DC: APA.

Amir RE, Van den Veyver IB, Schultz R, Malicki DM, Tran CQ, Dahle EJ, Philippi A, Timar L, Percy AK, Motil KJ, Lichtarge O, Smith EO, Glaze DG, Zoghbi HY (2000)

Influence of mutation type and X chromosome inactivation on Rett syndrome phe-notypes. *Annals of Neurology* 47(5):670–679.

Amir RE, Van den Veyver IB, Wan M, Tran CQ, Francke U, Zoghbi HY (1999) Rhett syndrome is caused by mutations in X-linked *MECP2*, encoding methyl-CpG-binding protein 2. *Nature Genetics* 23(2):185–188.

Armstrong DD (1992) The neuropathology of the Rett syndrome. *Brain Development* 14(Suppl):S89–98.

Armstrong DD (2001) Rett syndrome neuropathology review 2000. *Brain Development* 23(Suppl 1):S72–76.

Armstrong DD, Dunn K, Antalffy B (1998) Decreased dendritic branching in frontal, motor and limbic cortex in Rett syndrome compared with trisomy 21. *Journal of Neuro-pathology and Experimental Neurology* 57(11):1013–1017.

Armstrong DD, Dunn JK, Antalffy B, Trivedi R (1995) Selective dendritic alterations in the cortex of Rett syndrome. *Journal of Neuropathology and Experimental Neurology* 54(2):195–201.

Bailey A, Luthert P, Bolton P, Le Couteur A, Rutter M, Harding B (1993) Autism and megalencephaly. *Lancet* 341(8854):1225–1226

Bauman ML (1996) Brief report: neuroanatomic observations of the brain in pervasive developmental disorders. *Journal of Autism and Developemental Disorders* 26(2):199–203.

Bauman ML, Kemper TL, Arin DM (1995) Pervasive neuroanatomic abnormalities of the brain in three cases of Rett's syndrome. *Neurology* 45(8):1581–1586.

Belichenko PV, Dahlstrom A (1995) Studies on the 3-dimensional architecture of dendritic spines and varicosities in human cortex by confocal laser scanning microscopy and Lucifer yellow microinjections. *Journal of Neuroscience Methods* 57(1):55–61.

Belichenko PV, Fedorov AA, Dahlstrom AB (1996) Quantitative analysis of immuno-fluorescence and lipofuscin distribution in human cortical areas by dual-channel confocal laser scanning microscopy. *Journal of Neuroscience Methods* 69(2):155–161.

Belichenko PV, Hagberg B, Dahlstrom A (1997) Morphological study of neocortical areas in Rett syndrome. *Acta Neuropatholology* (Berl) 93(1):50–61.

Bienvenu T, Carrie A, de Roux N, Vinet MC, Jonveaux P, Couvert P, Villard L, Arziman-oglou A, Beldjord C, Fontes M, Tardieu M, Chelly J (2000) *MECP2* mutations account for most cases of typical forms of Rett syndrome. *Human Molecular Genetics* 9(9):1377–1384.

Brenner E, Mirmiran M, Uylings HB, Van der Gugten J (1983) Impaired growth of the cerebral cortex of rats treated neonatally with 6-hydroxydopamine under different environmental conditions. *Neuroscience Letters* 42(1):13–17.

Buccino MA, Weddell JA (1989) Rett syndrome—a rare and often misdiagnosed syndrome: case report. *Pediatr Dent* 11(2):151–157.

Courchesne E, Carper R, Akshoomoff N (2003) Evidence of brain overgrowth in the first year of life in autism. *JAMA* 290(3):337–344.

De Bona C, Zappella M, Hayek G, Meloni I, Vitelli F, Bruttini M, Cusano R, Loffredo P, Longo I, Renieri A (2000) Preserved speech variant is allelic of classic Rett syndrome. *European Journal of Human Genetics* 8(5):325–330.

Gillberg C (1986) Autism and Rett syndrome: some notes on differential diagnosis *Amer-ican Journal of Medical Genetics* Supplement 1:127–131.

Gillberg C (1987) Autistic symptoms in Rett syndrome: the first two years according to mother reports. *Brain Development* 9(5):499–501.

Gillberg C (1989) The borderland of autism and Rett syndrome: five case histories to highlight diagnostic difficulties. *Journal of Autism and Developmental Disorders* 19(4):545–559.

Gillberg C, Ehlers S, Schaumann H, Jakobsson G, Dahlgren SO, Lindblom R, Bagenholm A, Tjuus T, Blidner E (1990a) Autism under age 3 years: a clinical study of 28 cases referred for autistic symptoms in infancy. *Journal of Childhood Psychology and Psychiatry* 31(6):921–934.

Gillberg C, Ehlers S, Wahlstrom J (1990b) The syndromes described by Kanner and Rett-Hagberg: overlap in an extended family. *Developmental Medicine and Child Neurology* 32(3):258–261.

Gillberg C, Coleman M (2000a) Clinical diagnosis. *The Biology of the Autistic Syndromes (3rd ed.)* (pp. 4–38). London: Mac Keith Press. (Distributed by Cambridge University Press.)

Gillberg C, Coleman M (2000b) Double syndromes. *The Biology of the Autistic Syndromes (3rd ed.)* (pp.136–184). London: Mac Keith Press. (Distributed by Cambridge University Press.)

Gillberg C, Coleman M (2000c) The disease entities of autism. *The Biology of the Autistic Syndromes (3rd ed.)* (pp. 118–135). London: Mac Keith Press. (Distributed by Cambridge University Press.)

Hagberg B (1980) Infantile autistic dementia and loss of hand use: a report of 16 Swedish girl patients. *Paper presented at the Research Session of the European Federation of Child Neurology Societies*, Manchester, England.

Hagberg B, Aicardi J, Dias K, Ramos O (1983) A progressive syndrome of autism, dementia, ataxia, and loss of purposeful hand use in girls: Rett's syndrome—report of 35 cases. *Annals of Neurology* 14(4):471–479.

Hagberg B, Goutières F, Hanefeld F, Rett A, Wilson J (1985) Rett syndrome: criteria for inclusion and exclusion. *Brain Development* 7:372–373.

Hagberg B, Witt-Engerström I (1986) Rett syndrome: a suggested staging system for describing impairment profile with increasing age towards adolescence. *American Journal of Medical Genetics* 24:47–59.

Hammer S, Dorrani N, Dragich J, Kudo S, Schanen C (2002) The phenotypic consequences of *MECP2* mutations extend beyond Rett syndrome. *Mental Retardation and Developmental Disabilities Resource Review* 8(2):94–98.

Hammer S, Dorrani N, Hartiala J, Stein S, Schanen NC (2003) Rett syndrome in a 47,XXX patient with a de novo *MECP2* mutation. *American Journal of Medical Genetics* 122A(3):223–226.

Hoffbuhr K, Devaney JM, LaFleur B, Sirianni N, Scacheri C, Giron J. Schuette J, Innis J, Marino M, Philippart M, Narayanan V, Umansky R, Kronn D, Hoffman EP, Naidu S (2001) *MeCP2* mutations in children with and without the phenotype of Rett syndrome. *Neurology* 56:1486–1495.

Ishikawa A, Goto T, Narasaki M, Yokochi K, Kitahara H, Fukuyama Y (1978) A new syndrome (?) of progressive psychomotor deterioration with peculiar stereotyped movement and autistic tendency: a report of three cases. *Brain Development* 3:258.

Itoh M, Takashima S (2002) Neuropathology and immunohistochemistry of brains with Rett syndrome. *No To Hattatsu* (Japanese.) 34(3):211–216.

Jellinger K, Armstrong D, Zoghbi HY, Percy AK (1988) Neuropathology of Rett syndrome. *Acta Neuropatholology* (Berl) 76(2):142–158.

Jellinger K, Seitelberger F (1986) Neuropathology of Rett syndrome. *American Journal of Medical Genetics* (Suppl 1):259–288.

Johnston MV, Jeon OH, Pevsner J, Blue ME, Naidu S (2001) Neurobiology of Rett syndrome: a genetic disorder of synapse development. *Brain Development* 23(Suppl 1): S206–213.

Kashiwagi A, Meguro M, Hoshiya H, Haruta M, Ishino F, Shibahara T, Oshimura M (2003) Predominant maternal expression of the mouse Atp10c in hippocampus and olfactory bulb. *Journal of Human Genetics* 48(4):194–198.

Kemper TL, Bauman M (1998) Neuropathology of Infantile Autism. *Journal of Neuropatholology and Experimental Neurolology* 57(7):645–652.

Kohyama J, Ohinata J, Hasegawa T (2001) Disturbance of phasic chin muscle activity during rapid-eye-movement sleep. *Brain Development* 23(Suppl 1):S104–107.

Kojima J, Yamaji Y, Matsumura M, Nambu A, Inase M, Tokuno H, Takada M, Imai H (1997) Excitotoxic lesions of the pedunculopontine tegmental nucleus produce contralateral hemiparkinsonism in the monkey. *Neuroscience Letters* 226(2):111–114.

Lam CW, Yeung WL, Ko CH, Poon PM, Tong SF, Chan KY, Lo IF, Chan LY, Hui J, Wong V, Pang CP, Lo YM, Fok TF (2000) Spectrum of mutations in the *MECP2* gene in patients with infantile autism and Rett syndrome. *Journal of Medical Genetics* 37(12): E41.

Mazzocco MM, Pulsifer M, Fiumara A, Cocuzza M, Nigro F, Incorpora G, Barone R (1998) Brief report: autistic behaviors among children with fragile X or Rett syndrome: implications for the classification of pervasive developmental disorder. *Journal of Autism and Developmental Disorders* 28(4):321–328.

Miller S, van der Burg J (1973) The function of long propriospinal pathways in the coordination of quadropedal stepping in the cat. In Stein RB, Pearson KG, Smith RS, Redford JB (Eds.) *Control of Posture and Locomotion. Advances in Behavioral Biology (vol. 7)* (pp. 561–577). New Yord, London: Plenum.

Mori S, Matsuyama K, Kohyama J, Kobayashi Y, Takakusaki K (1992) Neuronal constituents of postural and locomotor control systems and their interactions in cats. *Brain Development* 14(Suppl):S109–120.

Morrison JH, Foote SL, Bloom FE (1984) Regional laminar, developmental and functional characteristics of noradrenaline and serotonin innervation patterns in monkey cortex. In Descarries L, Reader TR, Jasper HH (Eds) *Monoamine innervation of cerebral cortex* (pp. 61–75). New York: Alan R Liss.

Mount RH, Charman T, Hastings RP, Reilly S, Cass H (2003b) Features of autism in Rett syndrome and severe mental retardation. *Journal of Autism and Developmental Disorders* 33(4):435–442.

Mount RH, Hastings RP, Reilly S, Cass H, Charman T (2003a) Towards a behavioral phenotype for Rett syndrome. *American Journal of Mental Retardation* 108(1):1–12.

Nomura Y, Honda K, Segawa M (1987) Pathophysiology of Rett syndrome. *Brain Development* (Tokyo) 9:506–513.

Nomura Y, Segawa M (1986) Anatomy of Rett syndrome. *American Journal of Medical Genetics* 24:289–303.

Nomura Y, Segawa M (1990a) Characteristics of motor disturbances of the Rett syndrome. *Brain Development* (Tokyo) 12(1):27–30.

Nomura Y, Segawa M (1990b) Clinical features of the early stage of the Rett syndrome. *Brain Development* 12(1):16–19.

Nomura Y, Segawa M (2001) The monoamine hypothesis in Rett syndrome. In Kerr A, Engerström WI (Eds) *Rett Disorder and the Developing Brain* (pp. 205–225). New York: Oxford University Press.

Nomura Y, Segawa M, Hasegawa M (1984) Rett syndrome—clinical studies and pathophysiological consideration. *Brain Development* 6(5):475–486.

Nomura Y, Segawa M, Higurashi M (1985) Rett syndrome—an early catecholamine and indolamine deficient disorder? *Brain Development* (Tokyo) 7:334–341.

Nordin V, Gillberg C (1996a) Autism spectrum disorders in children with physical or mental disability or both I: clinical and epidemiological aspects. *Developmental Medicine and Child Neurology* 38:297–313.

Nordin V, Gillberg C (1996b) Autism spectrum disorders in children with physical or mental disability or both II: screening aspects. *Developmental Medicine and Child Neurolology* 38:314–324.

Olsson B, Rett A (1990) A review of the Rett syndrome with a theory of autism. *Brain Development* 12(1):11–15.

Olsson B, Rett A (1987) Autism and Rett syndrome: behavioural investigations and differential diagnosis. *Developmental Medicine and Child Neurology* 29(4):429–441.

Olsson B (1987) Autistic traits in the Rett syndrome. *Brain Development* 9(5):491–498.

Olsson B, Rett A (1985) Behavioral observations concerning differential diagnosis between the Rett syndrome and autism. *Brain Development* 7(3):281–289.

Orrico A, Lam C, Galli L, Dotti MT, Hayek G, Tong SF, Poon PM, Zappella M, Federico A, Sorrentino V (2000) *MECP2* mutation in male patients with non-specific X-linked mental retardation. *FEBS Letters* 481(3):285–288.

Percy A, Gillberg C, Hagberg B, Witt-Engerstrom I (1990) Rett syndrome and the autistic disorders. *Neurologic Clinics* 8(3):659–676.

Percy AK, Zoghbi HY, Lewis KR, Jankovic J (1988) Rett syndrome: qualitative and quantitative differentiation from autism. *Journal of Child Neurology* 3(Suppl):S65–67.

Piven J, Arndt S, Bailey J, Andreasen N (1996) Regional brain enlargement in autism: a magnetic resonance imaging study. *Journal of the American Academy of Child and Adolescent Psychiatry* 35(4):530–536.

Piven J, Bailey J, Ranson BJ, Arndt S (1997) An MRI study of the corpus callosum in autism. *American Journal of Psychiatry* 154(8):1051–1056.

Rapin I (2002) The autistic-spectrum disorders. *New England Journal of Medicine* 347(5): 302–303.

Raymond GV, Bauman ML, Kemper TL (1996) Hippocampus in autism: a Golgi analysis. *Acta Neuropatholology* (Berl) 91(1):117–119.

Rett A (1977) Cerebral atrophy associated with hyperammonaemia. In Vinken PJ, Bruyn GW (Eds.) *Handbook of Clinical Neurology* (vol. 29) (pp. 305–329). Amsterdam: North-Holland.

Rett A (1969) Hyperammonaemie und cerebrale Atrophie im Kindesalter. *Folia Hereditaria et Pathologica* 18:115–124.

Rett A (1966a) *Über ein cerebral-atrophisches syndrombei Hyperammonämie*. Vienna: Brüder Hollinek.

Rett A (1966b) Ueber ein eigenartiges hirnatrophisches Syndrom bei Hyperammoniämie in Kindesalter. *Wien Med Wochenschr* 116:723–738.

Samaco RC, Nagarajan RP, Braunschweig D, LaSalle JM (2004) Multiple pathways regulate *MeCP2* expression in normal brain development and exhibit defects in autism-spectrum disorders. *Human Molecular Genetics* 13(6):29–639.

Segawa M (1998) A neurological model of infantile autism. *Brain Science* (Japanese) 20: 169–175.

Segawa M (2003). Autism and serotonin. *Clinical Neuroscience* (Japanese) 21:693–695.

Segawa M (2001a) Pathophysiology of Rett syndrome from the standpoint of clinical characteristics. *Brain Development* 23(Suppl 1):S94–98.

Segawa M (2001b) Discussant—pathophysiologies of Rett syndrome. *Brain Develpoment* 23(Suppl 1):S218–223.

Segawa M (2001c) The role of genetic and environmental factors in brain development: development of the central monoaminergic nervous system. In Kerr A, Engerström WI (Eds) *Rett Disorder and the Developing Brain* (pp. 83–203). New York: Oxford University Press.

Segawa M (1979) Early infantile autism. *Japanese Journal of Neuropsychopharmacoly* (Tokyo) 1:189–200.

Segawa M (1982) Neurological approach to early infantile autism. *Hattatsu Shogai Kenkyu* (Tokyo) 4:184–197.

Segawa M (1980) Sleep mechanism and its development. *Pediatrics* (Tokyo) 21:441–453.

Segawa M, Nomura Y (1990) The pathophysiology of the Rett syndrome from the standpoint of polysomnography. *Brain Development* 1:55–60.

Segawa M, Nomura Y (1992) Polysomnography in the Rett syndrome. *Brain Development* 14(Suppl):S46–54.

Segawa M, Nomura Y, Hikosaka O, Soda M, Usui S, Kase M (1987) Roles of the basal ganglia and related structures in symptoms of dystonia. In Carpenter MB, Jayaraman A (Eds) *The basal ganglia II.* (pp. 489–504). New York: Plenum.

Shibayama A, Cook EH Jr, Feng J, Glanzmann C, Yan J, Craddock N, Jones IR, Goldman D, Heston LL, Sommer SS (2004) *MECP2* structural and 3'-UTR variants in schizophrenia, autism and other psychiatric diseases: a possible association with autism. *American Journal of Medical Genetics* 128B(1):50–53.

Tanaka S, Miyagawa F, Imai S, Hidano T (1987) Effets on learning of the lesion on the dorsal noradrenergic bundle. *Juntenndo Medical Journal (Tokyo)* 33:271–272.

Tao, J Van Esch H, Hagedorn-Greiwe M, hoffmann K, Moser B, Raynaud M, Sperner J, Fryns FP, Schwinger E, Gecz J, Ropers HH, Kalscheuer VM (2004) Mutations in the X-linked cyclin-dependent kinase-like 5 (CDKL5/STK9) gene are associated with severe neurodevelopmental retardation. *American Journal of Human Genetics* 75: 1149–1154.

The Rett Syndrome Diagnostic Criteria Word Group (1988) Diagnostic criteria for Rett syndrome. *Annals of Neurology* 23:425–428.

Thomas JA, Johnson J, Peterson Kraai TL, Wilson R, Tartaglia N, LeRoux J, Beischel L, McGavran L, Hagerman RJ (2003) Genetic and clinical characterization of patients with an interstitial duplication 15q11-q13, emphasizing behavioral phenotype and response to treatment. *American Journal of Medical Genetics* 119A(2):111–20.

Tranebjaerg L, Kure P (1991) Prevalence of fra(X) and other specific diagnoses in autistic individuals in a Danish county. *American Journal of Medical Genetics* 38(2–3):212–214.

Tuchman RF, Rapin I, Shinnar S (1991) Autistic and dysphasic children. I: Clinical characteristics. *Pediatrics* 88(6):1211–1218.

Valzelli L, Garattini S (1972) Biochemical and behavioural changes induced by isolation in rats. *Neuropharmacology* 11(1):17–22.

Veiga MF, Toralles MB (2002) Neurological manifestation and genetic diagnosis of Angelman, Rett and Fragile-X syndromes. *Journal of Pediatrics (Rio J)* 78(Suppl 1):S55–62.

Vourc'h P, Bienvenu T, Beldjord C, Chelly J, Barthelemy C, Much JP, Andres C (2001) No mutations in the coding region of the Rett syndrome gene *MECP2* in 59 autistic patients. *European Journal of Human Genetics* 9(7):556–558.

Wan M, Lee SS, Zhang X, Houwink-Manville I, Song HR, Amir RE, Budden S, Naidu S, Pereira JL, Lo IF, Zoghbi HY, Schanen NC, Francke U (1999) Rett syndrome and beyond: recurrent spontaneous and familial *MECP2* mutations at CpG hotspots. *American Journal of Human Genetics* 65(6):1520–1529.

Weaving LS, Christodoulou J, Williamson SL, Friend KL, McKenzie OL, Archer H, Evans J, Clarke A, Pelka GJ, Tam PP, Watson C, Lahooti H, Ellaway CJ, Bennetts B, Leonard H, Gecz J (2004) Mutations of CDKL5 cause a severe neurodevelopmental disorder with infantile spasms and mental retardation. *American Journal of Human Genetics* 75:1079–1093.

Witt-Engerström I (1992) Age-related occurrence of signs and symptoms in the Rett syndrome. *Brain Development* 14(Suppl):S11–20.

Witt-Engerström I, Gillberg C (1987) Rett syndrome in Sweden. *Journal of Autism and Developmental Disorders* 17(1):149–150.

World Health Organization (1992) *International Statistical Classification of Diseases and Related Health Problems* (10th rev.). Geneva:WHO.

Zappella M (1985) Rett syndrome: a significant proportion of girls affected by autistic behavior. *Brain Development* 7(3):307–312.

Zappella M, Meloni I, Longo I, Canitano R, Hayek G, Rosaia L, Mari F, Renieri A (2003) Study of *MECP2* gene in Rett syndrome variants and autistic girls. *American Journal of Medical Genetics* 119B(1):102–107.

Zoghbi HY (2003) Postnatal neurodevelopmental disorders: meeting at the synapse? *Science* 302(5646):826–830.

Chapter 8

The Question of Reversible Autistic Behavior in Autism

Michele Zappella

Autism is a long-lasting disorder in the great majority of cases. It is defined by behavior. This characterization of the disease entity by behavioral abnormalities may cause difficulties when describing the limited number of children who subsequently lose these features. For a long time, the potential of reversible autistic behavior was explored mostly on psychological grounds; while such studies initially claimed brilliant results, they subsequently were the object of severe criticism and turned out to be disappointing. These studies usually were conducted with the idea of autism as one disease that possibly misled their authors from searching in other directions. The potential for reversible autistic behavior is a research subject in which mistakes and a suspicion of quackery is a concern; it has been more recently explored from a neurological perspective by a few professionals. Recent data suggest that the latter approach can shed light on this controversial subject and add knowledge to other data obtained on different grounds.

Reversible autistic behavior concerns the following possibilities:

1. An improvement in the social and communicative abilities of the subject, notable through observation and the use of special skills that may, for example, allow him/her to interact better with other people and in some cases to have a more autonomous life, in spite of persisting significant core signs of the autistic spectrum disorder (ASD). Certain clinical features suggesting a more favorable outcome recently have been proposed; these especially concern subjects with high-functioning autism and the possibility for some of them to obtain an independent life in spite of the persistence of an autistic core (Wing 2004). The assets of such an individual include the following: (a) a certain level of linguistic and visuospatial abilities; (b) a quality of social interactions by persons who are socially active, though odd, do better than those who are passive and lonely; (c) the existence of special abilities that may be useful for some specific job; (d) an adequate insight associated with a positive view of themselves; and (e) the wish to relate with other persons. In contrast, the presence of various psychiatric comorbidities and of marked distress to sensory stimuli reduces the chances of a more positive outcome.

2. In children with syndromic autism, in which brain damage is usually relevant, autistic behavior can fade in time but other relevant disalibities persist. Transient autistic behavior is seldom the object of reported studies as in a child with Coffin-Lowry syndrome (Manouvrier-Hanu et al. 1999), but it can be noticed in a number of cases in which mental retardation, disorders of language development and dyspraxia are the final, permanent outcome. Disorders in which an autistic behavior can fade while profound disabilities persist include rare cases of diseases such as the Preserved Speech Variant (PSV) of Rett syndrome. These patients usually have autistic behavior; however, in 2 girls in whom IQ reached values near 50, with increasing intellectual abilities, autistic behavior decreased below the values usually accepted for the criteria of autism (Zappella et al. 2003). This condition (Zappella 1992) concerns girls with a disease initially similar to classic Rett syndrome but that subsequently shows signs of improvement both in manual abilities and in language.

In this population, the professional must be aware of these and similar possibilities that may require, in a given child, an appropriate change in educational measures and in rehabilitation. For example, children with profound oromanual dyspraxia may go through an initial phase where autistic behavior is prominent, followed by an improvement, and then by the disappearance of autistic symptoms, whereas dyspraxia remains as a main, central disturbance. Attention to an evolution of this kind mandates a change in the educational strategies, reducing environmental adaptations that have become inadequate and promoting, in contrast, a child's curiousity and communication.

3. There are some children who will show an initial positive response to therapeutic interventions but will remain autistic. An example is those with early onset [Gilles de la] Tourette syndrome (GTS) and an autistic disorder. This subgroup of young children, showing in some instances familial GTS, was originally described by Kerbeshian and Burd (1992, 1994) and these observations have been confirmed by Zappella (2002) who noticed an initial rapid improvement following the institution of a new treatment that subsequently became less marked and left the child still with autistic symptoms.

4. Finally, a radical change in behavior has been observed in some children whereby no more evidence of core autistic symptoms exists. Such a child resumes normal intellectual, social and communicative abilities that, in spite of the eventual presence of disturbances like tics, ADHD, etc., allow an independent and adequate social life.

Children who may experience a reversal of autistic symptoms include the following:

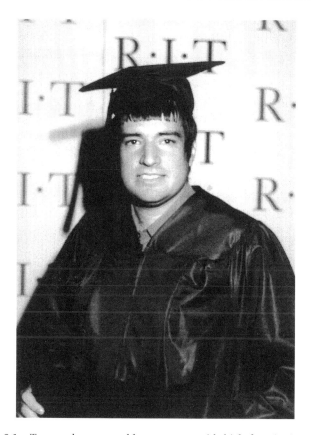

Figure 8.1   Twenty-three-year-old young man with high-functioning autism.

1. Those who experience profound deprivation in early infancy—frequently due to institutionalization in extremely poor conditions—of food, hygienic conditions, and an extensive absence and poor quality of human interactions. When this is likely the only cause of the autistic behavior, there is a possibility of partial or complete recovery. Observations of cases like these involve adopted children, initially reared in institutions from Eastern European countries, such as as Romania; it is likely, however, that similar outcomes were present also in western institutions in a more distant past. One very important variable for the potential reversal of autistic behavior in these children appears to be the duration of the deprivation; some of these children have reverted to normal behavior and intellectual abilities (Rutter et al. 1999; Rutter et al. 2001; Beckett et al. 2002). This population of adopted children with autistic behavior, however, is a mixed one, including cases of classic autism and, possibly, of depression (Gillberg 2004b).

2. Those with early onset bipolar disorders (BPD) with autism. Robert De-

Long and his coworkers have devoted a number of studies to the relationship between autism, affective disorders and the therapeutic use of fluoxetine (DeLong & Dwyer 1988; DeLong & Nothria 1994; DeLong et al. 1998). In a recent study of the use of fluoxetine in a population of children with autistic spectrum disorder (ASD) 2 to 8 years old, treated for 5 to 76 months (DeLong et al. 2002), they have reported a significant change in 22 children (17%) defined as "no longer identified as having autism." Most of these responders retained symptoms of attention-deficit-hyperactivity disorder, obsessive-compulsive disorder, and signs of immaturity in social interactions and praxis (which is the usual outcome also seen by recovered children with the dysmaturational syndrome). In 4 children the outcome was a bipolar disorder. These data are not entirely consistent with an early onset bipolar disorder where one would expect a subsequent evolution of the affective disorder in a higher number of cases. An additional problem is that some of these children may do well without the pharmacological help. I have observed a few cases of reversible autistic behavior. In these cases a family history of both mood disorders and GTS were initially interpreted as examples of early onset mood disorders (Zappella 1998). They were not treated pharmacologically, and at follow-up, in adolescence, they demonstrated full-blown GTS that, through a more careful anamnestic evaluation, could be traced back to their early years.

DeLong and coworkers (1994; 2002) identified the existence of a subgroup with high-functioning autism with familial BPD and high intellectual abilities that would benefit from this treatment: (a) children with autism who benefit from a fluoxetine treatment but remain autistic; and (b) children who recover entirely from autism and retardation through this medication. The latter possibility, although not yet confirmed by other professionals, should not be discarded, and it may concern a more limited number of cases.

3. Other individual rare cases of recovery can also be observed but are not easily classifiable (Perry et al. 1995).

4. Those with autism following intrauterine infections, such as rubella infection; following vaccination programs, this condition is now rare. During the last large rubella epidemic, it was noted that approximately a third of the children described as autistic by age 3 had lost these features at 7 years (Chess 1977).

In addition, the following two sets of disorders are of particular relevance to the clinician as, if appropriately identified, they can lead to profound behavioral changes in a given child.

EARLY ONSET EPILEPSY

Some patients with epileptic disorders where an autistic behavior or a dysintegrative disorder are present can show behavioral improvement following an appropriate pharmacological treatment; in these cases epilepsy originates in the brain networks responsible for communication and interactions. The autistic behavior is due to diffuse epileptic discharges from recognized or unrecognized seizures arising intermittently. Any partial epilepsy with a focus (or foci) in an area important for behavior can lead to disturbances. Repeated seizures often manifest as a continuous dysfunction when they originate in or spread to areas identified with key aspects of behavior and may leave no possibility for interictal recovery, as one seizure is followed by postictal state, followed by a new seizure.

These disorders include some cases of West syndrome, especially those with "late epileptic spasms"and those with early onset partial complex seizures; some of these patients may have a regression with autistic features reversible with appropriate treatment. Deonna and his coworkers have described a number of interesting cases with reversible autism in young epileptic children. In two young boys, both affected by tuberous sclerosis, autistic regression followed a period of apparent well-being. Surface EEGs initially did not reveal any abnormality (although subsequently there was evidence of frontal abnormalities in both) and, in one of the boys, no evidence of seizure was apparent. Following the administration of carbamazepine (CBZ), in both cases, most of the autistic features disappeared, although various degrees of disabilities remained (Deonna et al. 1993).

Subtle signs that may lead to the diagnosis and appropriate treatment are described in another case: a young child showed an autistic deterioration at 2 years accompanied by head and shoulder spasms. The patient's EEG revealed bursts of brief generalized polyspikes and spike-waves during these spasms that occasionally resembled hypsarrhythmia. Treatment with clonazepam led to a rapid, profound improvement both in the EEG and in behavior. The patient's score on the Child Autism Rating Scale (CARS) decreased in 2 months from 35 to 19. A subsequent analogous autistic deterioration occurred 6 months later, although EEG abnormalities were less evident, and again a pharmacological treatment with CBZ induced a complete reversal of autistic behavior and a IQ of 65 at 51 months (Deonna et al. 1995). The same author (Deonna 1995) has described an example of dysintegrative psychosis occurring in a 3½-year-old child. Fluctuation of symptoms led to the suspicion of epilepsy, although there were only equivocal anterior EEG changes and no clear-cut seizures. Treatment with CBZ led to a complete reversal of autistic symptoms and to almost normal development during the next 3 years.

Children with the Landau-Kleffner syndrome also may show autistic features in addition to limited or absent verbal comprehension; both can sometimes be recovered following an effective antiepileptic therapy with mental abilities reaching a level near to normal (Canitano & Zappella 2004; Deonna 2004). This syndrome, also called acquired epileptic aphasia, has a variable onset from to 2 to 9 years, most often subacute, progressive with spontaneous improvements and aggravations (fluctuations), usually with a verbal auditory agnosia but eventually with other types of aphasia. An EEG in such a case shows sharp and slow waves with a temporal predominance with an activation by sleep, sometimes quite marked (CSWS).

Early epilepsy can alter the dynamics of development, causing regressions with autistic behavior through different avenues, and while in some cases autistic behavior can fade following an appropriate antiepileptic treatment, some degree of delay or disability usually remains.

DYSMATURATIONAL SYNDROME (TOURETTE SYNDROME WITH REVERSIBLE AUTISTIC BEHAVIOR)

The dysmaturational syndrome (early onset GTS with reversible autism) occurs in children, almost all males, who after a normal development in their first year of life go through a profound regression with autistic features or a full-blown picture of autism accompanied by the appearance of multiple tics during the second year of life (Zappella 1994a). Appropriate intervention allows a rapid drop of the autistic behavior and a simultaneous recovery of a number of abilities. By age 5 to 6 years, these children have lost all traces of autistic behavior and their mental abilities fall in the normal range, but a different psychiatric dimension becomes clear in that most of them show the features of ADHD and Tourette syndrome, often with the corresponding comorbidities.

I have studied this disorder beginning in 1994 (Zappella 1994a, 1998, 1999, 2002; Zappella & Renieri 2005). The total number of children reported in these studies and/or various presentations is 85, but I observed many more clinically. Among the reported cases, only 3 girls were observed, with a male:female ratio of 28:1. A replication study is in progress with initial similar results (C. Gillberg personal communication).

Family Studies

Of two studies conducted with identical criteria on a total of 26 young children, motor tics were present in 61% of parents while features of ADHD were noticed in 27% of the fathers (Zappella 2002; Zappella & Renieri 2005). Family interactions were adequate in most cases; these families appeared as very close, with normal structure and communication; adverse family milieu events were few. In only one family, separation between parents occurred at the time of the regression; in the remaining families, parents were in harmony and apparently took an adequate care of their children. In one of these cases, the regression became more intense after the family moved abroad; but it had started before the move. In another case, the father's major depression occurred just before child's regression and was coincidental with the mother becoming relatively more absent for reasons related to her work. Among brothers and sisters, there are no examples of autism but occasional cases of disabilities such as congenital brain damage or deafness were noticed. Examples of brothers with ADHD and tics were present, but disorders of communication and social interaction were not identified in the families.

One set of homozygous twins and one set of heterozygous twins have been followed. (Zappella & Renieri 2005). The homozygous twins had the same dys-maturational syndrome: an autistic regression became apparent in both children at near 12 months, coincident with the appearance of tics. When seen at 3 years 6 months, one of the twins had already recovered from autistic behavior and showed no tics; the other still had both tics and autistic behavior. Subsequently, developmental abilities seemed to be equally recovered in both of them at 6 years 3 months with an IQ of 105 and 107, respectively, and no trace of autistic be-havior remained. In the heterozygous set, only one of the two was affected by this syndrome; the same was noticed in two other heterozygous sets observed personally but not reported in the literature.

These data give an interesting insight into the nature of the syndrome: the absence of brothers and sisters with autism or notable disorders of social inter-action and communication helps to place it somewhere separate from those syn-dromes with persistent autism, where one would expect a 3% occurrence, and examples of communication and social disabilities probably would be higher. The observations of the twins suggest the presence of a genetic component, and con-firm data on the high level of tics in parents and ADHD in fathers, as is usual in GTS, which is the real disorder at play.

Progress of the Disorder

The initial development of these children is usually reported as normal and par-ents' description is occasionally confirmed by the observations of videos con-ducted at home in the first year of child's life. They walk alone and say their first words between 10 and 18 months in most, but in a minority the appearance of language is delayed. The regression with autistic features and loss of previous abilities occurs between 1 and 2 years; subsequently, the improvement is moderate or absent. Multiple complex motor tics, and simple motor and vocal tics appear during the second year of life, and have been found to be of various intensity and frequency in the first evaluation visit. The physical appearance of these chil-dren is normal, including head circumference, with no relevant dysmorphic fea-tures. Laboratory evaluations such as chromosomes, fragile X, aminoacidemia, EEG, NMR, antistreptolysin titer are also normal.

The intensity of tics fluctuates over time and they often change in form; in some cases, they become less evident in the following years to become full blown at an age above 10 and more intense in adolescence. These usually include facial grimaces, eyes turned upward or laterally, sudden movements of the shoulders and upper limbs, hand movements in front of the face, hands clasped together, fingers squeezing, squatting, twirling when walking, and jumping. They are ac-companied by vocal tics in the form of belches, raspberries, grunts, and peculiar and repetitive sequences of noises or syllables. In all cases, both vocal and, sub-sequently, motor tics had always been present for more than a year.

At the first examination, some of these children may fulfil *DSM-IV* criteria for autistic disorder, confirmed by ABC or CARS data, but, in others, these data are less evident and diagnosis is within the atypical autism range. When seen at 2-3 years, after regression has already occurred, the children's abilities are below the norm, scoring correctly on no more than 70% of the items expected for their age and in many well below 50%; the majority are still unable to utter a word and have elements of inadequate oral motor coordination (for example, they cannot blow out a candle) and do not pinpoint. They show some signs of increased sensory feelings: reacting aversely either to intense, sudden noises or to drying their faces; if they are kissed; or protesting a haircut, a shower, or the texture of raw materials.

At the first evaluation, these children often enter into the office with pronounced avoidant behavior, but if the professional calls the child by name with a high voice and the child turns as surprised, if the doctor subsequently approaches the child and guides the child's hands in caressing him, and proposes to reciprocally touch various parts of the face, the child may accept this approach and, at the same time, become more sociable and varied in expressions. If the examiner then requests that the parents present interact physically with the child —tickle and toss the child in the air—all present may observe a rapid, profound change in the child's behavior: happy, friendly, ready to cooperate, and often able to do activities never done at home that come as a surprise to parents. This is a key point in a child's evaluation, that, coordinated with family data and with developmental reports, allows suspicion of this specific disorder. Moreover, the child has shown during the visit that this type of approach is beneficial to improving behavior and this approach can therefore be expanded and proposed to parents and to other persons who attend to the child.. The final diagnosis requires more time, based on repeated observations of a sharp reduction of autistic behaviors until they reach levels no longer compatible with a diagnosis of autism and are combined with a normal or quasi-normal level of recovered abilities. In the 26 children mentioned above, mean values of ABC in the first visit were 56 and, at follow-up, they were reduced to 4.

In the first year of treatment, often in the first months, recovery is rapid: the child gains more abilities than a normal child would in the same period of time. Some prolonged delay in improving praxic abilities—in the use of their mouth and their hands adequate to their general level of abilities, or in verbal understanding and expression—is, however, often observed during the treatment. These abilities become adequate at different ages, but most usually by 6 years of age.

Treatment

Initially, when the young child displays symptoms of autistic behavior, parents are coached to share their emotions with their sons, developing reciprocal bodily and emotional interactions along the lines of dual interactions that commonly occur within the first years of life in normal babies and young children (Trevarthen 1979). Within this context, an emphasis is placed on physical play: tossing the child in the air, piggyback riding, bouncing the child on the knee, chasing and tickling in which the adult may simulate an ant slowly moving on the child's body and suddenly reaching behind the neck pretending to bite him/her, giving kisses on the child's tummy, etc. These types of interactions are conducted by the adult with intense comic-dramatic expressions and postures and accompanied in the child by a high level of excitement, arousal, and amusement. The child may reciprocate this approach by assuming an attitude complementary to that of the parent: laughing and closing the arms around the body, or alternating this behavior with a reversed interaction where the child simulates an attack on the adult and the latter pretending to be afraid. Within these interactions, in part at least culturally determined, the adult and the child play a kind of comedy where the roles and their times alternate, and each often gives the other rapid, excited glances: happy screamings in the child and sudden muggling in the parent are the rule. The tactile component of this type of interaction is prevalent and this basic level of stimulation explains the intensity of the emotional response, but sight and vocal interactions also are an integral part of this dual amusement. There is evidence that the human voice is one of the more efficacious stimuli for eliciting social interactions in children (Mills & Melhuist 1974), a type of reaction usually not observed in children with autism (Klin 1991). This type of interaction is important in the development of social abilities and sex roles, subsequently developed with peers and including fragments of a number of behaviors such as the modulation of aggression, the development of verbal and preverbal language, exploration of the other, friendliness, sexuality, and so on (MacDonald & Parke 1984, 1986).

In their dual modality, as well as in the subsequent collective form with peers, interactions for fun have the immediate reward of supporting social interactions and cooperation: because it is fun, it is worthwhile to continue and expand the interaction, since every new proposal may carry promise for further fun! This type of interaction promotes further exploration and cooperation and has the cognitive advantage of making these children aware of the effect on other persons of their own emotional expressions and of understanding other persons' emotional behaviors.

Interactions for fun have seldom been the object of therapeutic strategies aiming to improve developmental disorders and, if suggested, often have been considered of marginal significance. I have been successfully using similar modalities in the treatment of elective mutism (Zappella 1979). It is interesting to make hypotheses on the rare use of physical play in therapies with these types of disorders. According to Sutton-Smith (1993), if we look at the earliest play theories of Western societies, until now they appear as part of a rationalization of an "irrational" childhood. This tendency toward a social control of the normal child is probably more marked in regard to those examples of severe deviance, such as autism, and may lead, on one side, to proposals of educational measures represented by an extensive structuring of the environment and, on the other, to ignoring the possibilities included in parent-child physical play, modalities that can be easily interpreted, albeit arbitrarily, as irrational. Instead, physical play also can be useful in a number of children with persistent autism, as a part of their rearing. These children enjoy it, their limited social and communicative abilities are fostered, their parents develop a more intense and emotionally richer attachment to them, and it may coexist well with other, more organized forms of interactions.

Children with the dysmaturational syndrome go through an experience of severe withdrawal with its concomitant profound sensory deprivation; they are not helped by a strictly structured program or by repetitive behavioral conditionings. They are, instead, in strong need of stimuli producing intensive motivations to interact and cooperate, and that is why interactions for fun have such a powerful effect in promoting their social and cooperative interactions, by giving a strong support to the learning of new abilities, as well as to gradually come out of the downward spiral of withdrawal behavior and, finally, to lose autistic symptoms.

Other concomitant interactive modalities are also useful and suggested to parents: relaxed interactions that favor the development of affiliation, friendliness, and exploration of the other person. For example, taking child's hands and guiding them to caress the face of the parent who reciprocates, continuing the interaction by a reciprocal touching and naming of various parts of the face (the nose, chin, ears, etc.), exchanging various grimaces, etc. These approaches belong to a larger category (approach behavior) and may reinforce each other and provide motivation for cooperation (Zappella 1994b, 1998). Additional interactions include also simple motor activations of the child, for example, joining hands and running together around the room for a few minutes, inducing a light amusement and relaxation, quickly followed by cooperation, eventually manually guided, in order to support the appearance of new abilities. Within this context, parents are encouraged to use the Portage method as one of the referral points for activities to engage with their children in order to guide them into resuming appropriate abilities. The Portage method has in this respect at least two principal advantages: first, it provides parents with a list of activities to be done with a child who went through a prolonged period when almost all aspects of development were profoundly slowed and therefore needs now both stimulation and active proposals; second, the gradual way of reaching an item, suggested in this method, is often useful because some of these children initially show elements of dyspraxia and, in these cases, splitting an item into simpler tasks and making use of manual or other supports, may be especially helpful. Motivation, however, is favored both through praise and the various types of interactions for pleasure listed above, instead of the traditional behavioral strategies, based on candies and other similar tools, which are not part of the treatment.

The child and family are seen every 2 months. Initially, when the child is still showing symptoms of the autistic series, these proposals are scattered throughout the day. Teachers in the nursery are asked to cooperate with parents using elements of the Portage method and favoring amusement and fun within the context of their school methods. Most of these children have ADHD and recommendations concerning this underlying disorder are slowly introduced. For example, not flooding the child with too many toys is among the first to be given, soon accompanied by the suggestion of having periods of time when the adult-child cooperation should occur with a few objects in a context with reduced stimuli, and by the suggestion of having the child free in the field some time every day. When the child is free from most autistic behaviors and has recovered many abilities, bringing behavior close to normality, the main remaining problem is often ADHD and the corresponding recommendations are those usual for children with this disorder (Barkley 1995). Similar indications are given to the nursery schools. Speech therapy is recommended and needs to occur regularly in those cases where it appears appropriate.

In the following years, as they grow up into the last part of the first decade and adolescence, the majority of these children have GTS, comorbid with ADHD and occasionally OCD and dyslexia. Social difficulties are sometimes present, but never in the form and level of Asperger syndrome or Multiple Complex Developmental Disorder. In a few cases, no comorbidities were noticed in spite of the persistent presence of GTS: examples, apparently, of "pure" GTS. A few children appeared entirely normal. A continuum of severity is therefore present both in the autistic phase and at follow-up. Tics tend to become less intense in the middle of the first decade and in the years immediately following it, but by 9–10 years of age and in the years of adolescence, they often become intense and a drug therapy for tics may be instituted.

The interaction with peers is usually among the last abilities to become adequate; the child becomes more and more interested in them, but lacks the social skills to engage them. These children need help from adults in dual situations with other children, guiding them in the exchange of friendly actions (bye-bye, give the hands, shake hands, etc.), alternated with guidance in constructive play of increasing interaction (for example, one child builds a train of red cubes, the other a train of blue cubes, making an angle with the previous one, etc.). Including the child in collective, ritual plays in the nursery may result in the spontaneous development of physical play with peers.

It also must be mentioned that there are families who spontaneously react appropriately to the withdrawal of their child, and implement their natural resources to stimulate him with modalities analogous to those described above. This is probably the reason why some cases go through a spontaneous recovery, as it is apparent in the history of some children with ADHD plus Tourette syndrome, seen later in their life when parents recall a period of regression during their second year of life.

Differential Diagnosis

In contrast, there are children with autism, GTS, and regression during the second year of life who, treated with this approach, will show a notable improvement in behavior in a first visit and make rapid improvements in the following months, but will subsequently remain autistic. Some of them have a family history of GTS. This subgroup, initially described by Kerbeshian and Burd (1992, 1994) is the most relevant in the differential diagnosis of the dysmaturational syndrome. The possibility of a Landau-Kleffner syndrome must also be considered; initial development is normal and regression affecting the comprehension of language with autistic features may well be accompanied by multiple motor tics, followed by some initial improvement, after the institution of physical play and appropriate education. In cases of this kind, there are two baseline evaluations that should be obtained as soon as possible: a complete EEG, possibly a video EEG, as well as family videos concerning the early development of the child where it may be possible to assess relevant elements of an initial normal development and, in some cases, tics that may have been not noticed by parents.

The appropriate diagnosis of dysmaturational syndrome requires caution, time, and a series of observational data. The dysmaturational syndrome should be proposed as a possibility that becomes probable with the appearance of adequate social interactions, initially within the family and then with peers, symbolic play and normally structured speech, and becomes true when the child has lost every aspect of autistic behavior and gained intellectual abilities within the normal range in spite of the frequent, persistent presence of hyperactivity and tics.

Possible Pathogenesis

In the present state of knowledge, some hypothesis can be advanced on what causes this initially severe disturbance in development. Tics and autistic regression occur almost at the same time and it is possible that the derangement concerning corticothalamostriatal-cortical pathways and/or the dopaminergic system as hypothesized for GTS as the neural basis for tics (Jeffreys et al. 2002; Singer et al. 2002; Berardelli et al. 2003) affects more specifically brain areas concerning the development of communication and social relationships, and makes the brain areas involved unavailable in a critical moment of child's development. The intensity and degree of the autistic regression is variable from case to case, as is the time required to recover normal relational, communicative, and intellectual abilities, suggesting different degrees of disruption in the corresponding brain areas by the dysfunctions causing tics and autistic behavior at the same time. In contrast with the early epilepsies where persistent, generalized or discrete foci of continuous or intermittent seizures can cause autistic behavior that may be reversible following appropriate drug treatment, here it appears as if possibly unstable, fluctuating dysfunctions of definite brain areas in a delicate moment of a young child's growth are susceptible to be modified by highly emotional interactions following along the lines of normal developmental relationships. It is also noteworthy that the dysmaturational syndrome, as well as in those institutional cases with reversible autism, one with an apparently genetic and the other with an environmental causal system, both appear to benefit from a similar relational approach where warm interactions, pedagogic guidance and, in some cases, speech therapy are in the forefront. They also share a rapid decline of the autistic features and a parallel rapid recovery of their abilities, once the environment changes in a positive direction, suggesting that in both cases transient, fluctuating dysfunctions in similar brain areas, possibly of a different nature, are at play.

The dysmaturational syndrome, where most parents had multiple tics, appears as a genetic anticipation of Tourette syndrome; the autistic behavior is a potentially transient symptom included in the former basic disorder. In other words, it is an entirely different condition from those currently included within the autistic spectrum disorders/autistic syndromes.

CONCLUSION

In a perspective based on child neurology and in evaluating developmental disorders according to their evolution (ADHD, GTS, etc.), it is no wonder that specific developmental disorders different from autism itself go through a phase of potentially transient autistic behavior, that some epileptic disorders with autistic features can be treated successfully with appropriate drugs and that some children with severe brain damage over time lose their initial autistic symptoms. Children reared in severely depriving institutions can improve and in some cases entirely recover if placed in normal families. It is also worth noting the characteristics of those subjects with high-functioning autism who can have an access to an independent life, in spite of retaining certain core autistic features.

Claims of complete recovery from autism have, however, long been made mainly in the field of behaviorism by personalities like I. Lovaas, and, on partly different grounds, by S. I. Greenspan. In the case of behavioral therapies, the initial suggestion by Lovaas (1987) was based on the intensity of the intervention as if working hard and following specific relational strategies would allow better results in term of complete healing, an assumption that has been subsequently refined in different manner and degree by other behaviorists. Greenspan and Wieder (1997) tend to distinguish children with ASDs/the autistic syndromes in subgroups according to sensory modalities (i.e., underreactive or hyperreactive to sound and touch) or to their capability for warm relating to others defined as Multisystem Developmental Disorder (Greenspan 1992). They suggest that those children most capable of learning to relate had specific early abilities in complex gestural interaction and islands of symbolic function. Greenspan's floor time and

Lovaas' behavioral approaches can be integrated in the view of this author: in both cases, the intensity of the intervention in addition to its quality remains a basic need. It requires daily, intense parental work focused on supporting attention and cooperation around child's actual interests, making use in addition of some behavioral interventions; preserved abilities plus other sensory and relational peculiarities are said to be important criteria for complete recovery to occur.

These two approaches seem to consider autism as a unitary condition that may have, in Greenspan's idea, a more benign variant in the Multisystem Developmental Disorder; it is difficult to compare them with the data reported above, because they lack the neurological analysis that to a large extent appears to be central for understanding most cases where autistic behavior is reversible.

In the present state of knowledge, it would be quite unusual for children belonging to the autistic syndromes to benefit from intensive treatments of any kind to the point of becoming normal.

REFERENCES

Barkley RA (1995) *Taking Charge of ADHD.* New York: Guilford.
Beckett C, Bredenkamp D, Castle J, Grootheues C, O'Connor TG, Rutter M, English and Romanian Adoptees (ERA) Study Team (2002) Behavior patterns associated with institutional deprivation: a study of children adopted from Roumania. *Journal of Developmental Behavioural Pediatrics* 23:297–303.
Berardelli A, Curra A, Fabbrini G, Gilio F, Manfredi M (2003) Pathophysiology of tics and Tourette syndrome. *Journal of Neurology* 250:781–787.
Canitano R, Zappella M (2004) Autistic epileptiform regression. *Functional Neurology,* submitted.
Chess S (1977) Follow up report on autism in congenital rubella. *Journal of Autism and Childhood Schizophrenia* 7:68–81.
DeLong GR (1994) Children with autistic spectrum disorder and a family history of affective disorder. *Developmental Medicine & Child Neurology* 36:674–688.
DeLong GR, Dwyer JT (1988) Correlation of family history with specific autistic subgroups: Asperger's syndrome and bipolar affective disorder. *Journal of Autism and Developmental Disorders* 18:593–599.
DeLong GR, Nothria C (1994) Psychiatric family history and neurological disease in autistic spectrum disorders. *Developmental Medicine & Child Neurology* 36:441–448.
DeLong GR, Ritch CR, Burch S (2002) Fluoxetine response in children with autistic spectrum diosrders: correlation with familial major affective disorder and intellectual achievement. *Developmental Medicine&Child Neurology* 44:652–659.
DeLong GR, Teague L, Kamram M (1998) Effects of fluoxetine treatment in young children with idiopathic autism. *Developmental Medicine&Child Neurology* 40:551–562.
Deonna T (2004) Autistic regression of epileptic origin. Presented at: MacKeith's meetings, The Royal Society of Medicine, February 23, 2004.
Deonna T (1995) Cognitive and behavioral disturbances as epileptic manifestations in children: an overview. *Seminars in Pediatric Neurology* 2:254–260.

Deonna T, Ziegler AL, Maeder MI, Ansermet F, Roulet E (1995) Reversible behavioural autistic-like regression: a manifestation of a special (new?) epileptic syndrome in a 28-month-old child. A 2-year longitudinal study. *Neurocase* 1:91–99.

Deonna T, Ziegler AL, Moura-Serra J, Innocenti G (1993) Autistic regression in relation to limbic pathology and epilepsy: report of two cases. *Developmental Medicine and Child Neurology* 35:166–176.

Gillberg C (2004) Institutional autism and aspects of autism in immigrants. Presented at: MacKeith's meetings, The Royal Society of Medicine, February 23, 2004.

Greenspan SI (1992) *Infancy and Early Childhood: The Practice of Clinical Assessment and Intervention With Emotional and Developmental Challenges.* Madison: International Universities Press.

Greenspan SI, Wieder S (1997) Developmental patterns and outcomes in infants and children with disorders in relating and communicating: a chart review of 200 cases of chidren with Autistic Spectrum Diagnoses. *The Journal of Developmental and Learning Disorders* 1:87–141.

Jeffries KJ, Schooler C, Schoenbach C, Herschovitch P, Chase TN, Braun AR (2002) The functional neuroanatomy of Tourette's syndrome: an FDG PET study III: functional coupling of regional cerebral metabolic rates. *Neuropsychopharmacology* 27:92–104.

Kerbeshian J, Burd I (1992) Epidemiology and comorbidity: the North Dakota prevalence studies of Tourette syndrome and other developmental disorders. In Chase TN, Friedhoff AJ, Cohen DJ (Eds) *Advances in Neurology* (pp. 67–74). New York: Raven Press, Ltd.

Kerbeshian J, Burd I (1994) Tourette's syndrome: a developmental psychobiologic view. *Journal of Developmental and Physical Disabilities* 6:203–218.

Klin A (1991) Young autistic children's listening preference in regard to speech: a possible characterization of the symptoms of social withdrawal. *Journal of Autism and Developmental Disorders* 21:29–42.

Lovaas I (1973) Behavioural treatment and normal educational and intellectual functioning in young autistic children. *Journal of Consulting and Clinical Psychology* 55:3–9.

MacDonald KB, Parke RD (1984) Bridging the gap: Parent-child play interactions and peer interactive competence. *Child Development* 55:1265–1277.

MacDonald KB, Parke RD (1986) Parent-child physical play: the effects of sex and age of children and parents. *Sex Roles* 7/8:367–378.

Manouvrier-Hanu S, Amiel J, Jacquot S, Merienne K, Norman A, Coeslier A, Labarrière F, Vallée L, Croquette MF, Hanauer A (1999) Unreported *RSK2* missense mutation in two male sibs with an unusually mild form of Coffin-Lowry syndrome. *Journal of Medical Genetics* 36:775–778.

Mills M, Melhuish E (1974) Recognition of mother's voice in early infancy. *Nature* 252:123–124.

Perry R, Cohen I, De Carlo R (1995) Deterioration, Autism and Recovery in Two Siblings. *Journal of the American Academy of Child and Adolescent Psychiatry* 34:232–237.

Rutter M, Andersen-Wood L, Beckett C, Bredenkampt D, Castle J, Groothues C, Kreppner J, Keayeney L, Lord C, O'Connor TG, the English and Romanian Adoptees (ERA) study team (1999) Quasi-autistic patterns following severe early global deprivation. *Journal of Child Psychology and Psychiatry* 40:537–549.

Rutter ML, Kreppner JM, O'Connor TG, English and Romanian Adoptees (ERA) Study

Team (2001) Specificity and heterogeneity in children's responses to profound institutional deprivation, *British Journal of Psychiatry* 179:371.

Singer HS, Szymanski S, Giuliano J, Yokoi F, Dogan AS, Brasic JR, Zhou Y, Grant AA, Wong DF (2002) Elevated intrasynaptic dopamine release in Tourette's syndrome measured by PET. *American Journal of Psychiatry* 159:1329–1336.

Sutton-Smith B (1993) Dilemmas in Adult Play with Children. In MacDonald E (Ed) *Parent-Child Play.* Albany, NY: State University of New York Press.

Trevarthen C. (1979) Instincts for human understanding and for cultural cooperation: their development in infancy. In von Cranach M, et al. (Eds) *Human Ethology: Claims and Limits of a New Discipline* Cambridge: Cambridge University Press.

Wing L (2004) Insight and other clinical predictors. Presented at: MacKeith's meetings, The Royal Society of Medicine, February 23, 2004.

Zappella M (1998) *Autismo Infantile: Studi Sulla Affettività e le Emozioni.* Roma: Carocci, 1996; spanish transl. Autismo Infantìl, Mexico: Fundo de Cultura Economica, 1998.

Zappella M (1994a) Bambini autistici che guariscono: l'esempio dei tic complessi familiari. *Terapia Familiare* 46:51–62.

Zappella M (2002) Early-onset Tourette syndrome with reversible autistic behaviour: a dysmaturational disorder. *European Child and Adolescent Psychiatry* 11:18–22.

Zappella M (1999) Familial complex tics and autistic behaviour with favourable outcome in young children. *Infanto-Revista de Neuropsiquiatria da Infancia e Adolescentia* 7: 61–66.

Zappella M (1979) *Il Pesce Bambino.* Milano: Feltrinelli, 1976; french transl. Paris: L'Enfant Poisson, Payot, 1979.

Zappella M (1994b) Shared emotions and rapid recovery in children with delayed development. In Forrest G (Ed.) *The Clinical Application of Ethology and Attachment Theory* Association for Child Psychology & Psychiatry, Occasional papers, No. 9.

Zappella M, Meloni I, Longo I, Canitano R, Hayek G, Rosaia L, Mari F, Renieri A (2003) Study of *MECP2* gene in Rett syndrome variants and autistic girls. *American Journal of Medical Genetics* 119B:102–107.

Zappella M, Renieri A (2005) Clinical and genetic observations in early onset Tourette syndrome with reversible autistic behaviour. Presented at: MacKeith's meetings, The Royal Society of Medicine, February 23, 2004; to be printed in Riva D et al. (Eds) *Autism and Pervasive Developmental Disorders.* New York: John Libbey, in press.

Chapter 9

The Problem of Alternative Therapies in Autism

Lorenzo Pavone
Martino Ruggieri

Autism continues to be a puzzling condition and thus lends itself to the most intriguing speculations. It is widely accepted that autism represents a comprehensive syndrome recognizing many different causes that have interfered (at very early stages) in the normal development of the central nervous system (Gillberg & Coleman 2000; Cohen & Volkmar 1997; Rapin 2002; Volkmar & Pauls 2003). The classic, original concept of autism as first introduced by Kanner in 1942-43 has rapidly expanded and today autistic disorder is but one of the variants of the behavioral symptoms constellation in the so-called autistic spectrum disorder (ASD) (Pervasive Developmental Disorders) (Gillberg & Coleman 2000; Rapin 2002).

Autism and allied ASD present several behavioral, clinical, and biochemical abnormalities. Classic autism is characterized by the following major defining features (Filipek et al. 2000; Gillberg & Coleman 2000; Volkmar & Pauls 2003):

1. There is a deficit in communicative and noncommunicative language, sociability and empathy.
2. There are so-called idiopathic forms (*nonsyndromic autism*) and forms where the specific cause is determined (*syndromic autism*).
3. The frequent association with behavioral disturbances (anxious disorders, obsessive compulsive disorder, aggressiveness, rage, attention deficit hyperactivity disorder, etc.) has a major overall impact on the social life of affected individuals.

Over the past decades, several methods have been used in the treatment of children with autism (reviewed in Gillberg & Coleman 2000; National Research Council 2001). In addition, various guidelines for diagnosis and treatment have

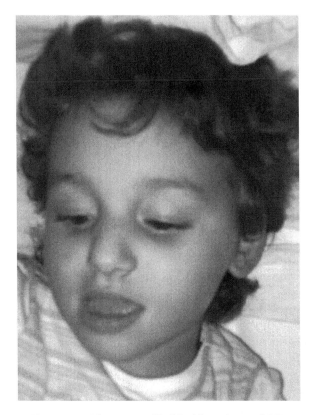

Figure 9.1   Three-year-old girl with autism and MR.

been published (Filipek et al. 2000). Parental participation, advanced testing protocols, and eclectic treatment strategies have driven progress toward a cure. Behavioral modification and structured education are beneficial but insufficient. Current pharmaceuticals fail to improve the primary symptoms and can have marked adverse effects (Howlin 1997; Baghdadli et al. 2002; Kidd 2002). Individualized, in-depth clinical and laboratory assessments and integrative parent-physician-scientist cooperation are the keys to successful ASD management (Filipek et al. 2000; Volkmar & Pauls 2003). Dietary restrictions, including removal of milk and other casein dairy products, wheat and other gluten sources, sugar, chocolate, preservatives, and food coloring have been tried (Ahearn et al. 2001; Ashwood et al. 2003; Bowers 2002; Garvey 2002; Knivsberg et al. 2001, 2002; No Authors Listed 2003; Raiten & Massaro 1986). Individualized IgG or IgE testing can identify other troublesome foods but not non–immune mediated food sensitivities. Gastrointestinal improvement rests on controlling *Candida* and other parasites, and using probiotic bacteria and nutrients to correct dysbiosis and decrease gut permeability (Ashwood et al. 2003; Brudnak 2002). Detoxification of mercury and other heavy metals by DMSA/DMPS chelation have been used (Holmes et al. 2003). Documented sulfoxidation-sulfation inadequacies call for sulfur-sulfhydryl repletion and other liver p450 support (McFadden 1996). Many nutrient supplements have been employed, including dimethylglycine (DMG) and a combination of pyridoxine (vitamin B6) and magnesium. Attempts with vitamins A, B3, C, and folic acid; the minerals calcium and zinc; cod liver oil; and digestive enzymes, have been tried (Nye & Brice 2002; Kidd 2003). Secretin, a triggering factor for digestion, is presently under investigation. Immune therapies (pentoxifyllin, intravenous immunoglobulin, transfer factor, and colostrum) and long-chain omega-3 fatty acids have been employed as well.

According to current knowledge, there is no established medical treatment that cures any group of patients with classic autism, with the exception of those with PKU or other metabolic diseases responsive to dietary therapy when started precociously. As mentioned above, numerous studies are aiming to improve or reduce the clinical dysfunctions of autism, especially problem behaviors that interfere with learning, and foster growth in areas including communication, cognition, and self-help skills (all those areas of deficit limiting the social life of affected persons).

Another important aspect is that as the basic mechanism for autism is still not defined a variety of treatments continue to be offered in everyday practice. It is very natural that families and therapists would seek out any therapy that sounds promising, especially for children (Aman et al. 2003). Physicians who work with autistic children must find a sensible balance between excessive criticism and passive acceptance of the wide variety of therapeutic options, not an easy task since many of the therapeutic options are not described or evaluated in the traditional scientific literature. Another practical issue is that many of these therapeutic strategies must deal with children who possess extraordinarily tuned sensory systems. Autistic children are also maturing and changing while the evaluation of the therapy is underway. In addition, many of these studies are plagued by the placebo effect and by a number of other possible misinterpretations due to lack of randomness, inappropriate or imprecise instrumentation, small samples or attrition of participants, and absence of long-term follow-up, and so on. For all these reasons it is not unusual for well-designed studies from excellent medical centres to disagree with each other (Gillberg & Coleman 2000).

Many alternative (nonspecific) treatments exist for which evidence of efficacy is limited or nonexistent. Such treatments are frequently proposed based on one case or an uncontrolled study; tremendous initial enthusiasm is followed by a more sober appraisal as controlled studies are done (Gillberg & Coleman 2000). In this chapter, we will review and comment on these topics.

Alternative therapies for autistic symptoms in general

Nonspecific therapies attempt to treat the core symptoms of the overall syndrome that we call autism, when it is not further defined. In the nonspecific therapies, although the drugs or the treatments are classified by a particular mode of action, it needs to be noted that the full impact of each drug on the brain usually involves other metabolic pathways and is far from being understood.

METABOLIC DISORDERS AND AUTISM: PHENYLKETONURIA (PKU)

Although the exact prevalence of metabolic abnormalities in ASD is unknown, some metabolic defects have been associated with autistic symptoms (McDougle 1993, 1996). These include phenylketonuria (PKU), histidinemia, adenylosuccinate lyase deficiency, dihydropyrimidine dehydrogenase deficiency, 5'-nucleotidase superactivity, and phosphoribosylpyrophosphate synthetase deficiency (Page 2000). When the metabolic consequences of an enzyme defect are well defined (e.g., PKU, 5'-nucleotidase superactivity), treatment with diet, drugs, or nutritional supplements may be able to prevent autism, or, when already present, to reduce the associated symptoms (Arnold et al. 2003). One such example is PKU.

PKU, one of the most common congenital disorders of amino acid metabolism, occurs in approximately 1/10,000 live births. It is inherited as an autosomal recessive trait and is caused by more than 200 different mutations affecting the functioning of the phenylalanine hydroxylase (PAH) enzyme or, more rarely, its essential cofactor tetrahydrobiopterin (BH4). If PAH (or BH4) is malfunctioning, the first amino acid (phenylalanine) is not converted into the second one (tyrosine) in the important pathway that produces catecholamines, dopamine, and norepinephrine in the brain. This results in phenylalanine going into minor pathways, some of which are toxic for the brain (hyperphenylalaninemia– HPA) by causing damage and reduction of myelin, neuronal loss and decreased levels of intraneuronal connections and neurotransmitter density. Early detection of PKU (by neonatal screening) allows very early dietary intervention and prevention of brain damage (which encompasses ASD) leading to a normal neuropsychological development. However, if infants with PKU are not started on the diet in the early weeks of life, they begin a deteriorating course that can result in the development of brain damage and, for some, in autistic syndromes (Dennis et al. 1999; Gillberg & Coleman 2000).

The association between PKU and ASD has been documented since the early 1960s (Benda 1960) and confirmed later on in larger ASD and/or PKU series (Friedman 1969; Bliumina 1975; Knobloch & Pasamanick 1975; Lowe et al. 1980; Reiss et al. 1986; Fombonne and du Mazaubrun 1992). The etiology of ASD in PKU is lack of early dietary intervention that in turn leads to abnormal brain development secondary to dysfunctional myelination and reduced neuronal connections with dopamine deficiency. Most children with PKU are severely retarded, epileptic, and hyperactive but not autistic; however, a significant subgroup of PKU meet ASD criteria (Friedman 1969; Reiss et al. 1986; Fombonne & du Mazaubrun 1992). The prevalence of ASD in untreated PKU, however, is low: 5.71% in the population of late diagnosed PKU sufferers in the province of Catania versus null in the population of early diagnosed PKU (Baieli et al. 2003). An important issue is that when children with PKU are treated after the diagnosis of PKU has been established for some time, ASD (as well as the spectrum of neurological dysfunction) does not improve (personal observation). It must be said, however, that it is the experience of other series (Lewis 1959; Lowe et al. 1980) and anecdotal cases (Williams 1998) to record improvement in functioning and developmental level in PKU/ASD children (Lewis 1959; Lowe et al. 1980) and adults (Williams 1998) when placed on a low-phenylalanine diet. However, major reversal of ASD symptoms is out of the question.

GLUTEN SENSITIVITY/GLUTEN SENSITIVE ENTEROPATHY (CELIAC DISEASE) AND AUTISM

Gluten sensitivity (GS) is an immune-mediated disease triggered by the ingestion of gluten (a protein that is found in some cereals such as wheat, oat, barley and rye) in genetically susceptible individuals (Ulshen 2004). Genetic susceptibility in GS is apparent by the fact that up to 90% of patients with gluten sensitive enteropathy (GSE) (celiac disease–CD) express the HLA class II molecules DQ2. The remaining 10% express HLA DQ8 (Maki et al. 2003; Ulshen 2004). Prevalence varies in different regions; its incidence is estimated around 1/100-1/200 in the general population (Maki et al. 2003). In its *classical infantile onset form* symptoms are caused by the involvement of the small bowel (GSE) and are characterized by irritability, apathy, diarrhoea, vomiting, abdominal distension, weakness, and weight loss. However, clinical manifestations can be diverse and *atypical forms* are also known with minimal or absent gastrointestinal symptoms: in these variants GS may pass unnoticed for a long period of time (Hadjivassiliou et al. 2002). It has been suggested that GS can be presented solely with nongastrointestinal manifestations (e.g., pruritic vescicular rash of dermatitis herpetiformis or neurological manifestations) (Gobbi et al. 1997; Hadjivassiliou et al. 2002). Even though GS is known to produce a variety of either neurological or psychiatric manifestations, particularly in the nonintestinal form in adults and children, the linkage between GS/GSE and ASD remains to be determined. The possibility has been raised of the symptoms of ASD being caused by the intake of specific foods, particularly gluten. Certainly in the overwhelming number of young children that present at a clinician's office with a diagnosis of ASD, careful history reveals that the symptoms began prior to age 18 months. This gives a limited period for the infant to have begun ingesting gluten-containing foods. In contrast, in the case of children whose symptoms start as late as 30 to 36 months, there may have been a sufficient time period of ingesting gluten-containing foods (Gillberg & Coleman 2000). However, population-based data indicates that only repetitive gluten challenges and long time elapses (in individuals unaware of GS or during phases of poor diet compliance) can put children at increased risk of developing or establishing any given neuropsychiatric manifestation in GS (M. Ruggieri et al. unpublished data). Thus, it seems unlikely that an early developmental disorder such as ASD can be caused by limited challenge with gluten.

GSE was first reported by Asperger (1961) in persons with his syndrome. Regarding autism as described by Kanner, the first report in the medical literature was in 1969 by Goodwin and Goodwin (1969) who later on followed the same case of a child with ASD (Goodwin et al. 1971) who improved after a gluten-free diet and exacerbated his symptoms with a normal diet, ordered in error. Since then, other case reports of children having both ASD and GSE have been published (Rimland 1972; Sullivan 1975; Reichelt et al. 1986; Shattock 1988; Braffet 1994). Two large studies have tried to identify the possibility of GSE in a subgroup of children with ASD. The first study (Walker-Smith et al. 1973) found a history of gastrointestinal symptoms in 7/18 children with autism; however, laboratory studies failed to demonstrate steatorrhea or antibodies to gliadin and results of jejunal biopsy in 3/8 gastrointestinal children were negative. The second study (McCarthy & Coleman 1979) reported behavioral improvement after gluten-free diet in 8 autistic children with a suspected GSE: all 8 children, however, had negative jejunal biopsies. According to the experience of one of us (Pavone et al. 1997) none of the children with antibody and biopsy proven GSE tested (by means of autism rating scales) at our institution was positive for ASD as compared to a control population. Thus, up to now, it appears that the occurrence of ASD and GSE in the same individual is likely to be a coincidence.

To determine the efficacy of gluten- and/or casein- free diets as an intervention to improve behavior, cognitive and social functioning in individuals with autism, Millward et al. (2004) searched for abstracts from the Cochrane Library (Issue 3, 2003), PsycINFO (1971-May 2003), EMBASE (1974-May 2003), CINAHL (1982-May 2003), MEDLINE (1986-May 2003), ERIC (1965-2003), LILACS (to 2003) and the specialist register of the Cochrane Complementary Medicine Field (January 2004) and examined also review bibliographies to identify all randomized, controlled trials involving programs that eliminated gluten, casein or both gluten and casein from the diets of individuals diagnosed with ASD: they reported a reduction in autistic traits with the combined gluten- and casein-free diet in one study only (Millward et al. 2004).

DIETARY INTAKE AND AUTISM

The hypothesis that the excessive dietary iron consumed by today's infants is the root cause of increased cases of autism, allergies and other childhood diseases was proposed (Padhye 2003). Iron is a powerful immune system modulator.

Excess iron creates a hyperactive immune system. This hyperactive immune system attacks undigested food peptides. The chemicals released during these intense allergic reactions can damage surrounding tissue. Neuronal degeneration is caused by combination of oxidative stress induced by free iron radicals and intense immune reactions. Iron chelators have been tried in autism and allergies.

In a recent case-control study from the UK General Practice Research Database (Black et al. 2002), 9 of 96 (9%) children with a diagnosis of autism and 41 of 449 (9%) children without autism (matched controls) had a history of gastrointestinal disorders (including chronic inflammation of the gastrointestinal tract, GSE, food intolerance, and recurrent gastrointestinal symptoms) before the index date (the date of first recorded diagnosis of autism in the cases and the same date for controls). The estimated odds ratio for a history of gastrointestinal disorders among children with autism compared with children without autism was 1.0 (95% confidence interval 0.5 to 2.2) thus indicating that no evidence could be found that children with autism were more likely than children without autism to have had defined gastrointestinal disorders (including food allergy or excess food intake) at any time before their diagnosis of autism.

Some organizations in the world known as Autism Intolerance & Allergy Network, Allergy-induced Autism Support or Self-Help Group (AIA) are pursuing the concept of an association between autism and food intolerances/allergy. They define allergy-induced autism as a subgroup of autism in which the autism symptoms appear to be triggered by intolerance to a variety of foods and chemicals, not the same in all cases. Deficiencies of detoxification enzymes (see below) have been suggested as pathogenic factors. In addition, children with ASD frequently reveal various gastrointestinal (GI) symptoms that may resolve with an elimination diet along with apparent improvement of some of the behavioral symptoms. Evidence suggests that ASD may be accompanied by aberrant (inflammatory) innate immune responses (Ashwood et al. 2003). This may predispose ASD children to sensitization to common dietary proteins (DP), leading to GI inflammation and aggravation of some behavioral symptoms. A recent study (Jyonouchi et al. 2002) has demonstrated that in ASD, individuals peripheral blood mononuclear cells (PBMCs) produced elevated IFN-gamma and TNF-alpha, but not IL-5 with common DPs at high frequency as observed in DPI (DP intolerance) PBMCs. ASD PBMCs revealed increased proinflammatory cytokine responses with LPS at high frequency with positive correlation between proinflammatory cytokine production with endotoxin and IFN-gamma and TNF-alpha production against DPs. Such correlation was less evident in DPI PBMCs. The authors concluded that immune reactivity to DPs may be associated with apparent DPI and GI inflammation in ASD children that may be partly associated with aberrant innate immune response against endotoxin, a product of the gut bacteria (Jyonouchi et al. 2002). Recent essays (Black et al. 2002) found no evidence that children with autism were more likely than children without autism to have had defined gastrointestinal disorders at any time before their diagnosis of autism and have also indicated that alterations in the diet of these affected children does not result in a cure of the autistic condition but rather a reduction in the severity of the symptoms. Although it is likely that food intolerance and/or allergies could increase behavioral changes, it seems somewhat unlikely that the full blown autistic syndrome would result. However, if a child is autistic and has obvious adverse reactions to some dietary products, then testing for metabolic or allergic problems should be considered (Ahearn et al. 2001).

VITAMINS

The use of mega-vitamin intervention began in the early 1950s with the treatment of schizophrenic patients (reviewed in Lerner et al. 2002; Nye & Brice 2002). Pyroxidine (vitamin B6) was first used with children diagnosed with "autism syndrome" when speech and language improvement was observed in some children as a result of large doses of B6. Vitamins would act via indirect pathways on neurotransmitters formation, serotonin in particular. A number of published studies attempted to assess the effects of vitamin B6 (Heeley & Roberts 1966; Bonisch 1968; Rimland 1988, 1998; Rimland & Ney 1974; Callaway 1977; Moss & Boverman 1978; Rimland et al. 1978; Sankar 1979). and vitamin B6/Mg (Mg was found to reduce undesirable side effects from B6) (Barthelemy et al. 1980, 1983; Findling et al. 1997; Lelord et al. 1981, 1982; Martineau et al. 1981, 1985; Tolbert et al. 1993) on a variety of characteristics—verbal communication, non-verbal communication, interpersonal skills, and physiological function—in individuals with autism. An extensive search of Cochrane Controlled Trials Register (Cochrane Library, 2004), MEDLINE (1966-July 2004), EMBASE (1980-July 2004), PsychINFO (1887-July 2004), Dissertation Abstracts International (1861-July 2004) revealed only two trials that used a double-blind crossover design. One study (Tolbert et al. 1993) provided insufficient data to conduct an analysis. The remaining study (Findling et al. 1997) yielded no significant differences between treatment and placebo group performances following the B6 intervention on measures of social interaction, communication, compulsivity, impulsivity, or hyperactivity. In conclusion, due to the small number of studies, the methodological quality of studies, and small sample sizes, no recommendation should be advanced regarding the use of B6-Mg as a treatment for autism. As regards to tolerability and side effects of vitamin B6/Mg compounds, they are generally well tolerated but sensory peripheral neuropathy, sun blisters and enuresis have been reported (Schaumberg et al. 1983; Coleman et al. 1985).

Another hypothesis is that autism may be a disorder linked to the disruption of the G-alpha protein, affecting retinoid receptors in the brain (Megson 2000). A study of 60 autistic children suggested that autism may be caused by inserting a G-alpha protein defect, the pertussis toxin found in the DPT vaccine, into genetically at-risk children. This toxin separates the G-alpha protein from retinoid receptors. Those most at risk report a family history of at least one parent with a preexisting G-alpha protein defect, including night blindness, pseudohypopar-athyroidism or adenoma of the thyroid or pituitary gland. Natural vitamin A may reconnect the retinoid receptors critical for vision, sensory perception, language processing and attention. Megson (2000) suggested that vitamin A could help persons with autism especially with vision, sensory perception, language processing, and attention problems. At present, however, that has not been tested either in case series studies or in double-blind, placebo-controlled studies.

The first studies on vitamin C started with Rimland studies in the 1960s and 1970s (Rimland 1972; Rimland et al. 1978; Gillberg & Coleman 2000) on administration of multivitamins (vitamins C, B3, B5, and B6) in children with autism. However, the positive effects of vitamin C were overshadowed by the apparent effectiveness of other vitamins; in addition, the dosage of vitamin C was very low (1 to 3 g per day). A second study presented the results of a 30-week double-blind, placebo-controlled trial exploring the effectiveness of ascorbic acid (vitamin C) (8g/70kg/d) as a supplemental pharmacological treatment for autistic children in residential treatment. Eighteen residential school children were randomly assigned to either ascorbate-ascorbate-placebo treatment order group or ascorbate-placebo-ascorbate treatment order group. Each treatment phase lasted 10 weeks and behaviors were rated weekly using the Ritvo-Freeman scale. Significant group by phase interactions were found for total scores and also sensory motor scores indicating a reduction in symptom severity associated with the ascorbic acid treatment (Dolske et al. 1993).

Initial observations on the use of folic acid and vitamin B12 in ASD were made by Lowe et al. (1981). Subsequent studies in boys (n=4) with the combination of infantile autism and the fragile-X syndrome tested oral folic acid and placebo, according to a double-blind crossover design. One boy's behavior appeared to improve on folic acid, but another boy did not seem to be affected at all. For the remaining two boys the results were equivocal (Gillberg et al. 1986) as in previous studies (Sankar et al. 1979).

Other food supplements that have been considered for autistic therapies are dimethylglycine (DMG), which is naturally found in some foods such as rice and liver although in small amounts. It has appeared to help in children with communication problems, particularly those with minimal speech. However, no controlled studies of any type have been conducted so far to test this hypothesis. Only Rimland (1972) and Rimland et al. (1978) noted these positive results on communication in autistic children who used the supplement. However, these children were under treatment with other compounds and supplements (Rimland 1972; Rimland et al. 1978; Gillberg & Coleman 2000).

KETOGENIC DIET AND AUTISM

This is a stringently controlled diet individualized for each child that provides nutrition predominantly as fats so that ketosis is maintained on a long-term basis

(Vioniong & Kessoff 2004). Wilder first introduced the ketogenic diet as a therapeutic method for epileptic seizures in the 1920s (Wilder 1921). The implementation of this method was based on clinical observations that fasting had beneficial effects in the control of epileptic seizures. The ketogenic diet was then abandoned because of the widespread use of antiepileptic drugs until the end of the 1970s, when interest in its use for the treatment of childhood epilepsies was rekindled (Evangeliou et al. 2003). Further progress in the basic sciences has established a clearer understanding of the ways in which ketone bodies affect the central nervous system: the diet, via alteration of the inhibitory-exalation balance, might change the energy metabolism of the brain, cell properties, meumoteous matter from action, neuromodulators, or the extra cellular environment of the brain (Vining & Kossoff 2004). As a result, the ketogenic diet has been used as one of a number of therapeutic means for epilepsy and other medical conditions (e.g., cancer). There have been also reports of application of a ketogenic diet for patients with Rett syndrome (Haas et al. 1986; Bujas-Petkovic et al. 1989): this method was used in Rett syndrome patients primarily for the control of seizures, but it was found that, in addition, the ketogenic diet was beneficial for mental behavior and hyperactivity. In view of these promising results Evangeliou et al. (2003) undertook a pilot follow-up study on 30 children (16 boys, 14 girls; aged between 4 and 10 years) with autistic behavior. The diet was applied for 6 months, with continuous administration for 4 weeks, interrupted by 2-week diet-free intervals. Seven children could not tolerate the diet whereas 5 other patients discontinued the diet. Of the remaining 18 children who adhered, the diet improvement was recorded in several parameters, including social behavior and interaction, speech, cooperation, stereotypy, and, principally hyperactivity that contributed significantly to their improvement in learning. Specifically, improvement was significant ($>$ 12 units of the childhood Autism rating Scale–CARS) in two patients, average ($>$ 8-12 CARS units) in eight, and was minor (2-8 units) in eight. Notably, improvement was more dramatic in the patients with mild autistic behavior while was minor or moderate in children with severe autistic behavior (Evangeliou et al. 2003). Such experience provides evidence that ketogenic diet may have its own place in the overall reserve for the treatment of ASD, in particular for less severe cases even though the small number of cases tested in the study could caveat the overall results; in addition it has a poor compliance in children.

NEUROTRANSMITTERS AND AUTISM

Recent studies suggested that serotonin reuptake inhibitors are helpful in reducing at least some symptoms of autism.

Inositol is a precursor of the second messenger for some serotonin receptors, and has been reported effective in depression, panic disorder and obsessive-compulsive disorder. However, a controlled double-blind crossover trial of inositol 200 mg/kg per day showed no benefit on 9 children with autism (Levine et al. 1997).

Secretin is a neurotransmitter in the neuropeptide group and is one of the hormones that control and regulate digestion (gastrin and colecystokinin [CKK] are the others). It is a polypeptide composed of 27 amino acids and is secreted by cells in the digestive system when the stomach empties. It stimulates (1) the pancreas to emit digestive fluids rich in water and bicarbonates, (2) the stomach to produce pepsin, and (3) the liver to produce bile. The secretin gene is located on chromosome 11p15.5 and the secretin receptors on chromosome 2.

Secretin has been found to have, besides gastrointestinal effects, various behavioral effects. For example, in experimental animals, it depresses the effects of single doses of morphine as well as respiration and increases the delay before animals jump to avoid adverse stimuli; in humans, it decreases approaches to novel items, movement in an open environment. As well as secreting bicarbonate, the pancreas secretes many other enzymes including lipases and especially peptidases. These peptidases will break down the peptides, which, according to proponents of the opioid excess theories of autism, may be responsible for the problems. Since secretin will stimulate the pancreas to produce these enzymes, it could ameliorate the symptoms by this mechanism. It could, also or alternatively, be acting in the brain itself or in the intestinal wall (if it acts at all).

Preliminary clinical trials on secretin administration in autistic persons began in 1997, and in 1998, Horwath et al. reported that secretin produced (within 5 weeks after infusion) a significant amelioration of gastrointestinal symptoms in three children with autistic spectrum disorders and a dramatic improvement in their behavior, manifested by improved eye contact, alertness, and expansion of expressive language. Anecdotal reports confirmed these findings. Results of further inquiries indicated that although treatment with secretin was reported to cause transient changes in speech and behavior in some children, overall it produced few clinically meaningful changes; placebo injections did not produce such effects (Chez et al. 2000). Further randomized, double-blind, placebo-controlled trials, however, demonstrated no evidence that either biological or synthetic secretin provided amelioration or reduction of any symptom in autism (Sandler et al. 1999; Chez et al. 2000; Dunn-Geier et al. 2000; Sandler and Bodfish, 2000; Carey et al. 2002; Molloy et al. 2002; Patel et al. 2002; Sponheim et al. 2002; Unis et al. 2002; Coplan et al. 2003; Levy et al. 2003; Welch et al. 2004). This held true when children with and without gastrointestinal problems were examined separately (Unis et al. 2002). Lack of evidence of methylation of the secretin gene was also found in lymphoblast cells from autistic patients or control individuals (Yamagata et al. 2002).

In conclusion, there is insufficient evidence to support secretin use as a therapy in autistic spectrum disorders and the use of secretin to treat autism is still "off label." Despite that, reports about using secretin-like substances to treat autism have appeared in many places, particularly the popular press. In addition, the costs for secretin doses lasting 2 weeks are very high.

GROWTH FACTORS AND AUTISM

Growth factors (GF) are well characterized, biologically active, small proteins that regulate normal cell growth development and cell death. GF are active within the body at very low physiological concentrations. Higher than normal concentrations of GF or inappropriately activated GF contribute to pathophysiologies of many diseases via aberrant cell signalling. Cell-signalling molecules, such as fibroblast growth factor-2 (FGF2), insulin-like growth factor-1 (IGF-1) and platelet-derived growth factor (PDGF) are part of the developmental stage GF that determine the timing of astrocytes and oligodendrocytes development and provide protective shields for environmental toxins.

It has been hypothesized that combinations of homeopathic GF could increase normal brain development and regulate nervous and immune system functioning in autism. FGF2 is a member of a large family of proteins that bind heparin sulfate and modulate the function of a variety of cells, especially in terms of growth and development, survival, stimulation of new blood vessel (neovascularisation) and cell specialization. Microinjections of FGF2 in the cerebral ventricles of rat embryos increases the proliferation of cortical progenitors in vivo, resulting in an increased cell number and surface volume. FGF2 is believed to have at least four main activities relevant to autism: (1) stem cell stimulation; (2) blood vessel regeneration; (3) bone marrow functioning; and (4) intestinal healing. Some parents of autistic children have used FGF2, with either positive reports or reports that it had made children hyperactive and regressed. There are, however, no randomized, double-blind or placebo controlled studies that can prove or disprove this hypothesis.

In addition to FGF2, other important GF participate in nervous system healing and protection. IGF-1 regulates and protects neuronal cell growth, healing and differentiation by playing critical roles in cortical, cerebellar and more in general neuronal live, death or specialization. PDGF is critical in the timing and differentiation or multi-potent steam cells into astrocytes and oligodendrocytes, especially during late foetal and post natal development. Transforming-growth factor-beta 1 (TGF_B1) pays key on/off regulatory roles and is expressed within the cerebellum, hippocampus, hypothalamus and midbrain.

Cerebrospinal levels of IGF-1 were statistically significantly lower in children with autism versus control children (Vanhala et al. 2001) and neurotrophic GF including neurotrophins nerve growth (NGF), brain-derived neurotrophic factor (BDNF), neurotrophin 3 (NT3) were over expressed in the first days of life (Nelson et al. 2001).

Combinations of these GF have been proposed ("Optimal Health Trio-liquid") and used in anecdotal reports of children with autism spectrum disorders with variable effects.

DETOXIFICATION OF MERCURY AND AUTISM

Mercury is ubiquitous in the global environment, ensuring universal exposure. Some forms of mercury are especially neurotoxic, including clinical signs at high doses. However, typical human exposures occur at low to moderate doses. Only limited data about neurotoxicity at low doses are available, and scientists differ in their interpretation of these data. Dose-response data on neurodevelopment are particularly limited. Despite or perhaps because of the lack of sufficient or consistent scientific data, public concern about a link between mercury exposure and developmental disabilities has been rising. After reviewing the data, the U.S. Environmental Protection Agency proposed a reference dose (an estimate of a daily dose that is likely to be without a risk of adverse effects over a lifetime) for methyl mercury that is substantially lower than previous guidelines from the World Health Organization, the U.S. Agency for Toxic Substances and Disease Registry, and the U.S. Food and Drug Administration. Some questions have been raised about the Environmental Protection Agency's guidelines, but the issue remains unresolved. Meanwhile, consumer groups have raised questions about the potential link between mercury exposure and ASD, as well as other adverse neurodevelopmental outcomes. This hypothesis has prompted some parents to seek regulatory, legal, or medical remedies in the absence of firm evidence. Anecdotal cases have reported that the effects of detoxification for heavy metals (such as mercury) are as dramatic as those found with secretin (see above).

The body of existing data, however, including the ecologic data presented herein, is not consistent with the hypothesis that increased exposure to mercury-containing substances (including vaccines) is responsible for the apparent increase in the rates of autism in young children being observed worldwide (Stehr-Green et al. 2003; Blaxill 2004; Blaxill et al. 2004). For instance, the discontinuation of thimerosal (mercury) containing vaccines in Denmark in 1992 was followed by an increase in the incidence of autism (Madsen et al. 2003); thus, the Danish ecological data do not support a correlation between mercury-containing vaccines and the incidence of autism (Madsen et al. 2003). No consistent significant associations were found between mercury-containing vaccines and neurodevelopmental outcomes in a U.S. study (Verstraeten et al. 2003).

THE "CANDIDA YEAST–AUTISM CONNECTION"

There is a great debate regarding the link between chronic candidiasis and autism. In general the medical community finds it hard to explain the association. The typical natural history of autism involves an increased awareness of atypical behaviors and communication difficulties around the toddler period, a time when children are often treated for middle ear infections with antibiotics that can upset the intestinal flora and possibly cause "yeast overgrowth." Some of the behavior problems have been linked to an overgrowth of *Candida albicans.* However, the existence of candidiasis in autistic children could very well be a coincidence rather than a cause. Rimland (1972), Rimland and Ney (1974) and Rimland et al. (1978) collected very interesting data from parents recording positive responses to Nystatin therapy; there seems to be little other confirmatory data. Some studies have been conducted in private pharmaceutical companies' laboratories testing a variety of interventions (including oral antibacterial and antifungal therapies, pancreatic enzymes, etc.).

AUDITORY INTEGRATION THERAPY AND AUTISM

Auditory integration therapy (AIT) was developed as a technique for improving abnormal sound sensitivity in individuals with behavioral disorders including autism. Other sound therapies bearing similarities to AIT include the Tomatis Method and Samonas Sound Therapy. To determine the effectiveness of AIT or other methods of sound therapy in individuals with ASD, Sinha et al. (2004) searched the Cochrane Central Register of Controlled Trials (Cochrane Library Issue 2, 2003), MEDLINE (1966-February 2002), EMBASE (1980-February 2002), CINAHL (1982-December 2001), PsycINFO (1887-February 2002), ERIC (1965-December 2001) and LILACS (1982-March 2002) including the reference lists of articles identified for further relevant publications. Treatment was auditory integration therapy (AIT) or other sound therapies involving listening to music modified by filtering and modulation. Control groups could be no treatment, waiting list, usual therapy or placebo equivalent. Outcomes sought were changes in core and associated features of ASD, auditory processing, quality of life and adverse events. All outcome data reported in included essays were based on long-term follow-up trials. They found no trials assessing sound therapies other than AIT. Six trials of AIT, including one cross-over trial, were identified with a total of 171 individuals aged 3-39 years. Four trials had fewer than 20 participants. Allocation concealment was inadequate for all the studies. Seventeen different outcome measures were used. Only 2 outcomes were used by 3 or more studies: Aberrant Behavior Checklist (ABC) (5) and Fisher's Auditory Problems Checklist (FAPC) (3). Meta-analysis was not possible due to very high heterogeneity (Aberrant Behavior Checklist subscores), or presentation of data in unusable forms. Three studies (Bettison 1997; Mudford et al. 2000; Sinha et al. 2004) did not demonstrate benefit (Mudford et al. 2000; Sinha et al. 2004) or demonstrated limited benefit (Bettison 1996) of AIT over control conditions. The remaining trials (Veale 1993, Rimland & Edelson 1995; Edelson et al. 1999) reported improvements at 3 months for the AIT group based on improvements of total mean scores for the ABC, which is of questionable validity. Rimland and Edelson (1995) also reported improvements at 3 months in the AIT group for ABC subgroup scores. No significant adverse effects of AIT were reported. The authors concluded that more research was needed to inform parents', carers' and practitioners' decision making about this therapy for individuals with autism spectrum disorders.

From a medical point of view, this therapy would not be harmful and therefore need not be discouraged even though it is still difficult to understand how such course of therapy could have such long-lasting results.

MUSIC THERAPY AND AUTISM

Groups of children with ASD have been investigated on the effect of a musical presentation of social story information on their behaviors. Social stories are a means of incorporating an individual with autism's propensity toward visual learning with educationally necessary behavior modifications. Participants in one study (Brownell 2002) were 4 first- and second-grade students with a primary diagnosis of autism attending an elementary school in eastern Iowa. A unique social story was created for each student that addressed a current behavioral goal. Subsequently, original music was composed using the text of the social story as lyrics. The independent variable for this study was one of three treatment conditions: baseline (A); reading the story (B); and singing the story (C). The reading and singing versions of the social stories were alternately presented to the students using the counterbalanced treatment order ABAC/ACAB. The dependent variable was the frequency with which the target behavior occurred under each condition of the independent variable. Data were collected for a period of 1 hour following presentation of the social story. Results from all four cases indicated that both the reading condition (B) and the singing condition (C) were significantly (p <0.05) more effective in reducing the target behavior than the no-contact control condition (A). The singing condition was significantly more effective than the reading condition only in Case Study III. For the remaining case studies, the mean frequency of the target behavior was smaller during the singing condition, but not significantly so.

DOMAN/DELACATO METHOD AND AUTISM

In the 1960s, psychomotor patterning was proposed as a new treatment modality for people with mental retardation, brain injury, learning disabilities, and other cognitive conditions. The concept of patterning was invented by Glenn Doman and Carl Delacato and is therefore often referred to as the Doman-Delacato technique (Delacato & Doman 1957; Doman et al. 1960). Their theories are primarily an extension of the outdated concept that ontogeny (the stages through which organisms develop from single cell to maturity) recapitulates phylogeny (the evolutionary history of the species). Thus the neurodevelopmental stages of crawling, creeping, crude walking, and mature walking through which normal children develop is directly related to the amphibian, reptilian, and mammalian evolutionary human ancestors. Doman and Delacato postulated that mental retardation represents a failure of the individual to develop through the proper phylogenetic stages. Their treatment modality supposedly stimulates proper development of these stages, each of which must be mastered before progress can be made to the next stage. This stimulation is done through what they call "patterning," in which the patient moves repeatedly in the manner of the current stage. In the "homolateral crawling" stage, for instance, patients crawl by turning their head to one side while flexing the arm and leg of that side and extending the arm and leg of the opposite side. Patients who are unable to execute this exercise by themselves are passively moved in this manner by 4-5 adults, alternating back and forth in a smooth manner. This must be repeated for at least 5 minutes, 4 times per day. This exercise is intended to impose the proper "pattern" onto the central nervous system. In the full treatment program, the exercises are combined with sensory stimulation, breathing exercises intended to increase oxygen flow to the brain, and a program of restriction and facilitation intended to promote hemispheric dominance. Advocates claim that patterning enables mentally retarded and brain injured children to achieve improved, and even normal, development in the areas of visuo-spatial tasks, motor coordination, social skills, and intellect. They also claim to promote superior development in a normal child. The theoretical basis of psychomotor patterning is therefore based on two primary principles, the recapitulationist theory of ontogeny and phylogeny, and the belief that passive movements can influence the development and structure of the brain.

In 1982, the American Academy of Pediatrics did not endorse the original program, at least partly because of lack of published data (American Academy of Pediatrics Policy Statement, 1982). During approximately 10 years in the late 1960s and early 1970s, dozens of clinical trials compared groups of developmentally delayed children given patterning treatment to comparable who received no treatment but similar amounts of attention (Joint Executive Board Statement 1967). None confirmed the claims of Doman and Delacato. Some found modest improvements in motor or visuo-spatial skills, but none showed improved intellectual development. The few positive studies were neither impressive nor reproducible. Doman, Delacato, and their associates incorporated the patterning technique into their *Institutes for the Achievement of Human Potential* (IAHP), which was established in Philadelphia in the 1950s and still operates today. A second facility, the National Academy of Child Development (NACD) in Huntsville, Utah, offers several patterning as part of their treatment program ranging from a home study program to an intensive treatment program.

OSTEOPATHY/CRANIOSACRAL THERAPY AND AUTISM

Craniosacral therapy is one of many terms used to describe a variety of methods based on the following claims: (1) the human brain makes rhythmic movements at a rate of 10 to 14 cycles per minute, a periodicity unrelated to breathing or heart rate; (2) small cranial pulsations can be felt with the fingertips; (3) restriction of movement of the cranial sutures (where the skull bones meet) interferes with the normal flow of cerebrospinal fluid (the fluid that surrounds the brain and spinal cord) and cause disease; (4) diseases can be diagnosed by detecting aberrations in this rhythm; (5) pain (especially of the jaw joint) and many other ailments can be remedied by pressing on the skull bones. Most practitioners are osteopaths, massage therapists, chiropractors or physical therapists. The other terms used to describe what they do include cranial osteopathy, cranial therapy, bio cranial therapy, and two chiropractic variants called craniopathy and sacro occipital technique (SOT).

Today's leading proponents have claimed that "craniosacral therapy is a gentle, non invasive manipulative technique. Seldom does the therapist apply pressure that exceeds 5 grams or the equivalent weight of a nickel. Examination is done by testing for movement in various parts of the system. Often, when movement testing is completed, the restriction has been removed and the system is able to self-correct." They infer that "the rhythm of the craniosacral system can be detected in much the same way as the rhythms of the cardiovascular and respiratory systems. But unlike those body systems, both evaluation and correction of the craniosacral system can be accomplished through palpation." Practitioners today rely on craniosacral therapy to improve the functioning of the central nervous system, eliminate the negative effects of stress, strengthen resistance to disease, and enhance overall health.

According to our opinion and experience in the field of autism, there is no scientific justification for this approach. Furthermore, this method could be harmful.

HOLDING THERAPY AND AUTISM

In the late 1970s, holding therapy gained wide-spread attention when Dr. Martha Welch, a child psychiatrist from New York, began using it as a means of working with children with autism. Holding therapy has many advocates, who claim remarkable results, as well as many detractors who disagree with its intrusive nature. The place of holding in changing autistic behavior is that it is one technique among many, and it is to be combined with baby play, treatment of specific learning difficulties, medical screening and exclusion of medical causes for associated behavioral problems, family support, and so on.

The therapy involves the forced holding of an autistic child through theoretical phases of acceptance, resistance and acquiescence. The rationale for this therapy is that a bond was not established with the affected child, perhaps because of problems with social reciprocity, and thus the child withdraws to defend himself against the perceived rejection. Dr. Welch reported very positive results.

One recent study aimed to analyze the use of holding, restraints, seclusion, and time-out in child and adolescent psychiatric in-patient treatment in Finland (Sourander et al. 2002). The study included 504 child and adolescent psychiatric in-patients in the year 2000. Time-out had been used for 28%, holding for 26%, seclusion for 8%, and mechanical restraints for 4% of the in-patients. In multivariate analysis, aggressive acts were the strongest factor associated with all kinds of restraint practices. Psychosis, suicidal acts and older age (13–18 years) were associated with seclusion and mechanical restraints. Younger age (< 13 years), attachment disorder and autism were associated with holding. The longer children had been in treatment, the more likely they were to have been restrained. The high prevalence of restraint techniques used indicates a need for guidelines for the use of restraint and seclusion that take into account the child's need for protection from his/her own impulses and the legal rights of the child.

From a medical viewpoint there should be no particular concerns regarding harmfulness and certainly hugging has its benefits. However, our personal concern is about the premise on which it is based and the possible adverse psychological effects on the parents, who had theoretically rejected their children.

HORSE AND PONY RIDING AND AUTISM

Hippotherapy, from the Greek word for "horse," is based on the idea that the rhythmic, repetitive movements of the horse work to improve cognitive skills, balance, posture, and strength in the disabled rider. Individuals claimed to benefit from this kind of therapy have had a variety of diagnoses, including cerebral palsy, stroke, and learning or language disabilities including autism. Horse riding and horse-related activities are claimed to assist successfully in the development and restoration of personal confidence, self-esteem, and communication skills. The effects of therapeutic riding have not been subjected to scientific scrutiny and there have been no case-control or double-blind studies so far to prove the efficacy of these methods in ASD. Conversely, injuries from riding horses are well-known complications.

DOLPHIN THERAPY AND AUTISM

Dolphin assisted therapy (DAT) is a therapeutic approach that claims to increase speech and motor skills in children and adults who have been diagnosed with developmental, physical, and/or emotional disabilities, such as mental retardation or ASD. The theory behind this controversial therapeutic approach is that when a child with special needs interacts with a dolphin, it increases his or her attention. The program is used to modify behavior; that is, reward the child, through dolphin interaction, when the child performs a desired function. Therefore, DAT can be seen as a motivational approach to accomplishing goals relating to speech, fine motor skills, gross motor skills, and cognitive thinking skills. In other words, DAT should encourage children to perform the more traditional types of therapy by rewarding the children with dolphin contact. There are several different programs providing DAT. Some programs also allow the children to participate in preparing the dolphin's food, feeding them, observing, interacting during training sessions, and giving rubs. With the new skills that the children learn in the program, the therapists claim that the children develop positive self-esteem and empowerment in all areas of their lives. Aside from actual contact with the dolphins, these programs may also include swimming and snorkelling lessons, and proper etiquette during dolphin encounters.

Critics of DAT argue that dolphin therapy does not do anything different for the child with special needs than work with other service animals, such as dogs and horses, can provide. They claim that any kind and gentle animal can break through the child's barrier and give successful results. We would be quite surprised if there was any validity to the notion that dolphins could target any particular area with their ultrasound. If there is any success, we would be much more inclined to attribute it to the general effects of the opportunity to interact with animals. In addition, these programs are expensive and short in duration. There is no scientific evidence at all that using dolphins is helpful. The reputable people in the field simply feel the kids like the dolphins, and it's a recreational thing.

DANCE/MUSIC THERAPY AND AUTISM

Many autistic patients love music. Several studies conducted by music therapists have shown that many children with autism respond more frequently, more appropriately, and with more pleasure to music than to any other auditory stimulus. In that respect, music therapy can be effective in working to improve motor coordination, communication skills, social and behavioral skills, attention span and sensory issues. Advocates of music therapy activities such as rhythm instrument playing and body movement claim that they aid in the development of fine- and gross-motor coordination skills, such as learning to use fingers to button clothes, to hold a pencil or use scissors in school, and to learn to identify and move body parts. Learning to share and take turns during rhythm instrument playing is also thought to build appropriate social and behavioral skills, both of which have important carry over into the school setting. The same applies to song singing activities believed to be effective in encouraging the child to develop listening skills, the ability to follow directions, and to develop and practice both verbal and nonverbal communication skills. Finally, it is not unusual to encounter music therapists who work with autistic children often collaborating in their treatment with other professionals, such as physical therapists, occupational therapists and speech-language therapists ("team-oriented" approach).

ARE RECOMMENDATIONS OF THE AMERICAN ACADEMY OF NEUROLOGY AND THE CHILD NEUROLOGY SOCIETY REGARDING LABORATORY INVESTIGATIONS IN ASD APPLICABLE TO ALTERNATIVE THERAPIES?

According to the panel of experts who produced the practice parameter guidelines for screening and diagnosis of autism (Filipek et al. 2000), there is insufficient evidence to support the use of other tests besides genetic testing (karyotype and DNA analysis of selected conditions) and selective metabolic testing (as indicated by clinical and physical findings). There is also inadequate evidence to support the use of hair analysis, celiac antibodies, allergy testing (including food allergies for gluten, casein, candida, and other molds), immunologic or neurochemical abnormalities, micronutrients, such as vitamin levels, intestinal permeability studies, stool analysis, urinary peptides, mitochondrial disorders (including lactate and pyruvate), thyroid function tests, or erythrocyte glutathione peroxidase studies. These conclusions seem to suggest that many of the experts on ASD do not give much credit to alternative therapies. Evaluation of the above parameters, however, may be necessary whenever a therapeutic trial is going to be undertaken at any level (practical daily therapeutic attempts or a research study).

CONCLUSION

Interventions considered to be alternative in ASD are in constant flux. New treatments emerge, older treatments become less popular, and the cycle recurs. Data supporting new treatments should be scrutinized for scientific study design, clinical safety, and scientific validity. Many families approach the clinician armed with brochures, handouts, and printouts from Web sites that are dedicated to the care and support of parents and children with ASD. A routine web search using "autism" and "alternative therapy" or "autism" and any of the above mentioned treatment strategies results in thousands of sites. The scientific validation and support for many interventions is incomplete and disparate from the recommendation in most of the world Academies of Pediatrics, Neurology or Psychiatry Policy Statements. Families should be encouraged to discuss all proposed investigations or treatments they wish to try with their primary care provider, so the practitioner can serve as the medical home (Levy & Hyman 2003). The clinician should communicate and collaborate with the family and educational professionals to encourage objective identification of what works. With increasing access to health information and societal pressure for families to actively participate in their health management, continued growth of interest in alternative therapies can be anticipated. Clinicians must remember that parents may have different beliefs regarding the effectiveness of treatment and different tolerance for treatment risks. Practitioners must keep avenues of communication open, remain open-minded, and not assume a "don't ask, don't tell" posture in the context of providing a medical home to the increasing number of children diagnosed with autism.

To the best of our current knowledge we have no data to establish if ASD may have to any extent a relation with allergy, food intolerance or toxins or any other compounds' adverse effects in predisposed subjects. To add vitamins to the daily diet or to substitute or avoid given aliments or substances so as to obtain certain therapeutic effects has so far no scientific basis in individuals with ASD.

Up to now there is no single etiology or given cause to explain ASD. A limited but given number of classical imaging and pathology studies has demonstrated mild neuronal developmental abnormalities, rather than specific lesions, in the cerebellum, limbic system and neocortex with anomalies of neuronal migration/ organisation in some patients. More recent imaging studies have demonstrated, by means of new and more sophisticated techniques, brain anomalies not only in the cerebellum and limbic system but also in the amygdala, frontal lobe, and hippocampus.

Neuronal cells in the central nervous system of children once committed and matured cannot be rebuilt, and become areas of permanent damage irresponsive to any treatment. Therefore it seems unlikely that a given compound or an aliment could exert a positive (or reversal) effect in these brains.

Somewhat different is the associated comorbidity that often accompanies ASD. It is possible that some substances or compounds, once eliminated from diet or pharmaceutically washed out, could reverse or ameliorate some of the comorbid symptoms in ASD. However, which are these substances? Are they the same for all individuals with ASD? Or are some specific ASD phenotypes influenced more or less by given compounds? Which are the pathogenic pathways involved?

So far there is no scientific evidence that any compound could influence in any respect the course of disease and/or could be responsible of any abnormality in ASD.

PERSONAL REMARKS

1. Autism is a neurological organic disorder manifesting early in life. When the diagnosis (even the earliest) is made, the brain has already been irreversibly damaged and therefore there are currently no means at all with proven efficacy that can interfere with the symptoms of ASD: pharmacological treatment therefore must be addressed toward the associated symptoms.

2. All types of treatments (established or alternative) should be assessed carefully before being undertaken in ASD. However, it should be remembered that these attempted treatments must be considered of outmost importance in helping the severely handicapped child and his or her family, who otherwise will collapse under the weight of a disabling and often enabling condition. Therapeutic attempts, however, are to be undertaken keeping in mind their overall efficacy versus tolerability and safety.

3. Rehabilitation and specific education therapy should be considered the current first choice treatment guidelines in the treatment of ASD.

4. Only in the future will we likely know what infective agents, substances or toxic compounds besides any other causes, such as genetic, may interfere with the brain functioning in ASD. Thus, only when we reach that level of knowledge we will be able to focus on a specific (dietary or pharmaceutical) therapy by introducing, adding or eliminating any cause from daily life of affected individuals at the earliest proven time.

REFERENCES

Ahearn WH, Castine T, Nault K, Green G (2001) An assessment of food acceptance in children with autism or pervasive developmental disorder-not-otherwise specified. *Journal of Autism and Developmental Disorders* 31:505–511.

Aman MG, Lam KS, Collier-Crespin A (2003) Prevalence and patterns of use of psychoactive medicines among individuals with autism in the Autism Society of Ohio. *Journal of Autism and Developmental Disorders* 33:527–534.

American Academy of Pediatrics (1982) Policy statement: The Doman-Delacato treatment of neurologically handicapped children *Pediatrics* 70:810–812.

American Academy of Pediatrics and American Academy of Neurology (1967) Joint executive board statement: Doman-Delacato treatment of neurologically handicapped children. *Neurology* 17:637.

Arnold GL, Hyman SL, Mooney RA, Kirby RS (2003) Plasma amino acids profiles in children with autism: potentials risk of nutritional deficiencies. *Journal of Autism and Developmental Disorders* 33:449–454.

Ashwood P, Anthony A, Pellicer AA, Torrente F, Walker-Smith JA, Wakefield AJ (2003) Intestinal lymphocyte populations in children with regressive autism: evidence for extensive mucosal immunopatholgy. *Journal of Clinical Immunology* 23:504–517.

Asperger H (1961) Die Psychopatologie des coeliank-iekranken Kindes. *Annales Paediatriae* 197:146–151.

Baghdadli A, Gonnier V, Aussilloux C (2002) Review of psychopharmacological treatments in adolescents and adults with autistic disorders. *Encephale* 28:248–254.

Baieli S, Pavone L, Meli C, Fiumara A, Coleman M (2003) Autism and phenylketonuria. *Journal of Autism and Developmental Disorders* 33:201–204.

Barthelemy C, Garreau B, Leddet I, Sauvage D, Domenech J, Muh JP, Lelord G (1980) Biological and clinical effects of oral magnesium and associated magnesium-vitamin B6 administration on certain disorders observed in infantile autism. *Therapie* 35:627–632.

Barthelemy C, Garreau B, Leddet I, Sauvage D, Muh JP, Lelord G, Callaway E (1983) Value of bahaviour scales and urinary homovanillic acid determination monitoring the combined treatment with vitamin B6 and magnesium in children displaying autistic behaviour. *Neuropsychiatrie de l'Enfance et de l'Adolescence* 31:289–301.

Benda CE (1960) Childhood schizophrenia, autism and Heller's disease. In *Proceedings of the First International Metabolic Conference, Portland, Maine.* New York: Grune & Stratton.

Bettison S (1996) The long-term effects of auditory training on children with autism. *Journal of Autism and Developmental Disorders* 26:361–374.

Bettison S (1997) The long-term effects of auditory training on children with autism. *Journal of Autism and Developmental Disorders* 27:347–348.

Black C, Kaye JA, Jick H (2002) Relation of childhood gastrointestinal disorders to autism: nested case-control study using data from the UK General Practice Research Database. *British Medical Journal* 325:419–421.

Blaxill MF (2004) Concerns continue over mercury and autism. *American Journal of Preventive Medicine* 26:91; reply 91–92.

Blaxill MF, Redwood L, Bernard S (2004) Thimerosal and autism? A plausible hypothesis that should not be dismissed. *Medical Hypotheses* 62:788–794.

Bliumina MG (1975) A schizophrenic-like variant of phenylketonuria. *Zhurnail Nevropthologii I Psikiatrii Imeni S S Korsakova* 75:1525–1529.

Bonisch E (1968) Ehrfarungen met Pyrithioxin bei hirgeschadigten kindern mit autistischen Syndrom. *Praxis de Kinderpsychologie* 8:308–310.

Bowers L (2002) An audit of referrals of children with autistic spectrum disorders to the dietetic service. *Journal of Human Nutrition and Dietetics* 15:141–144.

Braffet C (1994) No milk, no bread please. *Autism Society of Indiana Quarterly* 1:7–9.

Brownell MD (2002) Musically adapted social stories to modify behaviours in students with autism: four case studies. *Journal of Musical Therapy* 39:117–144.

Brudnak MA (2002) Probiotics as an adjuvant to detoxification protocols. *Medical Hypotheses* 58(5):382–385.

Bujas-Petkovic Z, Matjiasic R, Divcic B (1989) Rett's syndrome—differential diagnosis of autism in a case report. *Lijek Vjesn* 111:458–460.

Callaway E (1977) Response of infantile autism to large doses of B6. *Psychological Bulletin* 13:57–58.

Carey T, Ratliff-Scaub K, Funk J, Weinle C, Myers M, Jenks J (2002) Double-blind placebo-controlled trial of secretin: effects on aberrant behavior in children with autism *Journal of Autism and Developmental Disorders* 32:161–167.

Chez MG, Buchanan CP, Bagan BT, Hammer MS, McCarthy KS, Ovrutskaya I, Nowiski I, Cohen ZS (2000) Secretin and autism: a two-part clinical investigation. *Journal of Autism and Developmental Disorders* 30:87–94.

Cohen DJ, Volkmar FR (1997) *Handbook of Autism and Pervasive Developmental Disorders.* New York: Wiley.

Coleman M, Sobel S, Bhagavan HN, Coursin D, Marquardt A, Guay M, Hunt C (1985) A double blind study of vitamin B6 in Down's syndrome infants. Part I. Clinical and biochemical results. *Journal of Mental Deficiency Research* 29:233–240.

Coplan J, Souders MC, Mulberg AE, Belchic JK, Wray J, Jawad AF, Gallagher PI, Mitchell R, Gerdes M, Levy SE (2003) Children with autistic spectrum disorders, II: parents are unable to distinguish secretin from placebo under double-blind conditions. *Archives of Disease in Childhood* 88:727–739.

Delacato CH, Doman G (1957) Hemiplegia and concomitant psychological phenomena. *American Journal of Occupational Therapy* 11:186–197.

Dennis M, Lockyer L, Lazenby Al, Donnelly RE, Wilkinson M, Schoonheyt W (1999) Intelligence patterns among children with high-functioning autism, phenylketonuria, and childhood head injury. *Journal of Autism and Developmental Disorders* 29:5–17.

Dietary supplements seized after autism claims (2003) *FDA Consumer Magazine* 37:4.

Dolske MC, Spollen J, McKay S, Lancashire E, Tolbert L (1993) A preliminary trial of ascorbic acid as supplementary therapy for autism. *Progress in Neuropsychopharmacoly and Biological Psychiatry* 17:765–774.

Doman RJ, Spitz EB, Zucman E, Delacato CH, Doman G (1960) Children with severe brain injuries. Neurological organisation in terms of mobility. *JAMA* 174:257–262.

Dunn-Geier J, Ho HH, Auersperg E, Doyle D, Eaves L, Matsuba C, Orrbine E, Phubes G, Whiting S (2000) Effect of secretin on children with autism: a randomised controlled study. *Developmental Medicine and Child Neurology* 42:796–802.

Edelson SM, Edelson MG, Kerr DC, Grandin T (1999) Behavioural and physiological effects of deep pressure on children with autism: a pilot study evaluating the efficacy of Grand's hug Machine. *American Journal of Occupational Therapy* 53:145–152.

Evangeliou A, Vlachonikolis I, Mihailidou H, Spilloti M, Skarpalezotiou M, Makaronas N, Prokopiou A, Christodoulou P, Liapi-Adamidou G, Helidonis E, Sbyriakis S, Smeitink J (2003) Application of a ketogenic diet in children with autistic behaviour: a pilot study. *Journal of Child Neurology* 18:113–118.

Filipek PA, Accardo PJ, Ashwal S, Baranek GT, Cook EH, Dawson G, Gordon B, Gravel JS, Johnson CP, Kallen RJ, Levy SE, Minshew NJ, Ozonoff S, Prizant BM, Rapin I, Rogers SJ, Stone WL, Teplin SW, Tuchman RF, Volkmar FR (2000) Practice parameters: screening and diagnosis of autism. Report of the quality standards subcommittee of the American Academy of Neurology and the Child Neurology Society. *Neurology* 55:468–479.

Findling RL, Maxwell K, Scotese-Wojtila L, Huang J, Yamashita T, Wizniter M (1997) High doses pyridoxine and magnesium administration in children with autistic disorder: an absence of salutary effects in a double-blind, placebo controlled study. *Journal of Autism and Developmental Disorders* 27:581–578.

Fombonne E, du Mazaubrun C (1992) Prevalence of infantile autism in four French regions. *Social Psychiatry and Psychiatric Epidemiology* 27:203–210.

Friedman E (1969) The autistic syndrome and phenylketonuria. *Schizophrenia* 1:249–261.

Garvey J (2002) Diet in autism and associated disorders. *Journal of Family Health Care* 12: 34–38.

Gillberg C, Coleman M (2000) *The biology of Autistic Syndromes (3rd ed.).* Cambridge: Cambridge University Press.

Gillberg C, Wahlstrom J, Johansson R, Tornblom M, Albertsson-Wikland K (1986) Folic acid as an adjunct in the treatment of children with the autism-fragile X syndrome (AFRAX). *Developmental Medicine and Child Neurology* 28:624–627.

Gobbi G, Andermann F, Naccarato S, Banchini G (1997). *Epilepsy and Other Neurological Disorders in Coeliac Disease.* London: John Libbey.

Goodwin MS, Cowen MA, Goodwin TC (1971) Malabsorption and cerebral dysfunction. A multivariate and comparative study of autistic children. *Journal of Autism and Childhood Schizophrenia* 1:48.

Goodwin MS, Goodwin TC (1969) In a dark mirror. *Mental Hygiene* 53:550.

Haas RH, Rice MA, Trauner DA, Merritt TA (1986) Therapeutic effects of a Ketogenic diet in Rett syndrome. *American Journal of Medical Genetics* 1(Suppl):225–246.

Hadjivassiliou M, Boscolo S, Davies-Jones GAB (2002) The humoral response in the pathogenesis of gluten ataxia. *Neurology* 58:1221–1226.

Heely AF, Roberts GE (1966) A study of tryptophan metabolism in psychotic children. *Developmental Medicine and Child Neurology* 8:708–718.

Holmes AS, Blaxill MF, Haley BE (2003) Reduced levels of mercury in first baby haircuts of autistic children. *International Journal of Toxicology* 22:277–285.

Horwath K, Stefanatos G, Sololski KN, Watchel R, Nabors L, Tildon JT (1998) Improved social and language skills after secretin administration in patients with a autism spectrum disorders. *Journal of the Association for Academic Minority Physicians* 9:9–15.

Howlin P (1997) Prognosis in autism: do specialist treatments affect long-term outcome? *European Child and Adolescent Psychiatry* 6:55–72.

Jyonouchi H, Sun S, Itokazu N (2002) Innate immunity associated with inflammatory responses and cytokine production against common dietary proteins in patients with autism spectrum disorders. *Neuropsychobiology* 46:76–84.

Kanner L (1942–43) Autistic disturbances of affective contact. *Nervous Child* 2:217–250.

Kidd PM (2003) An approach to the nutritional management of autism. *Alternative Therapies in Health and Medicine* 9:22–31; quiz 32, 126.

Kidd PM (2002) Autism, an extreme challenge to integrative medicine. Part 2: medical management. *Alternative Medicine Review* 7:472–499.

Knivsberg AM, Reichelt KL, Hoien T, Nodland M (2002) A randomised controlled study of dietary intervention in autistic syndromes. *Nutritional Neuroscience* 5:251–261.

Knivsberg AM, Reichelt KL, Nodland M (2001) Reports on dietary intervention in autistic disorders. *Nutritional Neuroscience* 4:25–37.

Knobloch H, Pasamanick B (1975) Some etiologic and prognostic factors in early infantile autism and psychosis. *Journal of Pediatrics* 55:182–191.

Lelord G, Callaway E, Muh JP (1982) Clinical and biological effects of high doses of vitamin B6 and magnesium on autistic children. *Acta Vitaminologica Enzymologica* 4:27–44.

Lelord G, Muh JP, Barthelemy C, Martineau J, Garreau B, Callaway E (1981) Effects of pyridoxine and magnesium on autistic symptoms-initial observations. *Journal of Autism and Developmental Disorders* 11:219–230.

Lerner V, Miodownik C, Kaptsan A, Cohen H, Loewenthal U, Kotler M (2002) Vitamin B6 as add-on treatment in chronic schizophrenic and schizoaffective patients: a double-blind, placebo-controlled study. *Journal of Clinical Psychiatry* 63:54–58.

Levine J, Aviram A, Holan A, Ring A, Barak Y, Belmaker RH (1997) Inositol treatment of autism. *Journal of Neural Transmission* 104:307–310.

Levy SE, Hyman SL (2003) Use of complementary and alternative treatments for children with autism spectrum disorders is increasing. *Annales de Pediatrie* 32:685–691.

Levy SE, Sounders MC, Wray J, Jawad AF, Gallagher PR, Coplan J, Belchic JK, Gerdes M, Mitchell R, Mulberg AE (2003) Children with autistic spectrum disorders, I: comparison of placebo vs. single dose of human synthetic secretin. *Archives of Disease in Childhood* 88:731–736.

Lewis E (1959) The development of concepts in girls with dietary treatment of phenylketonuria. *Journal of Medical Psychology* 32:282–287.

Lowe TL, Cohen DJ, Miller S, Young JG (1981) Folic acid and B12 in autism and neuropsychiatric disturbances of childhood. *Journal of the American Academy of Child Psychiatry* 20:104–111.

Lowe TL, Tanaka K, Seashore MR, Young JG, Cohen DJ (1980) Detection of phenylketonuria in autistic and psychotic children. *JAMA* 243:126–128.

Madsen KM, Lauritsen MB, Pedersen CB, Thorsen P, Plesner AM, Andersen PH, Mortensen PB (2003) Thimerosal and the occurrence of autism: negative ecological evidence from Danish population-based data. *Pediatrics* 112:604–606.

Maki M, Mustalahti K, Kokkonen J (2003). Prevalence of celiac disease among children in Finland. *New England Journal of Medicine* 348:2517–2524.

Martineau J, Barthelemy C, Garreau B, Lelord G (1985) Vitamin B6, magnesium, and combined B6-Mg: therapeutic effects in childhood autism. *Biological Psychiatry* 20: 467–478.

Martineau J, Garreau B, Barthelemy C, Callaway E, Lelord G (1981) Effects of vitamin B6 on averaged evoked potentials in infantile autism. *Biological Psychiatry* 16:627–641.

McCarthy DM, Coleman M (1979) Response of intestinal mucosa to gluten challenge in autistic subjects. *Lancet* ii:877–878.

McDougle CJ, Naylor ST, Cohen DJ, Aghanjanian GK, Heninger GR, Price LH (1996) Effects of tryptophan depletion in drug-free adults with autistic disorder. *Archives of General Psychiatry* 53:993–1000.

McDougle CJ, Naylor ST, Goodman WK, Volkamr FR, Cohen DJ, Price LH (1993) Acute tryptophan depletion in autistic disorder: a controlled study. *Biological Psychiatry* 33:547–550.

McFadden SA (1996) Phenotypic variation in xenobiotic metabolism and adverse environmental response: focus on sulfur-dependent detoxification pathways. *Toxicology* 111: 43–65.

Megson MN (2000) Is autism a G-alpha protein defect reversible with natural vitamin A? *Medical Hypotheses* 54:979–983.

Millward C, Ferriter M, Calver S, Connell-Jones G (2004) Gluten- and casein-free diets for autistic spectrum disorder. The *Cochrane Database of Systematic Reviews* 2: CD003498.

Molloy CA, Manning-Courtney P, Swayne S, Bean J, Brown JM, Murray DS, Kinsman AM, Brasinghton M, Ulrich CD 2nd (2002) Lack of benefit of intravenous human secretin in the treatment of autism. *Journal of Autism and Developmental Disorders* 32:545–551.

Moss N, Boverman H (1978) Megavitamin therapy for autistic children. *American Journal of Psychiatry* 135:1425–1426.

Mudford OC, Cross BA, Breen S, Cullen C, Reeves D, Gould J, Douglas J (2000) Auditory integration training for children with autism: no behavioural benefits detected. *American Journal of Mental Retardation* 105:118–129.

National Research Council (2001) *Educating Young Children With Autism.* Washington, DC: National Academic Press.

Nelson KB, Grether JK, Croen LA, Dambrosia JM, Dickens BF, Jelliffe LL, Hansen RL, Phillips TM (2001) Neuropeptides and neurotrophins in neonatal blood of children with autism or mental retardation. *Annals of Neurology* 49:597–606.

Nye C, Brice A (2002) Combined vitamin B6-magnesium treatment in autism spectrum disorders. The *Cochrane Database of Systematic Reviews* 4:CD003497.

Padhye U (2003) Excess dietary iron is the root cause for increase in childhood autism and allergies. *Medical Hypotheses* 61:220–222.

Page T (2000) Metabolic approaches to the treatment of autism spectrum disorders. *Journal of Autism and Developmental Disorders* 30:463–469.

Patel NC, Yeh JY, Shepherd MD, Crismon ML (2002) Secretin treatment for autistic disorder: a critical analysis. *Pharmacotherapy* 22:905–914.

Pavone L, Fiumara A, Bottaro G, Mazzone D, Coleman M (1997) Autism and celiac disease: failure to validate the hypothesis that a link might exist. *Biological Psychiatry* 42:72–75.

Raiten DJ, Massaro T (1986) Perspectives on the nutritional ecology of autistic children. *Journal of Autism and Developmental Disorders* 16:133–144.

Rapin I. (2002) The autistic spectrum disorders. *New England Journal of Medicine* 347:302–303.

Reichelt KL, Sarlid G, Lindback T, Boler JB (1986) Childhood autism: a complex disorder. *Biological Psychiatry* 21:1279–1290.

Reiss AL, Feinstein C, Rosenbaum KN (1986) Autism in genetic disorders. *Sia Bulletin* 12:724–738.

Rimland B (1972) *Progress in research*. Proceedings of the Fourth Annual Meeting of the National Society for Autistic Children, Washington, DC.

Rimland B (1988) Controversies in the treatment of austistic children: vitamin and drug therapy. *Journal of Child Neurology* 3 Suppl:S68–S72.

Rimland B (1998) High dose vitamin B6 and magnesium in treating autism: response to study by Findling et al. *Journal of Autism Developmental Disorders* 28:581–582.

Rimland B, Callaway E, Dreyfus P (1978) The effect of high doses of vitamin B6 on autistic children: a double-blind crossover study. *American Journal of Psychiatry* 135:472–475.

Rimland B, Edelson SM (1995) Brief report: a pilot study of auditory integration training in autism. *Journal of Autism and Developmental Disorders* 25:61–70.

Rimland B, Ney PG (1974) Infantile autism: status of research. *Canadian Psychiatry Association* 19:130–135.

Sandler AD, Bodfish JW (2000) Placebo effect sin autism: lessons from secretin. *Journal of Developmental and Behavioral Pedriatrics* 21:347–350.

Sandler AD, Sutton KA, DeWeese J, Girard MA, Sheppard V, Bodfish JW (1999) Lack of benefit of a single dose of synthetic human secretin in the treatment of autism and pervasive developmental disorders. *New England Journal of Medicine* 341:1801–1806.

Sankar DVS (1979) Plasma levels of folates, riboflavin, vitamin B6 and ascorbate in severely disturbed children. *Journal of Autism and Developmental Disorders* 9:73–82.

Schaumberg H, Kaplan J, Windebank A, Vick N, Rasmus S, Pleasure D, Brown MJ (1983) Sensory neuropathy from pyridoxine abuse. *New England Journal of Medicine* 309:445–458.

Shattock P (1988) Autism: possible clues to the underlying aetiology. A parent's view. In Wing L (Ed) *Aspects of Autism* (pp. 1–18). London: Gaskell.

Sinha Y, Silove N, Wheeler D, Williams K (2004) Auditory integration training and other sound therapies for autism spectrum disorders. The *Cochrane Database of Systematic Reviews* CD003681.

Sourander A, Ellila H, Valimaki M, Piha J (2002) Use of holding, restraints, seclusion and time-out in child and adolescent psychiatric in-patient treatment. *European Journal of Adolescent Psychiatry* 11:162–167.

Sponheim E, Oftedal G, Helverschou SB (2002) Multiple doses of secretin in the treatment of autism: a controlled study. *Acta Paediatrica* 91:540–545.

Stehr-Green P, Tull P, Stellfeld M, Mortensen PB, Simpson D (2003) Autism and thimerosal-containing vaccines: lack of consistent evidence for an association. *American Journal of Preventive Medicine* 25:101–106.

Sullivan R (1975) Hunches on some biological factors in autism. *Journal of Autism and Child Schizophrenia* 5:177–184.

Tolbert L, Haigler T, Waits MM, Dennis T (1993) Brief report: Lack of response in an autistic population to a low dose clinical trial of pyridoxine plus magnesium. *Journal of Autism and Developmental Disorders* 23:193–199.

Ulshen M (2004) Malabsorptive disorders. In Behrman RE, Kliegman RM, Jenson HB (Eds) *Nelson Textbook of Pediatrics (17th ed.)* (pp. 1159–1171). Philadelphia: W.B. Saunders.

Unis AS, Munson JA, Rogers SJ, Goldson E, Osterling J, Gabriels R, Abbott RD, Dawson G (2002) A randomized, double-blind, placebo-controlled trial of porcine versus synthetic secretin for reducing symptoms of autism. *Journal of the American Academy of Child Psychiatry* 41:1315–1321.

Vanhala R, Turpeinen U, Riikonen R (2001) Low levels of insulin-like growth factor-I in cerebrospinal fluid in children with autism. *Developmental Medicine and Child Neurology* 43:614–616.

Veale D (1993) Classification and treatment of obsessional slowness. *British Journal of Psychiatry* 162:198–203.

Verstraeten T, Davis RL, DeStefano F, Lieu TA, Rhodes PH, Black SB, Shinefield H, Chen RT (2003) Vaccine Safety Datalink Team. *Pediatrics* 112:1039–1048.

Vining EPG, Kossoff EH (2004) The Ketogemic diet. In Wallace SS, Forrell K (Eds). *Epilepsy in Children.* London: Arnold: 405–408.

Volkmar FR, Pauls D (2003) Autism. *Lancet* 362:1133–1141.

Walker-Smith J (1973) Gastrointestinal disease and autism–the result of a survey. *Symposium on Autism, Sidney, Australia.* Abbott Laboratories.

Welch MG, Keune JD, Welch-Horan TB, Anwar N, Ludwig RJ, Ruggiero DA (2004) Secretin: hypothalamic distribution and hypothesised neuroregulation in autism. *Cellular and Molecular Neurobiology* 24:219–241.

Wilder RM (1921) The effects of ketonemics on the course of epilepsy. *Mayo Clinic Proceedings* 2:307–308.

Williams K (1998) Benefits of normalising plasma phenylalanine: impact of behaviour and health. A case report. *Journal of Inherited Metabolic Disease* 21:785–790.

Yamagata T, Aradhya S, Mori M, Inoue K, Momoi MY, Nelson DL (2002) The human secretin gene: fine structure in 11p15.5 and sequence variability in patients with autism. *Genomics* 80:185–194.

Chapter 10

An Integrated Approach to Therapy

Michele Zappella

Medical specialists, usually child neuropsychiatrists (or, in other countries, child neurologists/psychiatrists), more than any other professionals, have the opportunity to master the different aspects of situations connected with autism. They can deal with the general health of the subject affected by this disorder, the presence of specific additional somatic diseases, the diagnosis of autism and related conditions, the identification of specific subgroups within the autistic spectrum, and the diagnosis of comorbidities. They can prescribe the appropriate drugs or medical interventions. In addition, they are often requested to recommend educational avenues or rehabilitation approaches. They can also extend their attention to members of the family and, more extensively, to the society at large where the subject lives.

In every case, they should be aware that each of their choices, and the way they are conducted, may affect the above described variables and go beyond them, concerning, for example, such important aspects of human life as the psychic suffering of the patient or of family members. Some of these topics are the subject of extensive studies, others are relatively neglected, rarely are they considered together; these topics are, however, often closely related and the major aim of this chapter is to show a number of possibilities that we medical specialists encounter when dealing with our patients and their families.

EDUCATION AND THE FAMILY

An appropriate education is the most important support we can give to subjects with autism at every age; an adequate expression of his/her abilities and the quality of life of the person at school, in his family, and in the free time is strongly related to it. The number of articles that have appeared on autism in the past decade in the indexed literature is close to 3000 (Volkmar et al. 2004), excluding books and numerous other publications in languages other than English; a considerable number of these published studies are concerned with education. The paradoxical result of this increasing amount of material is that the avenues of appropriate education for autism have become a difficult labyrinth that may easily discourage the medical specialist from having appropriate and well-founded ideas on the subject. In every case, determination of the best educational option must include consideration of aspects of the child's family life, school and eventually work, with the possibility of reducing the therapeutic proposals for drugs.

The present chapter (written with a recognition of this unexpected result of dramatically increased global knowledge) will advance a possible model of therapies related to autism based both on assessed knowledge and direct experience. This is also an invitation to consider the real reasons why—in contrast with other disabling conditions such as Down syndrome and epilepsy, where therapies and education are universally the same—autism is muddled by innumerable educational and rehabilitation methods.

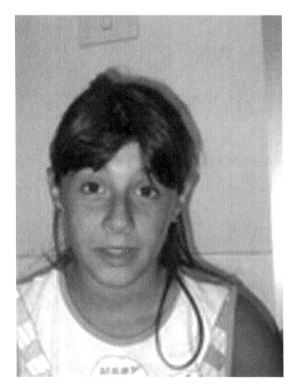

Figure 10.1   Thirteen-year-old girl with autism and MR.

Regarding education for the child with autism, the professional can pursue the two following aims: (1) Support and suggest a scholastic curriculum that can allow a reasonable expansion of his/her abilities; and (2) favor an appropriate and balanced development of the subject's family that supports an adequate structure and the family's internal and external communication, following the evolution of its needs along the years. This is important both for all the family members and for the child affected by autism for whom his family remains a basic, constant resource.

The Family

Medical specialists often encounter human pain when they first meet a family with a child affected by autism. If it is a young child, parents are often frantic, awaiting the weight of a diagnosis that may change their lives, as well as the imagined life of their beloved child. Eric Schopler, a leading psychologist in the education of persons with autism, has written a useful book, based on anecdotes derived from prolonged interactions with parents, that takes into account a number of their suggestions (Schopler 1995). A careful reading of his work, entitled *Parent Survival Manual*, is recommended for the medical specialist.

Depression and Anxiety in Parents

Parents, one or both, may become depressed and, in certain cases, there may also be a family history of mood disorder. An appropriate intervention with a medication such as a selective serotonin reuptake inhibitor (SSRI) might be indicated in such cases, plus psychological support if possible. An understandable depression in parents often occurs when the initial diagnosis is made, but it can appear at any age of the affected child; an appropriate use of medicines and care of the family environment may be important. A similar approach is often advisable in many other situations when parents are anxious and/or in several ways express a profound pain and alarm. Medical professionals should be aware that their power in these moments is great; they can foster hope or despair, can favor union and solidarity within the family or its opposite. Different results can occur based on how we physicians behave and speak, and from what we do. Psychic suffering, not necessarily coincident with depression or anxiety, makes people more fragile. It has been said that psychic pain can be an occasion to become more flexible and sensible. It can introduce a wisdom whereby the pretense of mastering knowledge appears fallacious and may render referral points more mobile (Roustang 2003). This outcome follows different stages, and it is more likely to happen if there is emotional support and extensive communication between the parents, among members of the extended family, and within the community.

Psychic Pain as a Trap

In contrast, prolonged psychic pain can be a trap, foster inappropriate views of the affected relative, and even lead to inappropriate therapies; it occasionally occurs today in cases of autism that parents may be offered a bewildering variety of therapeutic options. This kind of "closed" psychic suffering of the parents is not made lighter by apparent denial leading to choosing inappropriate activities for their children and on several occasions may induce an additional suffering, forcing children with autism beyond their real abilities and in some way losing them as real persons. The parents who choose this road may say that they attempt inappropriate methods to promote more dignity for their children; statements of this kind have been occasionally reported (E. Schopler, personal communication, 2002). A fragmented society where communication of personal suffering is rare and limited is the landscape that allows practices of this kind.

Agreeing to listen to a parent's sorrows is a delicate task, and the physician may not have a ready, adequate reply. This kind of incoming information from parents and patients might cast doubt on current approaches in the treatment of this disorder, such as some types of intensive early intervention, as well as hinder the opportunity to inform patients about their condition. For example, the mother of a 30-year-old comes to my office in tears: "He has now obtained a university degree but nobody will take him to work, he is entirely alone; was this the result of so many years supporting him, day by day, in the school and later in the university?" Some subjects with high functioning autism may ask their parents repeatedly: "Tell me I am not autistic" or "God is bad because he made me different." In contrast, an intelligent girl with Asperger syndrome will tell me that she pretends to have the diagnosis on her own, and will be pleased when I will confirm this diagnosis that she was able to make alone by reading about the subject. Autism is not only a heterogeneous disorder but also it includes many different situations; attention to recognizing psychic pain may be an appropriate guide to distinguish when a diagnosis may be felt as a stigma for the entire person, and when, instead, it might be the confirmation of personal intelligence by being able to guess one's own diagnosis.

Pretend Psychic Pain

There may be also false sufferings that can lead to a more accurate diagnosis and treatment as in the following example. I am visiting in a large outpatient clinic: before the next visit comes, I hear a child screaming as if he was terribly afraid. I walk out of my office and ask his parents to move to a large room full of attractive toys and stay there with their son until he is more relaxed. The child's screaming increases. I therefore ask the father to stay with his son while his mother gives me the child's history. The story is suggestive of a dysmaturational syndrome with early onset tics: the child is now 4½ years old and has improved considerably in the past year. Previous diagnosis by other specialists has been irreversible autism. The child says only two words, is fed by his mother, and refuses to do anything. The home is attended by members of the extended family, and the child behaves as a little tyrant, imposing his negative will on everybody. In the meantime the child, still screaming, has gone to the garden with his father. I go to the garden and ask the father to ask his son to take a rose, to pick up a small object on the ground, and to give a kiss to a person nearby. The child, continuing to scream, immediately accomplishes these requests in a precise way, revealing good verbal understanding. I begin to sense something "false" in this perpetual screaming and to suspect that it is more an attempt to control the situation than an expression of suffering. The hypothesis is soon made that, following the child's initial regression, a situation of alarm developed within the family, including the grandparents, that has made them fearful of contesting the child's will in any way. In particular, the child's mother feels that she must always stay near him. A prescription is made that, in the following month, both parents will disappear from home for some hours two times a week in the afternoon while another family member takes care of the child. A month later the child arrives at the visit smiling and speaking with several words and short phrases. His subsequent development was favorable and confirmed the diagnosis of a dysmaturational syndrome.

Mourning

As anyone else, a person affected by autism may lose persons of his family for whom attachment was great and go through a mourning process. In these cases, the peculiarities of autistic behavior must be taken into account; a young adult, for example, may be at times particularly disturbed by the new behavior exhibited by his relatives and by consequent changes in daily routine; this individual would be more ready to accept the loss of the beloved relative if everything else was unchanged and the loss was presented in a concrete, acceptable way.

Care for the Family

Care should also be taken for brothers and sisters; at times they avoid their sick relative, or alternatively they may become overinvolved. Parents care intensively for the individual with autism, who may become the only referral person for all difficulties and problems within that family and reduce the attention paid to siblings. Psychic suffering is one of the most common findings in a family of an individual diagnosed as autistic. Awareness and differential diagnosis on this topic together with elements of systemic therapy allow the clinician to diagnose and treat mood and anxiety disorders, avoid possible self damage in parents, prevent violence by or to children with autism, and locate an appropriate solution to complex family interactions. From these few examples, the reader can begin to consider how the use of medications, and/or working on family interactions, adding resources as needed such as the introduction of respite care, etc., should be a choice, changing from one situation to another.

It may be added that a medical specialist is often in charge of institutions, such as in-patient departments where parents stay with their children for a few days or departments with nearby communities where parents can have easy access to their children. In both cases, the staff's acknowledgment of the great magnitude of the task of these parents, analyzing the problems and helping them with community resources for education, and respite is essential to relieve family suffering. For the medical specialist, both in an office in front of a family or in a more extensive community setting, the physician can be a direct or latent guide to help family members to confront all the practical problems of rearing such a child and even difficult emotions such as family psychic pain.

Other Aspects of Education

The diagnosis of autism is usually obtained by 2–4 years of age; this often means taking care of the child's condition, initiating educational measures appropriate for him/her, as well as handling the family reaction to the diagnosis, all at the same time. Diagnosis of autism may require prolonged or repeated observation, should be supported by the use of tests commonly used in autism as ABC, CARS, ADI, ADOS, etc., and is usually accompanied by laboratory tests. The way the physician communicates the diagnosis to parents may contribute to soothing their pain and presenting a number of concrete problems, starting with an appropriate education and treatment for their child. Unfortunately parents are often confronted with too many methods, including inappropriate and very expensive strategies, whether recent or outdated (Herbert et al. 2002). They are, therefore, in need of clear guidance as how to proceed in helping their child.

In addition to making a diagnosis of autism and documenting the inabilities of the child in executive function, central coherence, theory of mind, and joint attention, the physician, in order to fully guide parents, must collect further data concerning the following: (1) general degree of abilities in various areas of development (cognitive, motor, autonomy, etc.); (2) verbal understanding and praxic abilities of mouth and hands, often abnormal in those with mental retardation; and (3) the presence and type of sensory abnormalities. In addition, it is relevant to find out if the child with autism belongs to an already known neurological syndrome, and therefore may eventually benefit from special treatments or drugs.

On the basis of these data, an adequate program can be organized in the home, in the nursery, and in eventual rehabilitation settings. Organization of this program should be guided by the one of the following two main paths of education now available: (1) Based on natural motivation whereby a child, normal or autistic, can be induced to do an activity either following spontaneous interests, increasing motivation through physical play, or obtaining an adequate and positive emotional tuning, or (2) Supported by artificial tools used in order to obtain an adequate motivation as, for example, in behavioral conditioning techniques.

This second pathway had the merit of opening the way to improve behavior even in very difficult situations in the 1960s and 1970s, an epoch when specialists were often disarmed in this respect. Presently, however, one of the main sources of interest for intensive behavioral therapies may be represented by the promise that through them some children can be cured of autism. It should be noted that classic autism appears to be caused by abnormalities in neural cell brain structure following a genetic defect occurring most often in the first two trimesters of pregnancy (see chapter 1); as a consequence it is highly unlikely that even very intense behavioral therapies can represent an adequate approach, inducing a complete reversal of autism and its neural basis. The same can be said of the use of drugs in young children with autism. However, if, autistic behavior is the expression of other separate conditions, such as early onset Tourette syndrome (GTS) as in the dysmaturational syndrome, or of early onset epilepsy, or of severely depriving early institutionalization, there is more evidence of positive results. This amelioration or reversal of autistic symptoms can be obtained either through an education based on natural motivation or with the specific use of drugs; apparently with more efficacy and less economic and human expense than the behavioral conditioning therapies (see chapter 8 on reversible autism).

An education based on natural motivation also is of help in treating successfully and inexpensively the cases of GTS/persistent Autistic Spectrum Disorder described by Kerbeshian et al. (1992) as noted by Zappella (2002). This type of education supports a general attitude to treat those affected by autism as persons, as subjects endowed by an active propensity towards their environment, with greater attention to their spontaneous initiatives. It may be an easier step towards a more adequate integration in the school and in adult life.

In persons with autism, the prevalent targets of interest for education are often determined by sensory peculiarities; in most cases, visual abilities are predominant, accompanied by a less efficient language comprehension with a wide range of difficulty from verbal agnosia to the slight but consistent difficulties found in high functioning autism. At the same time executive functioning, abilities related to sequencing activities, theory of mind (ToM), joint attention, and emotion may be altered, leaving the affected individual with difficulties in organizing himself. As a consequence, a structure based on visual images, sequencing the activities to attend each day may be recommended in school and to some extent at home, especially for children or older hyperselective individuals, with rigid behavior and more limited abilities. If the young child has additional disabilities such as a profoundly reduced verbal understanding or verbal agnosia and at the same time his executive abilities are poor, there is a greater need of structuring the environment in sequential activities. If oral and/or manual dyspraxia are present, care must be provided for these disabilities with appropriate remedial activities and Augmentative and Alternative Communication instituted. Even subjects with intelligence and language abilities closer to normal often require structure, clear order especially at work, taking care, and anticipating unexpected events.

Young children with autism are often retarded in their general abilities, and some follow a regression that has further hampered the level of their capacities, but that subsequently may be recovered. Therefore, some educational scales like the Portage method (Ross 1981) where items can be split in simpler elements and proposed every day, possibly in natural situations, in the family and in the nursery can provide an adequate support.

Interactional activities with large balls, bubbles, colored hoops, etc. can also be of help in promoting subjective modalities and joint attention with adults and other children (Xaiz & Micheli 2000), which can be appropriately integrated by other interactional strategies. Children with autism may enjoy and benefit from physical play and interactional exchanges at a body level (see chapter 8). In the home, in the school, and in various moments of adult life, attention must be given to sensory peculiarities such as hyperacusis, and overcrowded, noisy and chaotic situations avoided. Speech therapy to improve language deficits, pragmatics, and other aspects of communication is often beneficial.

Living and educating a young child with autism is an expensive enterprise, both in terms of the family economy, of time and of emotional resources. Frequently, one of the parents leaves work or chooses a part time job; therapies are expensive, and the economic status of the family may worsen. Social isolation and disruption of family ties can occur, although in some cases the reverse is true. In this context, where many risks are present, a balanced policy where the well-being of the affected child goes together with an adequate lifestyle for family members should be a main objective for the consulting physician. In this context, the opportunity of special methods, often claimed as favoring a better outcome, must be considered. Some of these have been the object of studies that denied their validity. For example, the NRC of the United States (NRC 2001) has reported more than fifty studies discarding the validity of Facilitated Communication. Also the Auditory Integration Therapy has been the object of negative evaluations (Gillberg et al. 1997). In a recent article, some Finnish authors (Kielinen et al. 2002) have reported the outcome of different therapies used in a large cohort of autistic subjects, including the use of TEACCH, the method suggested by Lovaas, and the Portage program and found no statistically significant difference between the outcome of these habilitation methods. Therefore, the economic and human weight of very expensive and time consuming treatments should be taken into account. It often occurs in clinical practice that children with autism with initial similar abilities obtain quite diverging results with the same educational method; some remain quite stable, others show notable improvements. It may be added that 20 girls with the Preserved Speech Variant of the Rett syndrome with *MECP2* mutation, all autistic, observed in my clinic in Siena, started to speak and to improve their general abilities to a level at times above an IQ of 50 after 5 years of age, certainly not because of a early intensive intervention that none of them had.

For children affected by autism, it seems more reasonable to educate them in an appropriate way both from a scholastic and a sociability point of view, giving credit essentially to what makes sense based on what we know. In the elementary school, problems may arise concerning education and interaction with peers. If the child with autism is mainstreamed, general intelligence is close to normal, and is followed by a special teacher experienced in the educational methods used in autism, he can enjoy a number of opportunities of structured interactions with peers within and outside the class. In these cases, this child needs some degree of structuring, must be protected regarding the sensory experiences, and follow a curriculum in part at least similar to that of peers. Medication to improve attention and reduce impulsivity and hyperactivity, when present, or other co-morbidities, may be helpful in some cases, as described later.

SELF/HETEROAGGRESSION, RAGE

Self and heteroaggression and fits of rage in subjects with autism are a frequent occasion for consulting a medical specialist. The differential diagnosis must include a number of possibilities:

1. There may be a somatic disease, for example gastroesophageal reflux, otitis media, appendicitis, a toothache, or another physical reason.

2. Many subjects with autism are mute or able to say only a few words. They often suffer from concomitant oral dyspraxia, eventually part of a more extensive dyspraxia. In some case they have a hypomobile, atrophic tongue. Some of these can in addition have deafness but others have a good hearing and a partial understanding. These persons may have some understanding of the more concrete aspects of verbal language but can be unable to make themselves well understood. Fits of rage in these cases may be caused by their inability to be understood by others. An appropriate assessment of disabilities of this kind is relevant for starting appropriate remedies in communication introducing Augmentative and Alternative Communication and/or, when it is possible, the use of gestures.

3. Others may be blind and have a profound abnormality concerning sleep rhythms. In some of them, melatonin, given at 10 PM for limited periods of time (2–3 months), can promote a more adequate sleep cycle and, secondarily, induce more relaxed behavior.

4. Environmental causes are a frequent cause of rage in autism. They may include a request the person with autism does not like and nevertheless is somehow obliged to do at home or in the school, attachment to a preferred, particular set of objects due to hyperselectivity, the interruption of an habitual pattern, an environment not adequately structured, confusion, unpleasant noises, hypersensitivity to touch, or imposed teaching aims that may be too distant from real abilities.

A 12-year-old boy with autism and mutism was recently brought to my attention for his fits of rage. It was soon evident that this boy, who was mainstreamed, was in general submitted to learning tasks inappropriate for his mental age. In addition he was doing facilitated communication and had broken 4 machines used for this approach, possibly because he was forced against his will to do this activity.

5. In some cases the interactions, otherwise positive within the family, may be altered in specific situations, causing a violent reaction.

A child aged 8 has systematic fits of rage when he comes home by car: if his parents, at the end of a short journey, say "let's go home," he will start a fit of rage that may be prolonged until the car enters the garden. In this case, parents were advised not to mention that they were going home, and the father was asked to stop his car at a distance from home and do some jogging with his son through different meadows, entering their house in a completely new way and through different avenues. Simple advice of this kind allowed the immediate disappearance of rage and subsequently the ability to resume a normal entrance by car.

In another family where no educational interventions had been conducted with their 3-year-old child affected by autism, fits of rage followed regularly the visual and verbal presentation of toys, as is usual with normal children. This child had limited verbal understanding that had not been assessed previously. Introducing physical playing with cognitive activities that included some physical guidance in the use of toys made this child happy to deal with toys offered by the family.

6. An environment not adequately structured for his specific needs.

7. Child abuse.

8. Partial complex seizures.

9. It may be part of a mood disorder. Self aggression in a mute autistic boy, especially if coupled with a sad face and other signs such as occasional weeping, with an altered sleep cycle and diminished interest in eating, can be suggestive of a depressive disorder; a treatment with SSRI, eventually coupled with mood stabilizers such as divalproex sodium or carbamazepine may be indicated (Hollander et al. 2001). As an example, paroxetine has been reported to bring dramatic cessation of severe self-biting of the arms in an adolescent with autism, after a long list of other drugs failed (Snead et al. 1994). In other cases, self and hetero-aggression and fits of rage are part of hypomanic episodes, usually marked by intense hyperactivity, occasional laughing episodes, reduced sleep. Mood stabilizers as reported above can initially be coupled with benzodiazepines in acute cases, or with risperidone, in older patients with olanzapine, and in more severe case with clozapine.

10. There are cases where pharmaceuticals cause side-effects that make their use dangerous. At the same time, proof of what causes this behavioral disorder is difficult to establish.

A 9-year-old girl with autism and reduced speech had started to act aggressively toward others, with increasing violence, attacking people in their eyes, tearing their hair, scratching their faces, kicking and beating them at home and in the school. Drugs commonly used in such situations had caused severe negative effects and could not be used. Fear and alarm prevented interactions with her at home and in the school. I suggested to the parents to take her regularly every day at a given time to a coach; one of them was supporting her from behind in a sitting position, holding her hands; in this way she could not cause harm. The other was nicely interacting with her with verbal and physical affectionate interactions; these were made reciprocal initially through physical guidance. If, during the day, fits of rage occurred, similar types of interactions were suggested. This approach allowed the disappearance of this disturbance in a few weeks, suggesting that aggression may reinforce loneliness that in turn may reinforce aggression. In this case blocking or redirecting aggression and fostering adequate interactions was a useful path.

11. Ocular self aggression, which can permanently damage the eye, is sometimes associated with hypocalcinuria in children with autism; there is a reasonable chance of stopping the self-abuse with calcium supplements given until the hypocalcinuria is corrected (Coleman 1994).

SLEEP DISORDERS

Sleep disorders are a frequent occurrence, especially in young children with autism, but may also be present in adults, and recent observations suggest an abnormal melatonin circadian rhythm may be the cause. Melatonin (MLT) is secreted by the pineal gland during darkness and suppressed by exposure to light. It acts on the suprachiasmatic nucleus that in turn regulates its secretion by sending information about light to the pineal gland. As a drug, it has soporific properties and has been successfully used in normal children with chronic sleep onset insomnia (Smits et al. 2003), as well as in children with autism and mental retardation aged 3 to 28 years at a dosage of 2.5 to 10 mg (Jan & O'Donnell 1996; Ishizaki et al. 1999). Side effects are rare and usually limited to residual drowsiness the next morning or excitement after awakening. It has been reported that suitable medication time postponed to late evening time (10 PM) improves the sleep-wake rhythm (Hayashi 2000). In a number of cases, treatment may be limited to 1 or 2 months and be followed by a general improvement in the health status and sleep. It must be noticed that benzodiazepines may block its production (Stores 2003). There are controversial suggestions, far from conclusive, on whether MLT can increase convulsions in neurodevelopmental disorders (Sheldon 1998) or reduce them drastically (Molino-Carballo et al. 1997). Niaprazine can also be tried for sleep disorders.

NONSPECIFIC SYMPTOMS OF AUTISM

The possibility of using new atypical antipsychotics drugs in young children with autism is supported by a few documented studies. Risperidone, a potent antagonist of dopamine D2, serotonin 2A, and other serotonin receptors was tried in an 8 weeks multisite, randomized, double-blind trial on children aged 5 to 17 years with positive effects on irritability, stereotypic behavior and hyperactivity (RUPP 2002). The medication schedule started with 0.5 mg at bedtime in children who weighed 20 to 45 kg, and gradually increased to a maximum of 1 mg in the morning and 1.5 mg at bedtime. Those with a weight above 45 kg could reach a maximal dose of 1.5 mg in the morning and 2 mg at bedtime. Common adverse events included increased weight and fatigue, but occasionally tremor, akathisia, dyskinesia, and constipation were reported. Masi et al. (2001; 2003) have conducted open studies in children with risperidone that has been found to positively affect symptoms in young autistic children, aged 3.6 to 6.6 years, at a dosage of 0.25 to 0.75 mg per day, improving in particular disruptive/hyperactive behavior and affective dysregulation (Masi et al. 2001). However, a trend towards a smaller treatment effect at follow up was found (Masi et al. 2003). EKG at baseline and as part of routine monitoring is recommended since a few children may experience tachycardia. Prolactin may increase at notable levels. Increased appetite and weight gain are frequently reported during treatment in children and adolescents (Armenteros et al. 1997).

Selective serotonin reuptake inhibitors (SSRIs) were originally studied to treat repetitive behaviors in autism because this class of drugs had established efficacy in treating similar symptoms in patients with obsessive-compulsion; the possibility of treating more than one symptom domain in autism has now been explored. Among the SSRIs, fluoxetine has been the object of extensive studies. DeLong and his coworkers have devoted a number of studies to the relationship between autism and affective disorders and to the effects of fluoxetine (DeLong & Dwyer 1988; DeLong & Nothria 1994; DeLong 1994; DeLong et al. 1998). In a recent study, DeLong et al. (2002) have reported their experience on a population of 129 young children 2 to 8 years old, treated for 5 to 76 months. The tolerated dosage (0.15 to 0.5 mg/kg) was found to be positive, especially at two levels: 4–8 mg per day or above 12 mg per day up to 20 and 40 mg per day. Adverse events were mostly limited to behavioral activation, irritability, and agitation, except single cases with diarrhea and cutaneous rash. Four children lost autistic features and evolved to a bipolar disorder. A good response was found in 52% of this children's population. An excellent response was found in 22 (17%), defined as "no longer identified as having autism." The excellent responders remained with attention-deficit-hyperactivity disorder, obsessive-compulsive disorder, anxiety, or immaturity. It is possible, however, that this population with favorable outcome overlapped with other disorders where reversible autistic behavior can occur without a pharmacological treatment (see chapter 8). These authors were able to identify a subgroup of children with regression, hyperlexia, high functioning autism, a family history of major affective disorder and unusual achievement that responded favorably to fluoxetine.

Fluvoxamine has also been tried with an inconsistent therapeutic response (Martin et al. 2003). These and other SSRIs may give excitement and irritability in subjects with ASD, especially if given without appropriate care for eventually existing comorbidities. Overall the body of available evidence for treating these individuals with these drugs remains devoid of an adequate body of data (Volkmar et al. 2004).

COMORBIDITIES

The study of psychiatric comorbidities in autism is relatively recent. During the eighties only occasional reports were given on mood disorders and TS and, only since the beginning of the '90s, have more descriptions been given of a substantial number of patients. It seems in fact that autism has a greater degree of comorbidities than most other brain disorders. Thus, Gillot et al. (2001) compared tests related to anxious behavior in children with high functioning autism with two control groups—one represented by children with specific language impairment and one by normal children—and found much higher values in the autistic group while the other two had similar values. These data, among others, suggest that the holistic damage of autism that includes cellular abnormalities spread over extensive parts of the cerebral cortex and other parts of the brain may well be the neurobiological basis of numerous comorbid disorders, in contrast with more localized, modular forms of brain damage as, for example, in specific language disorders.

Autism is often viewed essentially as one disorder: as a consequence behavioral and pharmacological therapies are evaluated in terms of target symptoms to confirm their validity. Within this context, comorbidities (i.e., other disorders with their symptom complexes and course), may be considered of marginal relevance and even ignored within controlled pharmacological studies. Alternatively, autism can be considered a disorder that not only is probably related to different diseases, but also has several dimensions related to the systems of human relations where the subject with autism spends his everyday activities (family, school, work, institutions, etc.), age, the possible existence of additional disabilities and comorbidities, as well as to other variables. This latter view tends to give relevance to elements that are reciprocally connected; for example, the depression of a young mother who has just been listening to the diagnosis for her son and has in addition given a family history of mood disorder, as well as the symptom complex and course of a comorbid condition appearing as a manic disorder in her son affected by autism. A sleep disturbance has a different meaning if connected or not to other symptoms, which taken together may render it a signal of depression. In a child with autism, hyperactivity may be part of an ADHD–like behavior or belong to a manic disorder. Both in normal and pathologic behavior, there are powerful biological constraints that combine different behaviors either relating them to common ontogenetic, motivational, and final systems, or to common pathologic pathways. Differences between these two perspectives may be profound in terms of diagnostic complexity and therapy: among them, the attention given to the presence, diagnosis and treatment of comorbid disorders is relevant.

Comorbidities are frequent within the autism syndromes and an appropriate pharmacological treatment is often required; for example, a subject with autism affected by depression must be rapidly identified and appropriately treated for this additional disorder. For this and other comorbidities, the main guidelines for diagnosis and therapy are those of classical child and adult psychiatry as described in *DSM-IV* and *ICD10*, although some peculiarities are at times present in subjects within the autistic syndromes. Within this range of disorders, in fact, the use of drugs requires caution since in a given child paradoxical reactions may occur, such as unexpected excitement with antiepileptic drugs or with an increasingly disturbed behaviour with risperidone. It is possible that these unexpected results obtained in some cases are related to the different genetic backgrounds of autistic subjects, as suggested by recent studies in this field. As a consequence the professional should begin treatment, especially in children, if this is possible, with very low doses and increase them slowly up to an appropriate and adequate value (Santosh & Baird 2003).

It has been noticed that the use of drugs in autism is increasing, and possibly they may be prescribed too often inappropriately. Aman et al. (1995) found an overall prevalence of 42.0% for psychotropics, AEDs and megavitamins in 1995, Martin et al. (1999) values of 55% and Aman et al. in a more recent study (2003) a prevalence of 65% with increased age being a relevant factor for receiving many psychotropic drugs. There can be many reasons why drugs are inappropriately used and it may well be that the prevalent concept of autism as one disorder favors the use of new drugs that at the time appear to be more promising. This trend can be exacerbated by pharmacological studies, where the presence of comorbid disorders is not taken in due account, that limit their attention to the targeting symptoms of autism. It should be noted, however, that the same problem can be found with some environmental therapies based on psychological or educational measures; inadequately given drugs may damage the subject in the short run while inappropriately intensive interventions of a psychological kind may in the long run leave parents economically and psychologically depleted, and be equally disturbing and of no help to the child.

The identification of comorbidities in a child with autism is a most important step where, when appropriate, pharmacological cures can be of substantial help, eventually coupled with appropriate interventions on the environment.

Attention Deficit Hyperactivity Disorder (ADHD)

In cases of attention deficit/hyperactivity disorder, the significance of symptoms must be interpreted with care. For example, it is a frequent occurrence to see young children with autism with devastating hyperactivity, continuously changing the scope of their activities; the same children may remain attentive looking to a cartoon for a prolonged period of time. In cases of this kind, a profound inadequacy in executive functioning and central coherence appears as a relevant cause of this behavior that is only superficially comparable to most ADHD patients. The same child may be relatively cooperative in a nursery where the special teacher has provided an adequate structure, but at home the same organization of life may not be possible. Or, alternatively, the young child might be difficult to manage in both situations. Cases of this kind are far from being a rare occurrence, and there is notable pressure on the professional to reduce the child's and caregivers' discomfort through use of drugs.

Rossi et al. (1999) in an open study proposed niaprazine, a relatively safe histaminic H1-receptor antagonist drug with sedative properties for short period of times at a dosage of 1mg/kg/day and found improvements in hyperactivity, attention deficit and disruptive behavior. Risperidone has been used in very young children with autism and, among the target symptoms, hyperactivity is apparently one of the most effected (Masi et al. 2001; 2003). Stimulants may easily cause increased irritability in young children—in older subjects, adverse effects may also occur—and it is possible that they are more efficacious in high functioning autistic subjects (Handen et al. 2000; Aman et al. 2003). In Asperger syndrome, in fact, ADHD appears to be the most frequent comorbidity (Ghaziuddin et al. 1998). It is likely that in this condition, as well as in high functioning autism, the ADHD symptoms are a consequence of related cognitive peculiarities and consequent disorganized random behavior; nevertheless, stimulants are considered helpful medications by some authors, such as Werry (2001), possibly through their nonspecific energizing effect.

In practice, treatment of a given subject with autism and other concurrent disorders can be quite complex; a child, for example, may be affected by epilepsy, well controlled by divalproex, show signs of attention deficit, that responds well to small doses of risperidone, (inducing, however, weight gain), and show an increase of complex motor and vocal tics as part of a GTS, more intense if he is not actively involved in some adequate activity. Behavioral suggestions in these cases can help in avoiding increasing dosages or the use of additional drugs.

Mood Disorders

The occurrence of mood disorders, like unipolar depression and bipolar disorders, in autism has been noticed since Kanner's original article (1943) and in a number of subsequent studies (Rutter, 1970; Komoto et al. 1984; Clarke, 1989; Ghaziuddin and Tsai, 1991; Ghaziuddin et al. 1992; DeLong 1994). Most cases of depression have been described in adolescents and adults, possibly more frequently in females (Lainhart & Folstein 1994), and more usually in high functioning autism and in Asperger syndrome, ranging in the latter approximately 30% of the cases (Wing 1981; Ghaziuddin et al. 1998). These data fit with clinical experience, but it is also true that, in cases of severe mental retardation, the diagnosis of depression may be difficult and probably is often missed. In persons with high functioning autism and with Asperger syndrome, depression may fit the criteria of *DSM-IV-R*. Depression in these individuals often results in increasing oppositional and aggressive behavior and can interfere with various kinds of social integration, including school placement. In some individuals, it may lead to catatonia. In persons where autism is associated with severe mental retardation, and in those who are or become mute, depression can be suspected when observing a profound change of mood with feature of sadness and a profound change in the sleep cycle, in appetite, and signs of fatigue. Self and hetero-aggression are frequently present. The history of mood disorders in the family is of help with the diagnosis.

Depression is frequently present in subjects with mental retardation (Glenn et al. 2003) that, in its turn, is present in approximately 70% of subjects with autism; the same can be said about epilepsy, recorded in approximately 30% of the autistic subjects. All these factors increase the risk for depression in this population. Additional multiple interacting factors, including poor social skills, unfavorable life events such as bereavement and parental discord (Ghaziuddin et al. 1995) and genetic factors are among the causes of this disorder. A family history of depression or of bipolar disorders has been noticed more frequently in autistic children who suffer from depression (Ghaziuddin & Greden 1998), and the existence of common genetic abnormalities accounting for both disorders in a specific subgroup has been advocated (DeLong 1999). Depression often has a negative impact on family life and, especially if reoccurs, it may be followed in adolescence and early adult life by a behavioral deterioration.

Treatment should be based on the use of antidepressant drugs; the first drugs of choice are selective serotonin reuptake inhibitors (SSRIs), like fluoxetine (DeLong et al. 2002), sertraline (McDougle et al. 1998), citalopram (Namerow et al. 2003), and eventually paroxetine and fluvoxamine in the appropriate age group. In bipolar disorders, depression requires administration of a SSRI and a mood stabilizer. Tricyclic antidepressants have been used in the past but their use is limited by possible cardiotoxic effects. Psychological support may be of additional value, especially in high functioning autism.

Bipolar disorders may affect subjects with high functioning autism, as well as those with mental retardation. Episodes of acute mania require hospitalization. First-line therapy includes monotherapy with a mood stabilizer or an antipsychotic drug, or the combination of two mood stabilizers or a mood stabilizer plus an antipsychotic medication. Combination therapy may offer an advantage over monotherapy and treatment could be based on antiepileptic drugs (AEDs) coupled with an atypical antipsychotic. In an international study, Yatham et al. (2003) found that risperidone given at a mean dosage of 4 mg in a population aged between 16 and 65 years added to AEDs was superior to the addition of a placebo. In adulthood, olanzapine, a potent 5-HT(2a/2c), dopamine D1, D2, D4 antagonist with anticholinergic activity, with a receptor affinity close to clozapine, in a dosage of 10–15 mg per day is often effective (Soutullo et al. 1999). Among AEDs, divalproex sodium (20 mg/kg per day) may be beneficial to patients with autistic spectrum disorders, particularly those with affective instability and impulsivity, as well as those with a history of EEG abnormalities or seizures (Hollander et al. 2001). Carbamazepine, lamotrigine, and topiramate are among the other AEDs used. As noted above, combination pharmacotherapy is often required in subjects with bipolar disorders irrespective of their age (Kowatch et al. 2003), which means making use in some cases of two AED or of lithium plus an AED or AED plus risperidone, and this attitude applies as well to autism comorbid with bipolar disorders. In some cases, the use of topiramate can be considered to counteract weight gain related to the use of risperidone, but the possibility of adverse effects must be considered (Canitano 2004).

Subjects with autism may, for example, be on a treatment with risperidone, when an episode of depression occurs, and the physician must be informed on corresponding drug interactions. Fluoxetine and paroxetine, potent inhibitors of the cytochrome P450 enzyme CYP2D8 and fluvoxamine, inhibitor of CYP1A2 and CYP2C19, can reduce the clearance of risperidone by inhibiting its active metabolite (9-OH-risperidone) or alternative metabolic pathways. As a consequence, the levels of risperidone may notably increase (Spina & Perucca 2002; Spina et al. 2003). Other antidepressants, as sertraline and citalopram, are weak inhibitors of different CYP isoforms and are therefore less likely to induce analogous metabolic interactions.

AEDs are a common adjunct therapy with atypical neuroleptics such as risperidone and olanzapine. In this respect, sodium valproate has been reported to have little or no interaction with risperidone (Spina et al. 2000). Carbamazepine can decrease the plasma concentrations of risperidone and olanzapine, as well as those of other neuroleptics like chlorpromazine and haloperidol, probably by inducing CYP3A3-mediated metabolism (Spina & Perucca 2002). Risperidone in its turn can lower carbamazepine plasma concentrations (Mula & Monaco 2002).

Tourette Syndrome

(Gilles de la) Tourette syndrome (GTS) is defined by the presence of multiple motor and vocal tics for a period of at least 12 months. In normal subjects, it usually starts by 6–7 years but, in those with autism, it may be more precocious. Familiarity for tics in the range of 70% is common, but it is less evident in persons with autism where, when tics appear, they seem to be apparently part of the same brain pathology. Simple motor tics may be clonic, dystonic, tonic, while complex motor tics may have or not an apparent aim like touching. Vocal tics can be simple like barking or complex with repetitive phrases. They change in time in their intensity, shape and location, and usually affect the head, neck and arms but may involve the whole body. In contrast, stereotypic activities are monotonous, often involve the whole body like rocking forward and backward or swinging on both sides.

GTS has been reported in approximately 6.5–8% of subjects with autism (Baron-Cohen et al. 1999) but it is more frequent in selected clinical populations such as in those with sensory abnormalities (Ringman & Jankovic 2000). GTS is more frequent in subjects with autism seen as in-patients in hospital settings where admission is related in some case to symptoms of the GTS series, such as frequent and high pitched vocal tics, which may disturb profoundly home and school settings. In cases of this kind, treatment of GTS is indicated and several drugs can be used. An atypical neuroleptic like risperidone and pimozide are among the drugs of first choice, followed in some cases by haloperidol. In older subjects, in late adolescence and adulthood, sulpiride and clonidine may be tried. In those cases refractory to a medical treatment, the possibility of injecting botulin toxin can be considered. GTS is often accompanied by the presence of ADHD and this is often the case also with subjects with autism.

Anxiety

Anxiety reactions, including separation anxiety and phobic reactions, are more easily defined in high functioning autism and Asperger syndrome, where they are fairly common. In those individuals with the autistic syndromes who also have severe mental retardation, behaviors typical of the autistic phenotype can be inappropriately related to anxiety. For example, avoidance behavior is commonly referred to anxiety (Edelman 1992), but it is also a typical autistic behaviour. Inner tension cannot always be verbalized by subjects with the autistic syndromes and mental retardation. It requires in some cases a pharmacological treatment. SSRIs are often the appropriate drugs (Lindsay & Aman 2003). Among them sertraline in low doses (25 mg–50 mg daily) has been studied in ASD children and improvement was reported in the acute symptoms of anxiety following changes in their routine or environment (Steingard et al. 1997). Fluvoxamine was successful in a single case where anxiety and repetitive behaviors were pronounced (Kauffman et al. 2001). Significant improvements were obtained with fluoxetine in anxiety and obsessive compulsive behaviors (Buchsbaum et al. 2001). In clinical practice, especially in young subjects with ASD and retardation, the use of fluoxetine and other SSRIs requires some caution; excitement can be induced and it may well be that the evaluation of mood in some of these subjects is often difficult. It has been suggested that abnormalities concerning the amygdala, noted in some cases studied postmortem by Bauman (1996), may contribute to abnormal fears and increased anxiety in subjects with autism (Amaral & Corbett 2003).

Epilepsy

The association between autism and epilepsy is the more frequent comorbidity that is documented; approximately one third of individuals suffer from seizures (see chapter 5). The prevalence appears to be higher with increasing age, with lower mental abilities and with severe language disorders; thus, while subjects with Asperger syndrome or high functioning autism have a low incidence, approximately evaluated approximately 5–10%, this percentage increases to 30% in classic autism and further increases in disintegrative disorder and Rett syndrome up to values of 90% (Tuchman & Rapin 2002). Moreover, in a significant number of autistic patients paroxysmal discharges on EEG, especially in sleep, are detected (Chez et al. 2004; Canitano et al. 2004); in these cases, there is no clear evidence that a treatment with AEDs should be undertaken. The frequency of epilepsy in the autistic syndrome shows two peaks: one before 5 years of age and another in early adolescence. All types of seizures can occur, usually complex partial, partial secondarily generalized, atypical absences, generalized tonic-clonic seizures. It can be noticed that, in patients with ASDs, evidence of cellular maldevelopment has been found in the neocortex, cerebellum, limbic system, including the temporal lobe and the hippocampus, an organ frequently involved in epilepsy (Kemper & Bauman 1993; Casanova et al. 2002). It has also been reported that ASD, epilepsy and affective disorders tend to occur together (Di Martino & Tuchman 2001). Treatment follows the general guidelines applied in epilepsy.

SPECIFIC TREATMENTS IN AUTISM

Since most children with the autistic syndromes have yet to have a specific diagnosis, specific treatments remain rare. Even in the group of patients with syndromic autism, specific medical therapies are usually lacking. Most children with syndromic autism have a multiple congenital anomaly (MCA/MR) syndrome, modifiable by early infant education. Known medical treatments in syndromic autism include a special nonphenylalanine diet or BH4 in PKU autism (see chapter 9) and thyroid in infantile hypothyroid autism (both forms of autism are now virtually nonexistent wherever there is newborn screening). Research treatments are underway in purine autism. There are two disease entities identified so far: adenylosuccinate lyase deficiency and nucleotidase-associated pervasive developmental disorder (NAPDD). Uridine therapy has been suggested for both, but whether it really helps is unknown since there is only one double-blind, crossover trial of uridine in NAPDD in just four children (Page et al. 1997).

The overwhelming majority of children with autism have what is known as nonsyndromic autism. Most of these children have no specific diagnosis; research therapies await better diagnostic criteria. In fact most reports of attempts at treatment in nonsyndromic autism are anecdotal or are in series without planned study design or double-blind confirmation at this time. However, the future is not necessarily so bleak. For example, in children who have alteration of mitochondrial function, there are possible strategies for medical treatment (Gold & Cohen 2001); this may include a significant subgroup of children with autism. There is a report in two children with duplication of the maternally derived chromosome 15q11–q13 region who are having trials of carnitine and mitochondrial cofactor supplements (Filipek et al. 2003).

SUMMARY

Medical treatment is generally hampered in the autistic syndromes from the lack of an underlying diagnosis. But there are many tools available today: rational educational planning, family support, non-specific pharmaceuticals, and therapy for symptom complexes that can be very helpful.

REFERENCES

Aman MG, Kristen SLL, Collier-Crespin A (2003) Prevalence and patterns of use of psychoactive medicines among individuals with autism in the Autism Society of Ohio. *Journal of Autism and Developmental Disorders* 33:527–534.

Aman MG, Van Bourgondien ME, Wolford PC, Sarphare G (1995) Psychotropic and anticonvulsant drugs in subjects with autism: prevalence and patterns of use. *Journal of the American Academy for Child and Adolescent Psychiatry* 34:1672–1681.

Amaral DG, Corbett BA (2003) The amigdala, autism and anxiety. *Novartis Foundation Symposium* 251:177–187.

Armenteros JL, Whitaker AH, Welikson M, Stedge DJ, Gorman J (1997) Risperidone in adolescents with schizophrenia: an open pilot study. *Journal of the American Academy of Child and Adolescent Psychiatry* 36:694–700.

Baron-Cohen S, Scahill VI, Izaguirre J, Hornsey H, Robertson MM (1999) The prevalence of Gilles de la Tourette syndrome in children and adolescents with autism: a large scale study. *Psychological Medicine.* 29:1151–1159.

Bauman ML (1996) Brief report: neuroanatomic observations of the brain in pervasive developmental disorders. *Journal of Autism and Developmental Disorders.* 26:199–203.

Buchsbaum MS, Hollander E, Haznedar MM, Tang C, Spiegel-Cohen J, Wei TC, Solimando A, Buchsbaum BR, Robins D, Bienstock C, Cartwright C, Mosovich S (2001) Effect of fluouxetine on regional cerebral metabolism in autistic spectrum disorders: a pilot study. *International Journal of Psychopharmacology* 4:119–125.

Canitano R (2004) Clinical experience with topiramate to counteract neuroleptic weight gains in ten individuals with autistic spectrum disorder. *Brain and Development,* in press.

Canitano R, Luchetti A, Zappella M (2004) Epilepsy, EEG abnormalities and regression in children with Autism. *Journal of Child Neurology*, in press.

Casanova MF, Buxhoeveden DP, Switala AE, Roy E (2002) Minicolumnar pathology in autism. *Neurology* 58:428–432.

Chez MG, Buchanan T, Aimonovitch M, Mrazek S, Krasne V, Langburt W, Memon S (2004) Frequency of EEG abnormalities in age-matched siblings of autistic children with abnormal sleep EEG patterns. *Epilepsy Behaviour* 5:159–162.

Clarke DJ, Littlejohns CS, Corbett JA, Joseph S (1989) Pervasive Developmental Disorders and psychoses in adult life. *British Journal of Psychiatry* 155:692–699.

Coleman M (1994) Clinical presentation of patients with autism and hypocalcinuria. *Developmental Brain Dysfunction* 7:104–109.

DeLong GR (1994) Children with autistic spectrum disorder and a family history of affective disorder. *Developmental Medicine and Child Neurology* 36:374–688.

DeLong GR (1999) Autism: new data suggests a new hypothesis. *Neurology* 52:911–916.

DeLong GR, Dwyer JT (1988) Correlation of family history with specific autistic subgroups: Asperger syndrome and bipolar affective disease. *Journal of Autism and Developmental Disorders*, 18: 593–599.

DeLong GR, Nothria C (1994) Psychiatric family history and neurological disease in autistic spectrum disorders. *Developmental Medicine and Child Neurology* 36:441–448.

DeLong GR, Teague L, Kamram M (1998) Effects of fluoxetine treatment in young children with idiopathic autism. *Developmental Medicine and Child Neurology* 40:551–562.

DeLong GR, Ritch C, Burch S (2002) Fluoxetine response in children with autistic spectrum disorders: correlation with familial major affective disorder and intellectual achievement. *Developmental Medicine and Child Neurology* 44:652–659.

Di Martino A, Tuchman RF (2001) Antiepileptic drugs: affective use in autistic spectrum disorders. *Pediatric Neurology* 25:199–207.

Edelman RJ (1992) Anxiety. *Theory, Research and Intervention in Clinical and Health Psychology*. Chichester: Wiley.

Filipek PA, Juranek J, Smith M, Mays LZ, Ramos ER, Bocian M, Masser-Frye D, Laulhere TM, Modahl C, Spence MA, Gargas JJ (2003) Mitochondrial dysfunction in autistic patients with 15q inverted duplication. *Annals of Neurology* 53:801–804.

Ghaziuddin M, Alessi N, Greden J (1995) Life events and depression in children with pervasive developmental disorders. *Journal of Autism and Developmental Disorders* 25:495–502.

Ghaziuddin M, Greden J (1998) Depression in children with autism/pervasive developmental disorders: a case-control family-history study. *Journal of Autism and Developmental Disorders* 28:111–115.

Ghaziuddin M, Tsai L (1991) Depression in autistic disorder. *British Journal of Psychiatry* 159:721–723.

Ghaziuddin M, Tsai L, Ghaziuddin N (1992) Comorbidity of autistic disorder in children and adolescents. *European Child and Adolescent Psychiatry* 1:209–213.

Ghaziuddin M, Weidmer-Michail E, Ghaziuddin N (1998) Comorbidity in Asperger syndrome: a preliminary report. *Journal of Intellectual Disability Research* 4:279–283.

Gillberg C, Johansson M, Steffenburg S, Berlin O (1997) Auditory integration training in children with autism, brief report in an open pilot study. *Autism* 1:97–100.

Gillot A, Furniss F, Walter A (2001) Anxiety in high functioning children with autism. *Autism* 5:277–286.

Glenn E, Bihm EM, Lammers WJ (2003) Depression, anxiety, and relevant cognition in persons with mental retardation. *Journal of Autism and Developmental Disorders* 33: 69–76.

Gold DR, Cohen BH (2001) Treatment of mitochondrial cytopathies. *Seminars in Neurology* 21:309–325.

Handen BL, Johnson CR, Lubensky M (2000) Efficacy of methylphenidate among children with autism and symptoms of attention-deficit hyperactivity disorder. *Journal of Autism and Developmental Disorders* 30:245–255.

Hayashi E (2000) Effect of melatonin on sleep-wake rhythm: the sleep diary of an autistic male. *Psychiatry Clinical Neuroscience.* 54:383–384.

Herbert JD, Sharp IR, Gaudiano BA (2002) Separating facts from fiction in the etiology and treatment of autism: a scientific review of evidence. *Scientific Review of Mental Health Practice* 1:23–43.

Hollander E, Dolgoff-Kaspar R, Cartwright C, Rawitt R, Novotny S (2001) An open trial of divalproex sodium in autism spectrum disorder. *Journal of Clinical Psychiatry* 62: 530–534.

Ishizaki A, Sugama M, Takeuchi N (1999) Usefulness of melatonin for developmental sleep and emotional/behavior disorders-studies of melatonin trial on 50 patients with developmental disorders. *No To Hattatsu* 5:428–437.

Jan JE, O'Donnell ME (1996) Use of melatonin in the treatment of pediatric sleep disorders. *Journal of Pineal Research* 21:193–199.

Kanner L (1943) Autistic disturbances of affective contact. *Nervous Child* 2:217–250.

Kauffman C, Vance H, Pumariega AJ, Miller B (2001) Fluvoxamine treatment of a child with severe PDD: a single case study. *Psychiatry* 64:268–277.

Kemper TL, Bauman ML (1993) The contribution of neuropathologic studies to the understanding of autism. *Neurologic Clinic* 11:175–187.

Kerbeshian J, Burd L (1992) Epidemiology and comorbidity: the North Dakota prevalence studies of Tourette syndrome and other developmental disorders. In Chase TN, Friedhoff AJ, Cohen DJ (Eds) *Advances in Neurology* (pp. 67–74). Raven Press: New York.

Kielinen M, Linna SL, Moilanen I (2002) Some aspects of treatment and habilitation of children and adolescents with autistic disorder in Northern Finland. *International Journal of Circumpolar Health* 61(Suppl 2):69–79.

Komoto J, Usui S, Hirata J (1984) Infantile autism and affective disorders. *Journal of Autism and Developmental Disorders* 14:81–84.

Kowatch RA, Sethuraman G, Hume JH, Kromelis M, Weinberg WA (2003) Combination pharmacotherapy in children and adolescents with bipolar disorders. *Biological Psychiatry* 53:978–984.

Lainhart JE and Folstein SE (1994) Affective disorders in people with autism: a review of published cases. *Journal of Autism and Developmental Disorders* 24:587–601.

Lindsay RL, Aman MG (2003) Pharmacologic therapies aid treatment for autism. *Pediatric Annals* 32:671–676.

Martin A, Koenig K, Anderson GM, Scahill L (2003) Low-dose fluvoxamine treatment of children and adolescents with pervasive developmental disorders: a prospective, open-label study. *Journal of Autism and Developmental Disorders* 33:77–85.

Martin A, Scahill L, Klin A, Volkmar FR (1999) Higher functioning pervasive developmental disorders: rates and patterns of psychotropic drug use. *Journal of the American Academy of Child and Adolescent Psychiatry* 38:923–931.

Masi G, Cosenza A, Mucci M, Brovedani P (2001) Open trial of risperidone in 24 children with pervasive developmental disorders. *Journal of the American Academy of Child and Adolescent Psychiatry* 40:1206–1214.

Masi G, Cosenza A, Mucci M, Brovedani P (2003) A 3-year naturalistic study of 53 preschool children with pervasive developmental disorders treated with risperidone. *Journal of Clinical Psychiatry* 64:1039–1047.

McDougle CJ, Brodkin ES, Naylor ST, Carlson DC, Cohen DJ, Price LH (1998) Sertraline in adults with pervasive developmental disorders: a prospective open-label investigation. *Journal of Clinical Psychopharmacology* 18:62–66.

Molino-Carballo A, Munoz-Hoyas A, Reiter R, Sancheq-Fonte M, Moreno-Madrid F, Rufo-Campos M, Molina-Font JA Acune-Castroviejo D(1997) Utility of high doses of melatonin as adjunctive anticonvulsant therapy in a child with severe myoclonic epilepsy. *Journal of Pineal Research* 23:97–105.

Mula M, Monaco F (2002) Carbamazepine-risperidone interactions in patients with epilepsy. *Clinical Neuropharmacology* 25:97–100.

Namerow LB, Prakash T, Bostic JQ, Prince J, Monuteaux MC (2003) Use of citalopram in Pervasive Developmental Disorders. *Journal of Developmental Behavioural Pediatrics* 24:104–108.

National Research Council (NRC) (2001) *Educating Children with Autism.* Washington DC: National Academy Press.

Page T, Yu A, Fontane J, Nyhan WL (1997) Developmental disorder associated with increased cellular nucleotidase activity. *Proceedings of the National Academy of Sciences* 94:11601–11606.

Research Units in Pediatric Psychopharmacology (RUPP) Autism Network (2002) Risperidone in children with autism and serious behavioural problems. *New England Journal of Medicine* 347:314–321.

Ringman JM, Jankovic J (2000) Occurrance of tics in Asperger's syndrome and autistic disorder. *Journal of Child Neurology* 15:394–400.

Ross T (1981) Portage system: programmed for success. *Nursing Mirror* 152:20–21.

Rossi Giovanardi P, Posar A, Parmeggiani A, Pipitone E, D'Agata M (1999) Niaprazine in the treatment of autistic disorder. *Journal of Child Neurology* 14:547–550.

Roustang F. (2003) Quoi faire de nos propres souffrances? Round Table on "The Psychic Suffering." *Accademia di Terapia di Famiglia,* Rome.

Rutter M (1970) Autistic children: infancy to adulthood. *Seminars in Psychiatry* 2:435–450.

Santosh PJ, Baird G (2003) Pharmacotherapy of target symptoms in autistic spectrum disorders. *Indian Journal of Pediatrics* 68:427–431.

Schopler E (1995) *Parent survival manual.* New York: Plenum Press.

Sheldon SH (1998) Pro-convulsant effects of oral melatonin in neurologically disabled children (letter). *Lancet* 351:1254.

Smits MG, Henk F, Kristiaan van der Heijden, Meijer AM, Anton ML Coenen, Kerkhof GA (2003) Melatonin improves health status and sleep in children with idiopathic sleep-onset insomnia: a randomized placebo-controlled trial. *Journal of the American Academy of Child and Adolescent Psychiatry* 42:1286–1293.

Snead RW, Boon F, Presberg J (1994) Paroxetine for self-injurious behaviour. *Journal of the American Academy of Child and Adolescent Psychiatry* 33:909–910.

Soutullo CA, Sorter MT, Foster KD, McElroy SL, Keck PE (1999) Olanzapine in the treatment of adolescent acute mania: a report of seven cases. *Journal of Affective Disorders* 53:279–283.

Spina E, Avenoso A, Facciola G, Salemi M, Scordo MG, Giacobello T, Madia A (2000) Plasma concentrations of risperidone and 9-hydroxysperidone: effects of comedication with carbamazepine or valproate. *Therapy Drug Monitor* 22:481–485.

Spina E, Avenoso A, Scordo MG, Ancione M, Madia A, Gatti G, Peruce E (2003) Inhibition of risperidone metabolism by fluoxetine in patients with schizophrenia: a clinically relevant pharmacokinetic drug interaction. *Journal of Clinical Psychopharmacology* 22:419–423.

Spina E, Perucca E (2002) Clinical significance of pharmacokinetic interactions between antiepileptic and psychotropic drugs. *Epilepsia* 43(Suppl 2):37–44.

Steingard RJ, Zimnitzky B, DeMaso DR, Bauman ML, Bucci JP (1997) Sertraline treatment of transition-associated anxiety and agitation in children with autistic disorder. *Journal of Child and Adolescent Psychopharmacology* 7:9–15.

Stores G (2003) Medication for sleep-wake disorders. *Archives of Diseases of Children* 88:899–903.

Tuchman R, Rapin I (2002) Epilepsy in autism *Lancet Neurology* 1(6):352–358.

Volkmar FR, Lord C, Bailey A, Schulz RT, Klin A (2004) Autism and pervasive developmental disorders. *Journal of Child Psychology and Psychiatry* 45:135–170.

Werry JS (2001) Pharmacological treatments of autism, attention deficit hyperactivity disorder, oppositional defiant disorder, and depression in children and youth—commentary. *Journal of Clinical Child Psychology* 30:110–113.

Wing L (1981) Asperger syndrome: a clinical account. *Psychological Medicine* 11:115–119.

Xaiz C, Micheli E (2000) *Giochi e Attività Sociali Nell'Autismo.* Trento: Erickson.

Yatham LN, Grossman F, Augustyns I, Vieta E, Ravindran A (2003) Mood stabilizers plus risperidone or placebo in the treatment of acute mania. *British Journal of Psychiatry* 182:141–147.

Zappella M (2002) Early-onset Tourette syndrome with reversible autistic behavior: a dysmaturational syndrome. *European Child and Adolescent Medicine* 11:18–22.

Glossary

The words defined below are limited to their use in this book; many of these words have other meanings.

Agnosia   loss of ability of the brain to recognize the import of incoming sensory stimuli.

Allele   (allelomorphic gene) one of two contrasting genes situated at the same locus in homologous chromosomes, concerned with the same category of information, with a very slight difference in sequence from each other. A null allele fails to produce the gene product, a protein.

Aphasia   inability to comprehend or express language.

Apoptosis   programmed cell death that is usually a normal process. It is energy-dependent and plays a critical role in development and homeostatic processes.

Apraxia/dyspraxia   an inability or diminished ability to carry out purposive, useful, or skilled motor acts, especially if complicated; a loss of the capacity to use objects correctly.

Autosomes   autosomal chromosomes, in pairs, are chromosomes numbered 1 to 22 (in contrast to the gonosomes).

Chromosomes   the carriers of the genes, they are single linear duplex DNA molecules complexed with numerous proteins. When systematically arranged, they form a karyotype of 46 human chromosomes. The parts of a chromosome are the following: the *centromere* the constricted middle section of a chromosome that divides it into long and short arms; the *long arm*, called 'q'; the *short arm*, called 'p'; the *telomeres* the ends of the arms

Chromosomal errors   *Deletion* part of a chromosomal arm is missing.

Duplication, interstitial a segment of a chromosome duplicated inside the chromosome, *supernumerary marker* duplicated material outside the chromosome.

Ring chromosome chromosome bent around upon itself to form a ring.

Mosaicism two or more cell populations, each with a different chromosomal karyotype.

Translocation a piece of one chromosome is transferred to another chromosome. If two nonhomologous chromosomes exchange pieces, the translocation is said to be balanced.

Trisomy two sets of 23 chromosomes plus one extra chromosome: a total of 47 chromosomes instead of the usual 46.

Tetrasomy two extra chromosomes. Total of 48 chromosomes.

Uniparental disomy two copies of a chromosome are derived from only one of the parents.

Codon in the coding sequence of the gene, each set of three DNA bases forms a codon, a triplet of the bases in a DNA molecule that codes for one amino acid. This is the genetic code for creating one of the 20 amino acids found in proteins.

Comorbidities additional diseases or symptom complexes occurring simultaneously along with the primary disease entity in the patient.

Color anomia inability to learn the names of colors.

Contiguous gene syndrome recognizable patterns of malformation associated with loss of several genes that are physically adjacent to each other on a critical chromosome segment. An example is the velocardiofacial/DiGeorge syndrome (deletion 22q11.21).

Cranial circumference the tape measurement of the size of a person's head.

Macrocephaly it measures too large, above 2 standard deviations for age.

Microcephaly it measures too small, below 2 standard deviations for age.

DNA a sequence of nucleotides, usually double-stranded. A nucleotide can have any of four bases: (A) adenine, (T) thymine, (G) guanine, or (C) cytosine. These nucleotides, in sets of three called trinucleotides or DNA triplets, are the alphabet of inheritance.

Genes units of genetic information consisting of the double-stranded macromolecule DNA with two complimentary strands that wrap around one another to form a double helix.

Genetic studies *Association* when a disease is statistically related to a particular allele of a gene. *Linkage* when the presence of a disease is statistically related to the presence of a marker in a particular locus on a chromosome. *Locus* specific region of a chromosome that contains a gene (its location or its address).

Genetic patterns *Mendelian*

Autosomal: dominant traits that are expressed in the heterozygous state.

Autosomal: recessive traits that are only expressed in the homozygous state.

X-linked: traits expressed in sons, inherited from the X chromosome of the mother. There is no father-to-son transmission. Daughters may (X-linked dominant) or may not (X-linked recessive) be affected.

Non-Mendelian

mitochondrial (mtDNA): the disease follows maternal inheritance patterns.

trinucleotide repeat expansion: the nucleotides in DNA come in sets of three called trinucleotides or DNA triplets. When they expand (or contract) beyond the usual number, they cause malfunction of the gene and a subsequent genetic disease. An example is the excessive number of C (cytosine) G (guanine) G (guanine) sequences in the fragile X syndrome.

Genome all of the genes in an organism, organized into chromosomes.

Genomic imprinting a transcriptional operation in which inactivation of genes or chromosomal regions of one of two matched chromosomes occurs. This leads to preferential expression of an allele depending upon its parental origin. An example is the Angelman syndrome (suppression of the maternal allele).

Gonosomes   the chromosomes that determine the sex of the individual, the 23rd pair of chromosomes, called X and Y. XX = female; XY = male.

Heteroplasmy   a mixture of DNA in a mitochondrion, some of which contain mutant DNA while other mitochondria contain normal, also known as wild-type, DNA. Such a mixture allows otherwise lethal mutations to persist. (Homoplasmy is the presence of either consistently normal or consistently mutant DNA.)

Hypocalcinuria   levels of calcium in the urine are too low.

Hypsarrhythmic EEG   a distinctive EEG pattern of high-voltage slow waves and spikes observed in infants with infantile spasms.

Kyphoscoliosis   backward and lateral curvature of the spine.

Macroorchidism   enlarged testes.

Megaloencephaly   brain that is too large.

Microencephaly   brain that is too small.

Mitochondria   the organelles in the cytoplasm of each cell that generate energy for cellular processes. They have their own unique extrachromosomal DNA that is distinct from the DNA in the nucleus of the cell, called mtDNA.

Monogenetic disease   a disease in which a single gene is necessary and sufficient to cause the disease.

Monotherapy   treatment limited to a single drug.

Mutations in a gene   a mutation can be defined as any change in the primary nucleotide sequence of DNA. Mutations involving single nucleotides are known as point mutations.

Myelin   formed by oligodendroglia, myelination of the brain is largely a postnatal event.

Pectus excavatum   known as "funnel chest," this is a midline restriction of the thoracic cavity.

Phenotype   visible or measurable characteristics of an individual.

Phonology   vocal sounds, phonetics.

Polymorphisms   a DNA sequence alteration that is found at a frequency of >1% in a given population; they are particularly common in noncoding regions of the genome and are inherited according to Mendelian law.

Prosody   the variation in pitch and rhythm of speech.

Prosopagnosia   face recognition deficit (a visual agnosia).

Semantic   the meaning of words; the rules of their use.

Syndactyly   webbing between adjacent fingers or toes.

Ventriculomegaly   enlarged ventricles in the brain.

Appendix

A Targeted Neurological Examination in Autism/Asperger

Mary Coleman, MD
Christopher Gillberg, MD, PhD

Name_____ Sex_____ Birth date_____ Date of exam_____
On the child's date of birth, the mother's age_____, the father's age_____
Height_____ percent for age/sex_____% Weight_____ percent for age/sex_____%
Cranial circumference_____ percent for age/sex_____% (*Do this measurement last!*)

HISTORY

    1. Bleeding during the first trimester?   YES NO
    2. Bleeding during the second trimester?
    3. Hypotonia in infancy (floppy baby) or later?
    4. Toe walking or other signs of hypertonus?
    5. Late walking, after 15 months? (*If YES, write age in months*)_____months
    6. Ataxic, off-balance walking?
    7. General clumsiness?
    8. Speech absent?
    9. Expressive and receptive speech present but age delayed?
  10. Difficulty swallowing?
  11. Difficulty breathing?
  12. Major hearing impairment (*deafness, more than 30dB*   YES NO
      any ear)? *Explain*_____
  13. Major vision impairment (*blindness, under 0.4 corrected*)?
      *Explain*_____
  14. Infantile spasms?

15. Myoclonic jerking?
16. Epilepsy, other than infantile spasms?
17. Tics or facial grimacing? (*underline which*)
18. Perceptual peculiarity—oversensitivity to sound or touch? (*Underline which ones*)
19. Perceptual peculiarity—relative insensitivity to pain, cold, or heat? (*Underline which ones*)
20. Perceptual peculiarity—oversensitivity to smell. Describe_____
21. Hands/fingers flapping, clapping, clasping, twirling, flickering? (*underline which*)?
22. Thumb or finger sucking? (*underline which*)
23. Whirling self or objects, rocking? (*underline which*)
24. Fascinated by water?
25. Drooling or protruding tongue? (*underline which*)
26. Abnormal eating behavior (pica, food fads, food refusal, hoarding, overeating, anorexia)? (*underline which*)
27. Bowels abnormal—often severe constipation?
28. Bowels abnormal—increased frequency/often   YES   NO
    severe diarrhea?
29. Abnormal activity level—hyperactive?
30. Abnormal activity level—hypoactive?
31. Inappropriate laughter?
32. Self-injurious behavior (SIB) – head, eyes, hands, other sites? *Explain*_____
33. Sleep disturbance? *Explain*_____
34. Explosive behaviors? *Explain*_____
35. Autistic regression? (*If YES, age*_____*months*)

STIGMATA EXAMINATION

36. A definite dysmorphic face?
37. Hypertelorism (widely spaced eyes)?
38. Ear anomalies (low set, asymmetrical, malformed or adherent lobes, extremely soft and pliable?) (*underline which*)
39. Mouth anomalies (high palate, cleft palate, submucous cleft soft palate, tongue furrow or smooth/ rough spots? (*underline which*)
40. Fingers unusual (tapered, ring or index fingers as long or longer than the middle finger) (*underline which*)

41. Partial or full syndactactyly (partial or full fusion) of 2nd and 3rd toe?
42. Other stigmata?_____

NEUROLOGICAL OBSERVATION

YES   NO

43. Abnormalities of the skin (self-mutilation, areas of hypo-pigmentation, hyperpigmentation such as café au lait, acne-like lesions, scaly lesions, or others)? *Explain*_____

_____

44. If speech is present, is it echolalic, formal, slurred, scan-ning, dysarthric, dysprosodic, or have other abnormali-ties? *Explain*_____

_____

45. Abnormality of posture, including catatonia? *Explain*_____
46. Abnormality of gait (wide-based, unsteady, feet dragging, shuffling, arms not moving, other)? *Explain*_____
47. Ptosis (drooping) of eyelids?
48. Nystagmus or strabismuss?
49. Tics?
50. Tremor—resting? *Where?*_____
51. Tremor—intention/action? *Where?*_____
52. Chorea (abrupt, jerky, brief, explosive involuntary move-ments of arms or body)?
53. Athetosis (slower, writhing, coarse involuntary move-ments of hands or body)?

NEUROLOGICAL TESTING

YES   NO

54. Ask child to smile—*NO, if symmetrical; YES, if asymmet-rical, describe*_____
55. Ask child to raise eyebrows—*NO, if symmetrical; YES, if asymmetrical, describe*_____
56. Movement of eyes when following?—*NO, if normal; YES, if abnormal, then describe*_____
57. Dysdiadochokinesia? (*impairment of rapid alternating movements?*)

58. Astereognosis? (*inability to identify hidden object placed in the hand by feel alone)?*

59. *Deep tendon reflexes, biceps & patellar?—NO if normal; YES, if abnormal, explain*_____

60. Extensor plantar response—Babinski sign? (*stimulation of the plantar surface of foot is followed by NO: plantar toes flexion or YES: extension/dorsiflexion of toes with separation and fanning*).

DON'T FORGET THE CRANIAL CIRCUMFERENCE TESTING.

Citation Index

Subject Index

Page references in italics represent illustrations, those in bold indicate tables.